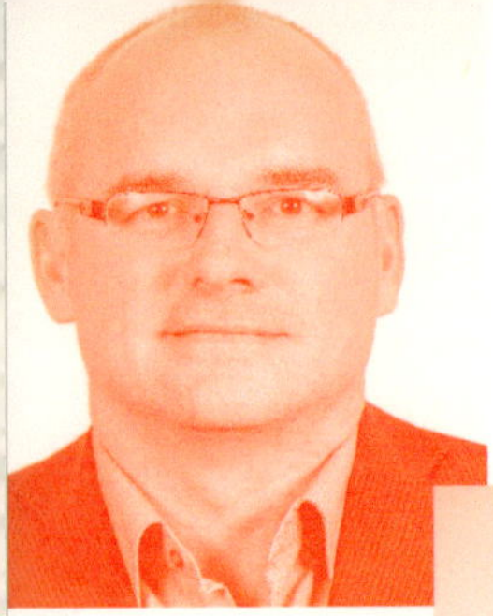
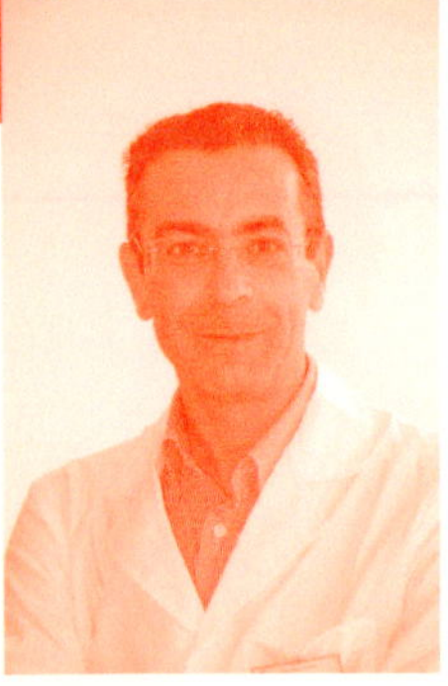
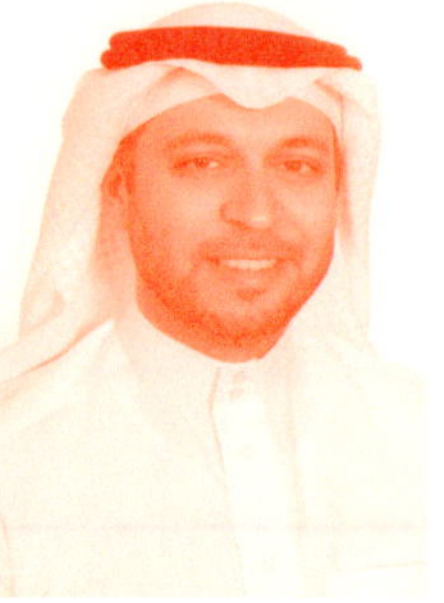
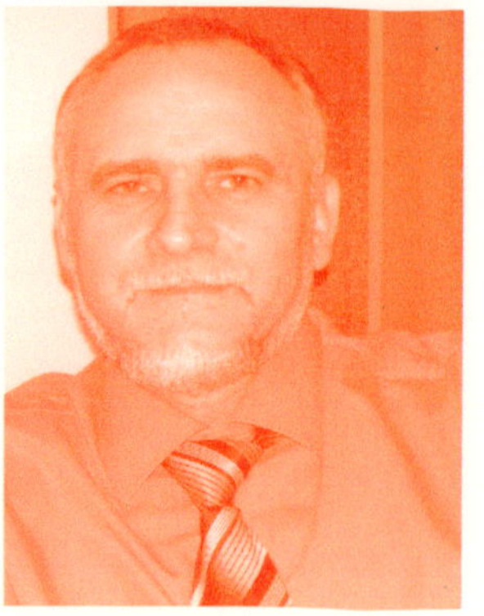
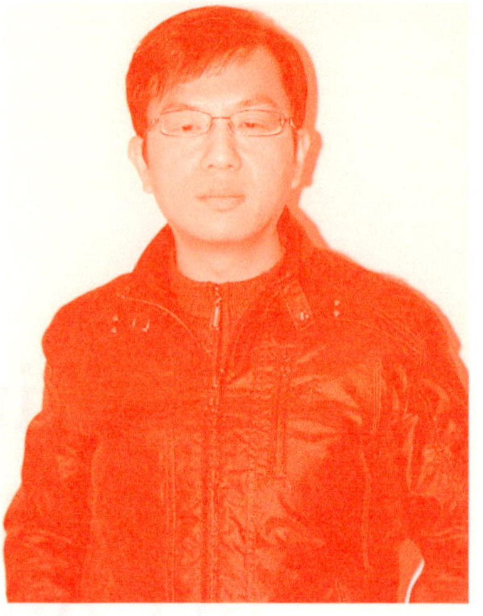
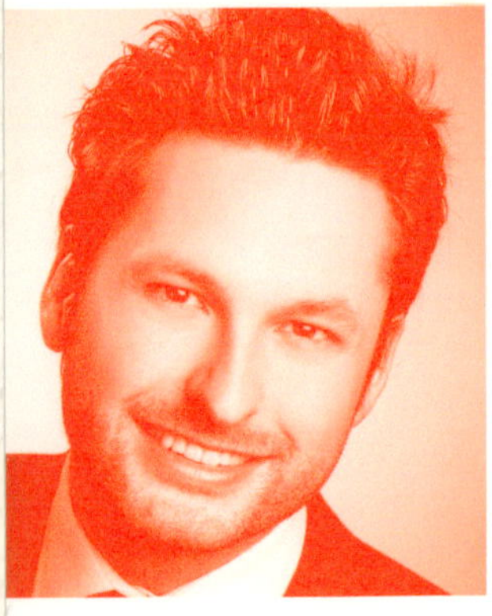
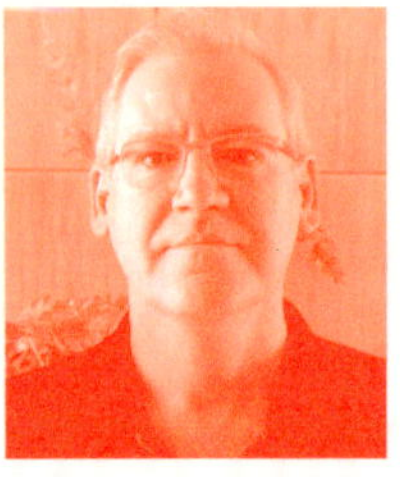

IntechOpen

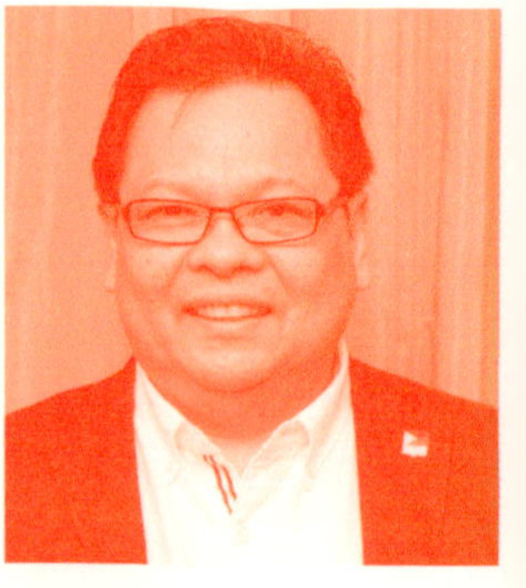
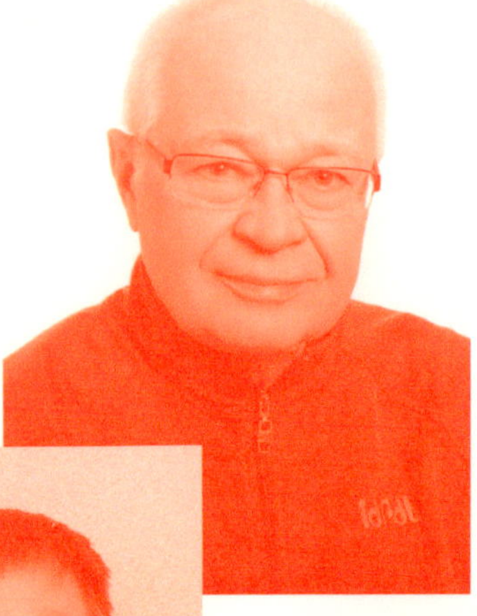
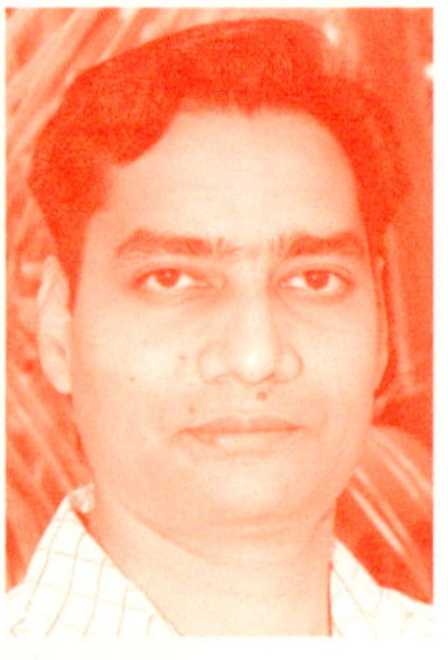
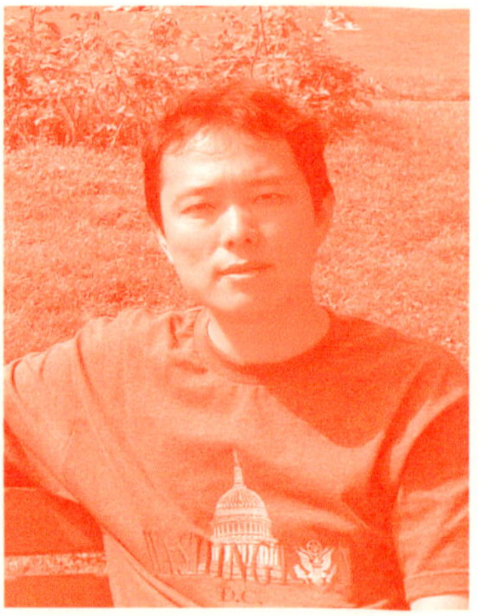
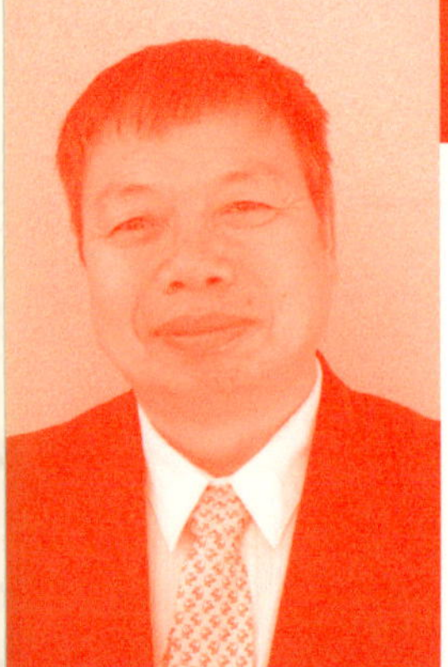
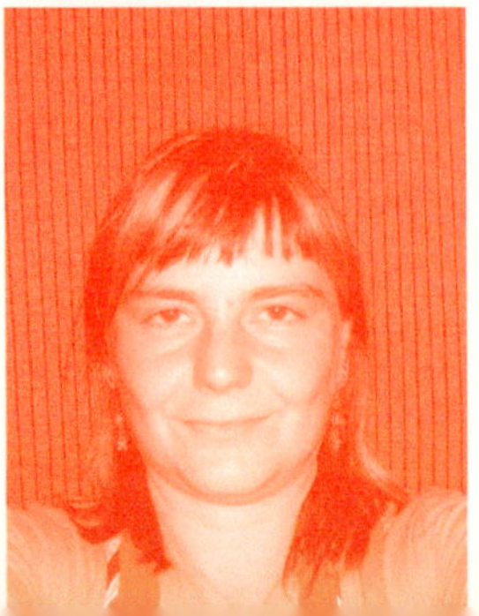

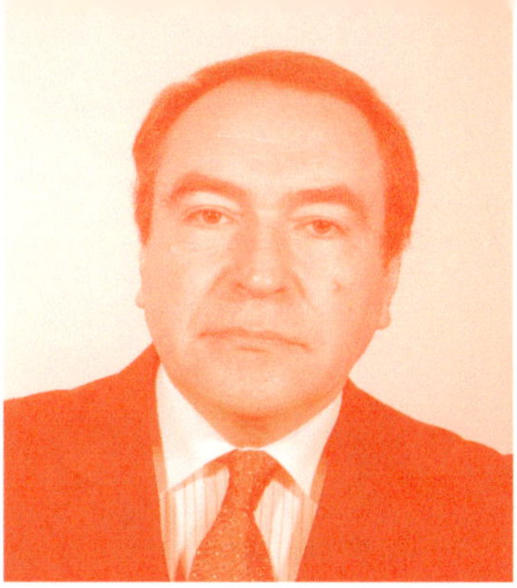
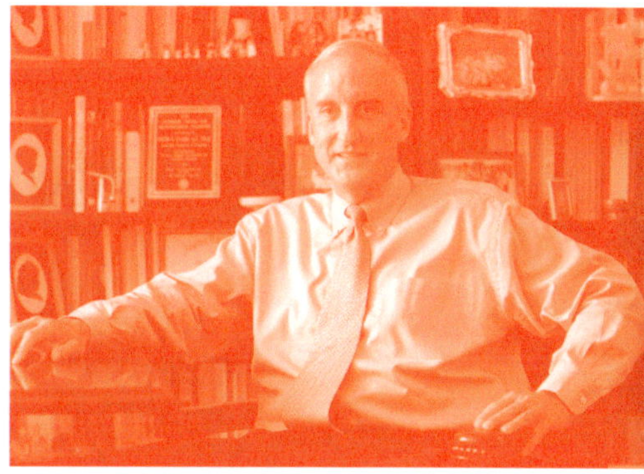
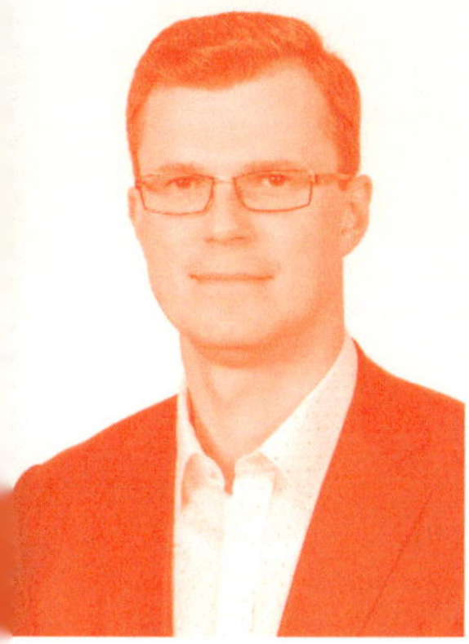
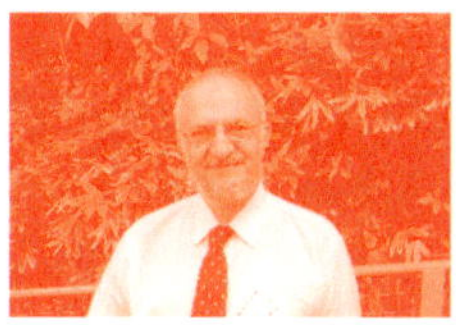
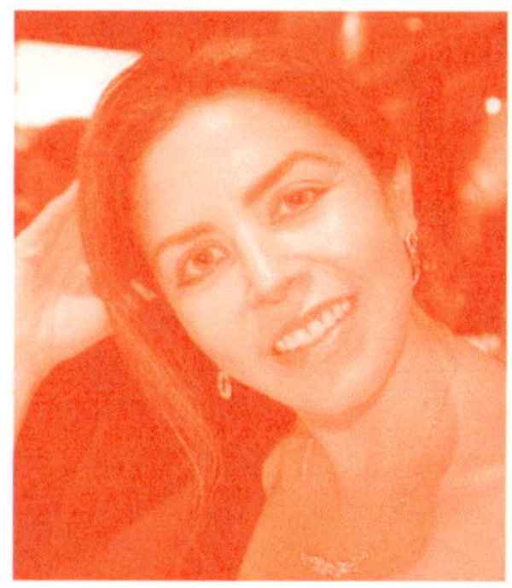

Supporting open minds since 2005

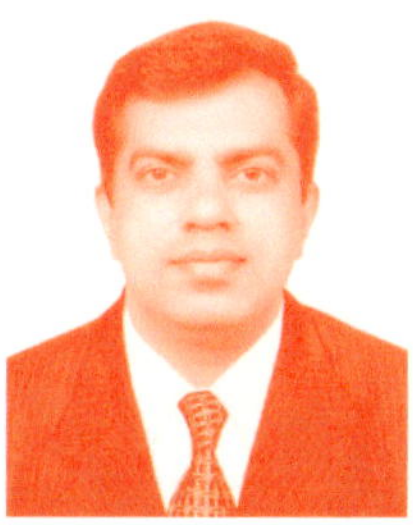
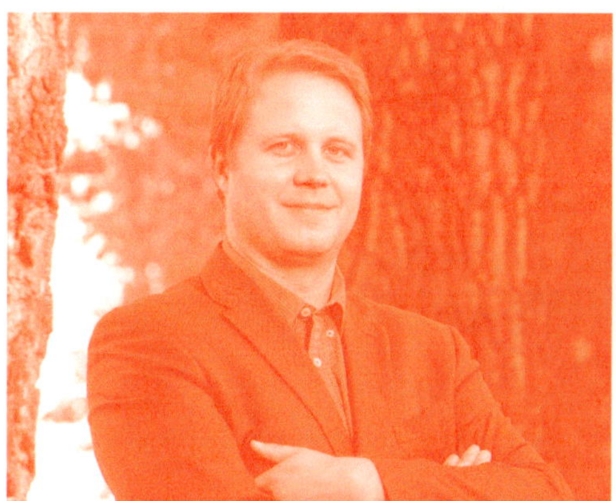
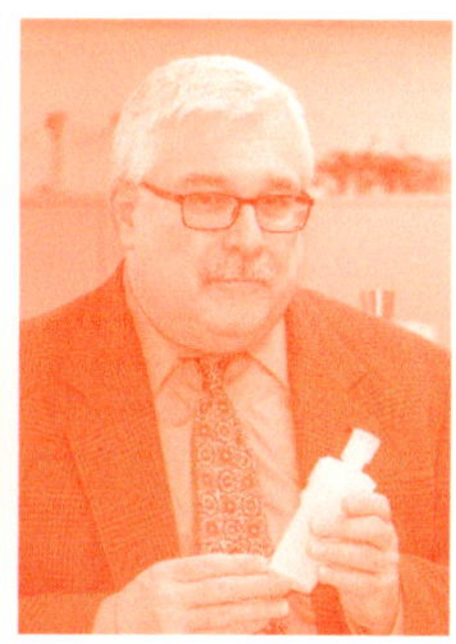
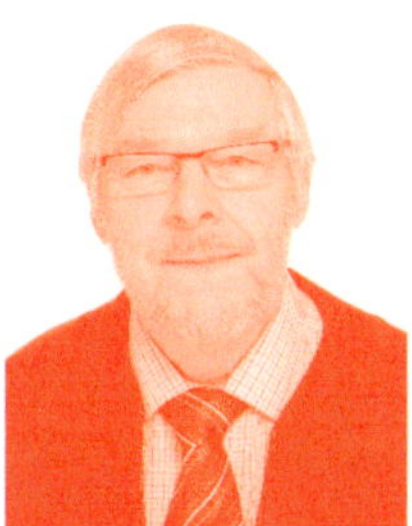
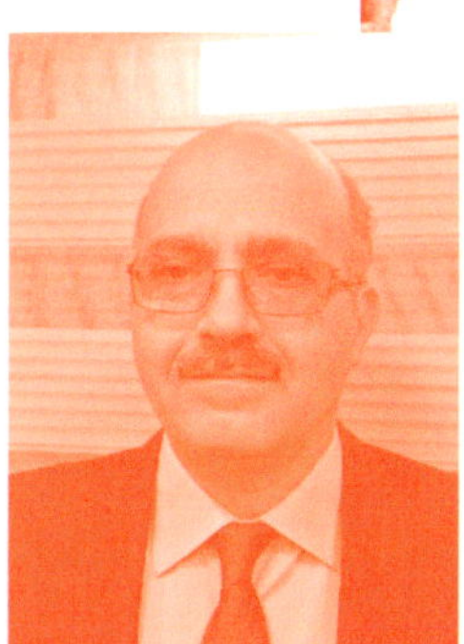
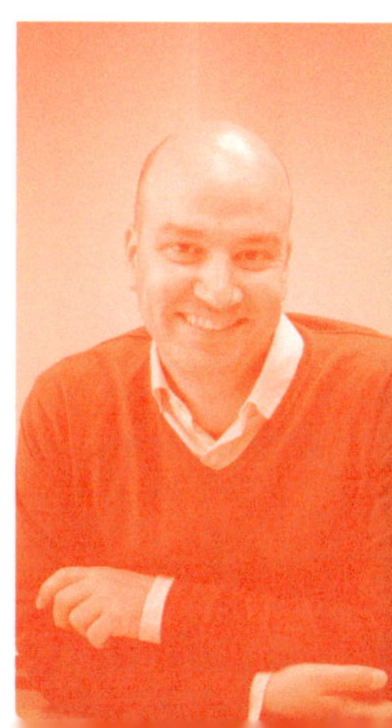
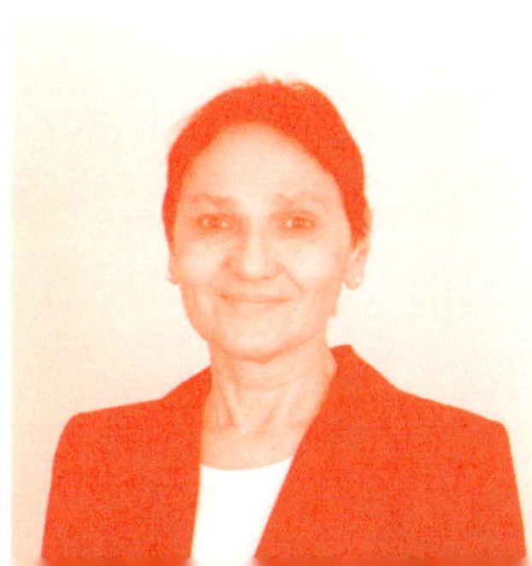

Neurostimulation and Neuromodulation in Contemporary Therapeutic Practice
http://dx.doi.org/10.5772/intechopen.77890
Edited by Denis Larrivee and Seyed Mansoor Rayegani

Contributors
Vladimira Vuletic, Darko Chudy, Nenad Bogdanovic, Valentino Racki, Ferdinando Sartucci, Tommaso Bocci, Horia Salca, Miguel Royo-Salvador, Marco Fiallos-Rivera, Alexandr Kovalenko, Viktor Misikov, Valeriy Shamigulov, Konstantin Sinelnikov, Dmitrii Iskra, Priya Dev, Abhishek Pathak, Sara Schatz, Francesco Patti, Vincenzo Cimino, Clara Grazia Chisari, Alice G. Witney, Said M. Yaiesh, Tariq F. Al-Shaiji, Abdullatif Al-Terki, Seyed Mansoor Rayegani, Marzieh Babaee, Seyed Ahmad Raeissadat, Mohammad Hossein Khosravi, Meisam Hoseinyazdi, Reza Jahankhah, Sara Haseli, Denis Larrivee, Svetlana E. Khatkova, Denis V. Kovlen, Roberta Ferrucci, Alberto Priori, Massimiliano Valeriani

First published in London, United Kingdom, 2020 by IntechOpen
IntechOpen is the global imprint of INTECHOPEN LIMITED, registered in England and Wales, registration number: 11086078, 5 Princes Gate Court, London, SW7 2QJ, United Kingdom
Printed in Croatia

British Library Cataloguing-in-Publication Data
A catalogue record for this book is available from the British Library

Additional hard and PDF copies can be obtained from orders@intechopen.com

Neurostimulation and Neuromodulation in Contemporary Therapeutic Practice
Edited by Denis Larrivee and Seyed Mansoor Rayegani
p. cm.
Print ISBN 978-1-83880-291-2
Online ISBN 978-1-83880-292-9
eBook (PDF) ISBN 978-1-83968-772-3

For EU product safety concerns:
IN TECH d.o.o., Prolaz Marije Krucifikse Kozulić 3, 51000 Rijeka, Croatia, info@intechopen.com or visit our website at intechopen.com.

Meet the editors

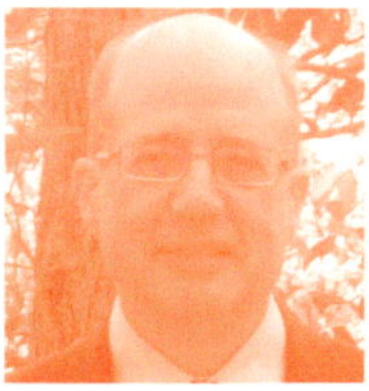

Dr. Denis Larrivee is a visiting scholar at the Mind and Brain Institute, University of Navarra Medical School and Loyola University, Chicago. He has held professorships at the Weill Cornell University Medical College, NYC, and Purdue University, Indiana. A former fellow at Yale University's Medical School, Dr. Larrivee received the Association for Research in Vision and Ophthalmology's first place award for studies on photoreceptor degenerative and developmental mechanisms. He is the editor of *Brain Computer Interfacing* and an editorial board member of the *Annals of Neurology and Neurological Sciences* (USA) and *EC Neurology* (UK). He is also the author of more than eight-five papers and book chapters in such varied journals/venues as *Neurology and Neurological Sciences*, *Journal of Neuroscience*, *Journal of Religion and Mental Health*, and *IEEE Xplore*. In 2018, he was a finalist for the international Joseph Ratzinger Expanded Reason award sponsored by the Francis Vittorio University of Madrid.

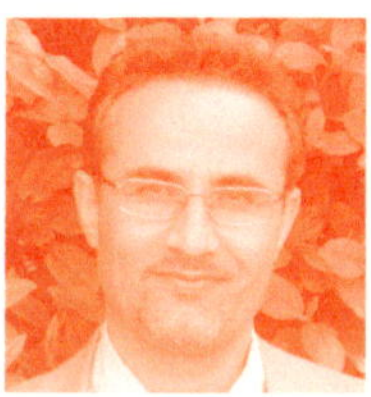

Professor S. Mansoor Rayegani is an academic physiatrist who completed his residency training in Physical Medicine & Rehabilitation (PM&R) at Shiraz University of Medical Sciences, Iran, in 1992. In 1994, he began his academic career as Assistant Professor of PM&R at Shohada Medical Center, Shahid Beheshti University of Medical Sciences, just after passing the Iranian Board of PM&R in which he gained first rank. He is one of the founding members of a PM&R residency program in Tehran. Professor Rayegani's fields of interest include electrodiagnostic medicine, pain, spinal cord injury, neurorehabilitation, and medical education. He supervises and coordinates a neurorehabilitation and hypertonicity clinic. He has supervised more than forty postgraduate residency theses and published about 130 indexed medical articles. He is also an editorial board member for the *Journal of the International Society of Physical and Rehabilitation Medicine* (JISPRM) and a member of the journal's education and publication committee. Professor Rayegani is currently president of the Iranian society of PM&R, editor in chief of *Physical Medicine, Rehabilitation, and Electrodiagnosis* (PMRE), director of the Iranian Board of PM&R, and chief of the PM&R Research Center at Shahid Beheshti University of Medical Sciences.

Contents

Preface

For centuries, electrical stimulation has been employed for treating neural disorders. As early as the Egyptian period, for example, medical records cite the use of electric eel shock therapy for pain, while during the eighteenth century it was used for treating paralysis and psychiatric symptoms. Enthusiasm for electrotherapy waned somewhat in the late 1800s and early 1900s as psychotherapies came to acquire greater prestige for treating psychiatric symptoms. In recent decades, however, interest in neurostimulation for therapy has again reignited, beginning chiefly with applications for motor disorders and pain treatment. High-frequency stimulation of the subthalamic nucleus or globus pallidus in patients with Parkinson's disease (PD) was notably found to produce clinical effects that were similar to surgical ablation, yet were reversible, unlike surgery, making them an appealing therapeutic strategy.

For the most part, the mechanisms elicited by neurostimulation are unknown. One widely acknowledged proposal is that neurostimulation somehow affects the electrical patterning that enables information transfer, since electrical activity is known to be fundamental to brain communication. The understanding of how patterning is structured, however, has been both evolving and vigorously debated, with the result that mechanisms of neurostimulation are themselves poorly understood. In the 1990s, though, Singer proposed a new thesis premised on the combinatorial properties of brain oscillations, which were intrinsic to neural operation. This provided for virtually unlimited freedom of expression in neural communication, unlike earlier models. Impelled in part by the prospect of an improved understanding of underlying mechanisms that may modulate, facilitate, or disrupt brain activity, as well as successes in symptomatic and long-term therapeutic relief, neurostimulatory and neuromodulatory protocols have since seen rapid growth in domains other than the motor diseases. Additionally fueling recent growth are the intrinsic advantages of neurostimulation over the more commonly used pharmaceutical agents. Unlike pharmacological approaches, which are difficult to target to specific brain regions and whose temporal distribution is usually prolonged, neurostimulation is inherently better suited to address the discrete spatial and temporal variation that characterizes individual dysfunctions.

The need for surgical intervention with its risk of secondary complications has spawned, moreover, an additional and equally broad group of non-invasive applications, including transcranial magnetic stimulation (TMS), transcranial direct current stimulation (tDCS), and repetitive TMS (rTMS), among others, which can be used both therapeutically as well as diagnostically. Diagnostically, for example, TMS can be a surrogate marker of recovery that is both sensitive and quantitative for cranial vascular disorders. TMS has also proven to be a useful tool for examining cortical and corticospinal physiology and enabling the understanding of motor dysfunction. When physiologic data are correlated with clinical function, they can assist diagnosis of underlying motor dysfunction. Operant conditioning with TMS, for instance, has been used both to assess the weakness of corticospinal connections and to promote targeted neuroplastic change.

In view of the promise of these new methods, this book documents their expanding panorama, with particular emphasis on their evolution in medical care. The wide variety of medical applications presented in the text is intended not only to document the latest advances but also to evidence that their development is servicing more than the epiphenomenal; that is, neurostimulation and neuromodulation are not simply providing symptomatic care but involve substantive effects on dysfunctional physiology within the nervous system. Accordingly, the chapters illustrate the versatility of the technology and the generality of the physical and biological principles evoked in various treatments.

The book is divided into four sections that sequentially cover theory and breadth, a focal exploration of neurostimulation in motor diseases, new and ancillary treatments for diseases of neural degeneration, and, finally, novel applications likely to see future growth.

Keeping in mind the factors propelling the evolution of these approaches, Section 1 considers a trio of topics, including theoretical issues governing neurostimulatory influence, ancillary methodological support for enhancing efficacy, and the range of circumstances encountered in application. Specifically, Chapter 1 speaks to how neurostimulation is likely to influence the structure of global brain activity in disease, with epilepsy used as a paradigmatic case. Chapter 2 features ancillary methodological issues involving the targeting of neurostimulation that are fundamental to therapeutic efficacy. Chapter 3 then surveys the diversity of neurological diseases and impairments for which neurostimulation has achieved therapeutic success, illustrating the common principles evoked in each treatment.

Section 2 explores how neurostimulation therapies evolve in medical management, with motor diseases as an exemplar, since these applications have had the longest interval within which to develop. Focusing on spasticity and dystonia, the section provides an in-depth examination of how neurostimulation can be merged successfully with pharmacological and rehabilitative methods in medical management regimes. Chapter 4 emphasizes the medical management of rehabilitation in spasticity and how adjunct treatments using neurostimulation or pharmacology can promote rehabilitative practices. Reversing this approach, Chapter 5 considers the now prevailing use of pharmacological intervention for spasticity and how approaches that rely primarily on pharmaceutical reagents can be enhanced through supplementary treatments that include neurostimulation. Chapter 6 closes this section with a review of the diagnostic tools needed for selecting among these options.

An especially significant new field for neurostimulation and neuromodulation is the neurodegenerative diseases, discussed in Section 3. Given the increased prevalence and chronic nature of cognitive diseases characterizing the elderly and a worldwide upward trend in elderly demographics, there is great need for new approaches to the treatment of these diseases. The chapters in this section discuss two strategies for approaching treatments of these diseases: the delay of their temporal progression and the mitigation of their effects on quality of life. Chapter 7 explores a novel neuromodulatory option for treating Alzheimer's dementia (AD) using improved long-term insulin delivery protocols that can delay neuron loss in degenerating brain tissue. Chapter 8 reviews how neurostimulation can overcome debilitating side effects like insomnia and somatosensory dysfunctions that greatly impact quality of life.

Finally, Section 4 explores the current diversity of applications for which neurostimulation is increasingly resorted to. These applications target not only the brain but also major tracts that course through the spinal cord. Chapters 9 and 10 explore the use of non-invasive neurostimulation for pain. The significance of this work becomes apparent when one considers that chronic pain affects billions of people yearly. Chapter 9 reviews the clinical use of neurostimulation, often employed for intractable circumstances, while Chapter 10 explores potential mechanisms evoked by stimulation. Finally, Chapters 11 and 12 discuss therapeutic applications of neurostimulation in spinal dysfunctions.

This is an exciting time for therapies used to treat CNS disorders, when traditional rehabilitative and neurotransmitter-based pharmacological approaches are being supplemented or even supplanted by the new methods of neurostimulation and neuromodulation, which can intervene more precisely and on shorter time scales in regions specifically affected by the disorders. This book seeks to convey the therapeutic prospects of these new methods as well as the details of medical praxis. It is hoped that the excitement of these developments will induce their use in wider clinical settings and inspire the evolution of an even broader range of regimes that can engage the brain in the brain's own language.

Denis Larrivee
Professor,
Mind and Brain Institute,
University of Navarra Medical School,
Spain

Loyola University Chicago,
USA

Seyed Mansoor Rayegani, M.D
Professor of Physical Medicine and Rehabilitation,
Physical Medicine and Rehabilitation Research Center,
Shahid Beheshti University of Medical Sciences,
Tehran, Iran

Section 1

Neurostimulation in Theory and Practice

Chapter 1

Introductory Chapter: Neurostimulation and the Structural Basis of Brain Activity

Denis Larrivee

1. Introduction: neurostimulation and global organization

Despite its remarkable clinical efficacy and several decades of use, neurostimulation remains a therapy whose neurophysiological basis is yet undetermined [1]. This lack of basic scientific understanding has imposed a conceptual barrier that has broader implications for therapeutic efficacy. Nonetheless, an improved understanding of the mechanisms of brain activity, observations on the etiological basis of neurological diseases, and insights from diverse therapeutic applications offer hope for understanding how the therapy physiologically impacts neural impairments.

Because the form of neurostimulation is rhythmic, it has been suggested that neural mechanisms responding to stimulation are similarly rhythmic [2]. Rhythmic activity is notably ubiquitous in brain operation, and has been observed in single neurons that display patterned spiking, as well as at network levels, where variable inhibitory and excitatory feedback configure repetitive activity [3]. Increasingly, these are proposed to be oscillatory [4]. Significantly, oscillators are prone to pairing and can combine in an indefinite number of permutations to recreate encoded feature representations. The therapeutic role played by neurostimulation thus plausibly entails oscillatory interactions, where neurostimulation could modify dysfunctional oscillations, presumably by altering their intrinsic features, like patterning, synchronization, and desynchronization. Recent studies show in fact that brain activity is globally structured through oscillatory interactions, with key elements distributed throughout the brain. Such elements would be expected to be similarly perturbed in various impairments; hence, restoring normal function would require that they be reconstructed.

Consistent with this proposal, it is known that global brain activity is coordinated by slow frequency oscillations that resonate between subcortical and cortical regions [4]. These activity structures mediate organismal functions, which are cohesively ordered to the good of the individual; hence, their investigation can be expected to provide a basis for understanding the higher order organization that underlies brain dynamics at global scales. Indeed, without such understanding, the effects induced by neuromodulation and neurostimulation remain anecdotal and their utility to therapeutic design uncertain.

How then is global brain activity affected by neurostimulation? Some insight into this question can be expected from the study of diseases known to disrupt global brain events. One candidate is epilepsy, which has been treated by neurostimulation for several decades. Significantly, a characteristic feature of epilepsy is the occurrence of epileptogenesis outside initial seizure foci. The processes associated with this distribution are not known, but current evidence implicates contributions from both higher order cognition and homeostatic mechanisms, that is, top-down and bottom-up factors that amplify and spread local seizures. This chapter will review current work on these processes, some of which associate with consciousness and default mode network operation, with the expectation that they are also likely to be found in other disease states. Their characterization is thus likely to inform intervention in other medical disorders and so enhance the efficacy of neurostimulation for an increasingly diverse range of cognitive impairments.

2. Epilepsy as a paradigm for global perturbation

Epilepsy is a widely occurring, common neurological disorder. After stroke, it is the second leading brain impairment, affecting nearly 50 million people worldwide [5]. Epilepsy has been defined by the International Bureau for Epilepsy (IBE) as a "disorder of the brain characterized by a persistent predisposition to generate at least one epileptic seizure and by the neurobiological, cognitive, psychological and social consequences of this condition" [6]. Seizures may also cause various sequelae that can entail brief changes in perception and behavior, mild convulsions, and temporary loss of consciousness, which appear to relate to seizure origin and the degree of their intensity. The neurophysiological factors leading to these sequelae are currently unknown. On the other hand, it is known that epileptogenesis affects brain areas well beyond the epileptogenic foci [7]. The domains affected, their mechanisms of spatial distribution, and the nature of disturbance are thus likely to be significant factors in generating the variability observed in epilepsy's symptoms. Among the often profound changes occurring during epileptic episodes, for instance, are altered states of consciousness, which are likely to involve major networks outside the region of seizure origin. Consistent with such observations, functional connectivity is impaired in large-scale brain networks that extend both bilaterally and via subcortical structures [8]. For recurring seizures, therefore, large-scale interactions could be major pathogenic factors contributing to symptom severity.

Findings from patients resistant to treatment with anti-epileptic drugs, in fact, strongly suggest this. Because the probability of resistant patients to achieve complete remission with new antiepileptic drugs is less than 10%, surgical intervention is often considered the best option for treating intractable epilepsy [9]; however, after temporal lobe and/or localized neocortical resections, only 29–65% of the patients are free of seizures. This relatively low success rate has prompted a number of studies on the mutual, excitatory, and inhibitory interrelations of brain structures participating in epileptogenesis, which have converged on a proposal of epileptic systems that develop in the brains of these patients. The existence of such complex epileptic systems could explain the intractability of epilepsy and the lack of success of resective surgery.

2.1 Impaired homeostasis and the globalizing of epilepsy

How extra-focal, ictal activities emerge in the epileptic brain is still unknown. However, since many of the factors contributing to epileptogenesis, such as stroke or trauma, likely affect homeostatic mechanisms, it has been suggested that included among the chief etiological factors are those related to impaired preservative or homeostatic processes [10]. Fasting, notably, has long been known to have an anticonvulsant effect. The discovery in the 1920s that the anticonvulsant activity was due to ketosis led to treatments using strictly altered diets, for example, the ketogenic diet. Consistent with the results of these dietary studies, conditions precipitating epilepsy like traumatic brain injury, and diseases with which epilepsy is often comorbid, like Alzheimer's, exhibit a chronic loss of energy homeostasis. Moreover, energy levels are acutely impaired during seizures or their precipitating events. Since energy homeostasis is clearly a global requirement, its impairment is likely to contribute to the spread of epileptic foci.

Since the discovery of the effect of fasting on epilepsy, many studies have confirmed the essential participation of metabolic dysregulation and the imbalance of energy metabolites in the disease. During seizures, for instance, the rates of glucose and oxygen consumption rise [11], requiring more energy than that produced by oxidative phosphorylation via the TCA cycle. Glycolysis, consequently, replaces oxidative phosphorylation as the main supply of neuronal ATP. Enzymes involved in the TCA cycle, such as aconitase, malate dehydrogenases, and succinate dehydrogenases decrease their activity during seizures, whereas those involved in anaerobic glycolytic metabolism, such as phosphofructokinase and glucose kinase, increase. The fall in oxygen levels occurring during seizure hyperactivity also induces the expression of hypoxia-inducible factors (HIFs), further exacerbating the inhibition of the mitochondrial TCA cycle and the preferential activation of glycolysis. Glycolysis, however, is insufficient to sustain the hypo-polarization required for preventing spontaneous axonal firing, which is mediated by the energy-demanding sodium-potassium-ATPase (Na^+/K^+-ATPase) enzyme. Na^+/K^+-ATPase malfunctioning, for example, has been shown to result in neuronal hyperexcitability, and to be involved in post-seizure extracellular K^+ clearance and in neonatal seizures [12].

Additionally, with the onset of seizures, the rapid drop in ATP results in a corresponding elevation of adenosine that can exceed baseline levels by more than 40 times [13]. Adenosine, significantly, is a key regulator for energy homeostasis in cells. Its rise, due to ATP depletion, serves as a negative feedback regulator that attenuates cellular activities that consume energy. The rise in adenosine in neurons, particularly, has been shown to attenuate cellular ATP-consuming processes directly related to neural function. Among its effects is a receptor-mediated inhibition of synaptic transmission in the brain [14]. The presynaptic adenosine-1 receptors (A1R), for instance, inhibit synaptic release of most neurotransmitters, especially those used for excitatory transmission. Significantly, a pathological hallmark of epilepsy is astrogliosis, which has been linked to the overexpression of adenosine kinase (ADK) and the consequent adenosine deficiency. Consistent with this observation, a fall of 25% in adenosine is measured by microdialysis in epileptogenic zones. Increased ADK expression, furthermore, results in the spontaneous occurrence of seizures, whereas ADK reduction in the cortex and hippocampus of transgenic mice confers resistance to seizures and to epileptogenesis. Cumulatively, impaired adenosine metabolism—and the specific impairments to aerobically generated energy metabolites appear as key factors leading to epileptogenesis.

2.2 Epileptogenic recruitment and energy impairment

An important aspect of the generation of epileptic seizures is the recruitment of substantial regions of cortical tissue into pathological activity. Given a progressive spreading of metabolic impairment, recruitment can be expected to consecutively engage nearest neighbor, neuronal circuits. On this basis Wang et al. [15] posited a model of interacting minicolumn arrays distributed across a cortical tissue sheet, which sequentially evoked epileptogenic activity. Their model generated focal zones of hyperactivity within the simulated sheet, an observation consistent with microperiodic epileptiform discharges seen during interictal intervals in epilepsy. The high activity zones recruited first neighboring and, later, distant sites, eventually leading to abnormal activity throughout the whole sheet. The time required to recruit the whole sheet depended on the number of hyperexcitable clusters, with earlier recruitment occurring when more clusters were present. Together, the model's predictions were consistent with some notable observations seen during epileptogenesis.

Among the chief mechanisms likely to account for the global activation seen in these results is that of spike timing-dependent plasticity (STDP), where units neighboring epileptic zones experience localized and synchronous depolarizations coinciding with the depolarization occurring within the zones [3]. With STDP, epileptogenesis would be expected to initiate synchronized activity focally, followed by a progressive advance to larger and larger cortical areas. Indeed, it has been presumed that ictal episodes lead to recruitment through processes of synchronization.

Such synchronization has been shown to occur during the late phases of seizure discharge. Seizure initiation and interictal epileptiform events, however, are not consistently associated with synchronous activity, as would be expected if synchronization were chiefly due to localized effects of spike timing-dependent plasticity. One of the most common neurophysiological patterns observed in focal seizures is characterized by low-voltage fast activity at seizure onset, followed by irregular spiking that only subsequently develops into periodic bursting, interspersed with post-burst depressions. This pattern is nearly always seen in human temporal lobe epilepsy [16], in neocortical focal epilepsy, and in acute models of focal seizures. Moreover, there is also a fragmentation of the low amplitude, fast activity, which becomes substituted with a variety of novel background rhythms. Interictal events, additionally, vary in amplitude, pattern, and duration, and are characterized by spikes, sharp waves, and short spike bursts, with rhythmic activity in theta/delta frequency range that can be recorded both within the epileptic zone and around it. In fact, observations of interictal and ictal patterns from epileptic patients showed that synchronization and enhanced excitation were not likely to occur in specific phases of ictogenesis and that synchronous neuronal bursting was not observed during interictal spikes and seizures. Intracranial recordings during the early phase of seizures instead showed that neurons in the epileptic zone and in surrounding areas reduce their firing activity and synchronization, as measured by spiking heterogeneity indices. Transitions into seizure activity due to a localized synchronous enhancement, thus, were relatively rare making them unlikely to contribute to seizure spread. Cumulatively, the data (variability of spiking patterns, the temporal and spatial nonuniformity of foci, and the lack of neighboring recruitment) are therefore caveats to explanations invoking metabolic impairment as a chief vehicle for epileptic globalization, implicating other mechanisms in seizure spreading.

2.3 Globalizing epileptogenesis through higher order cognitive structure: consciousness and the DMN

Unlike the contribution from metabolic impairment, these additional mechanisms likely include interactions with structured cognitive activity [4], including global brain states that govern higher order cognition. Evidence for such influence on two higher order states is considered here, consciousness, and default mode network activity. Both have been shown to be impaired in epilepsy.

2.4 Relating changes in consciousness to epileptogenic spreading

In the most commonly occurring type of chronic, drug-resistant epilepsies, the temporal lobe epilepsies (TLEs), alterations of consciousness (AOC) constitute a particularly dramatic clinical manifestation [17]. Video-EEG recordings reveal that some 60–80% of patients suffering from TLE exhibit AOC during seizures. Due to the frequency of AOC in these patients, the international classification of epileptic seizures has identified impaired consciousness as a framework within which the main categories of partial seizures, simple and complex, can be differentiated. The association between epilepsy and consciousness, a global, higher order brain state, suggests that specific processes associated with consciousness are factors that may contribute to how epileptogenesis spreads to various brain regions.

Consistent with this, temporal lobe seizures are characterized by epileptic discharges originating from one or several regions of the temporal lobe and propagating through apparently interconnected networks located between cortical and subcortical structures [18]. Among the features that have been shown to contribute to a spreading epileptogenesis during AOC are those involving long-range increases in neural synchrony (as opposed to localized influences of synchronization), that is, between the temporal lobes and regions outside the temporal lobe. Studies of severely affected patients, those exhibiting a complete loss of consciousness, could be distinguished from less severely affected subjects on the basis of synchronization differences seen in long-range measurements. Within the temporal zone, differences during seizures were not markedly different between the two groups but differed significantly when measurements were also made of more distant regions, including the thalamus and parietal cortex. Since the group displaying complete loss of consciousness exhibited a specific increase in synchronization between these widely separated regions, the results suggest that extra-temporal structures are associated with increases in long-range synchrony during AOC [18].

2.5 Changes in default mode network connectivity during epileptogenesis

Another key, higher order structure, the default mode network (DMN), has also been shown to be impaired by epilepsy [8]. The DMN is a major resting network that enables transitioning between task-negative and task-positive states, with functional communication occurring through the basal ganglia. Significantly, several experimental and clinical studies show that the putamen and other BG nuclei are likely to modulate epileptic seizures, with changes in functional connectivity between the DMN and ganglia apparently the source of this modulation. The changes observed in these studies occurred in nuclei of the DMN in epileptic patients even during rest, a task-negative state. Within the DMN, functional connectivity in the left superior, frontal gyrus, left postcentral gyrus, and the right superior temporal gyrus was decreased in epilepsy patients compared with normal controls. Between the basal ganglia and DMN, including the regions belonging to the left lingual gyrus, left and right putamen, right insula/inferior frontal gyrus, and left inferior frontal gyrus, connectivity was increased; that is, the connectivity between the DMN and basal ganglia regions was no longer anticorrelated as in controls, but was instead either insignificant or even slightly positive. Thus, the data suggest that the putamen operates in a manner that is quasi-independent of the DMN during epilepsy, a feature that may relate to changes within nuclei of the DMN itself. Although these studies do not show the emergence of ictal episodes in the DMN, as a group they demonstrate that epileptogenesis can modify functional connectivity in a major neural network at long distances from seizure sites.

3. Mechanisms of neurostimulation: beyond functional inhibition

3.1 Oscillations and spreading regimes in epileptogenesis

The effect of epilepsy on global, higher order cognition suggests that these distributed associations could comprise therapeutic targets. Crucially, neurostimulation has been found to decrease seizure frequency in medically resistant epilepsy, apparently through mechanisms affecting extended epileptogenic systems [9]. However, details of these mechanisms, like those for motor diseases, remain to be clarified. For example, the proposal of functional inhibition for PD does not explain all functional changes observed in the basal ganglia [19].

Instead of functional inactivation, by mechanisms such as local depolarization block, inactivation of neuronal voltage-dependent channels, or functional deafferentation, functional activation has also been observed in PD. Most of the cells inhibited by high-frequency stimulation still preserve spontaneous activity, for instance. Moreover, tremors in Parkinson's are most prominent during wakefulness, when motions are most frequent, a state characterized as disassociated, but are much reduced in sleep, when down states, which are characterized by associations with large amplitude slow oscillations, are present [4]. These observations indicate that neurostimulation is likely to exert a much more complex influence on neural activity in PD, and, by extension, in epilepsy as well.

The complexity of this influence is likely to be due to several properties known to characterize neural oscillations that are intrinsic to the principle oscillatory patterns seen in normal brain operation [3]. Disease states are known to alter these properties, modifying oscillatory behavior and affecting how neurostimulation can in turn reverse the effects of the disease. The intrinsic ability of oscillators to combine through synchronization, for example, can be evoked via a number of mechanisms such as phase and amplitude coupling [20] and various forms of cross-frequency coupling that configure the conditions for synchrony in which oscillators align and then resonate in unison. Due to their ubiquity throughout the brain they are capable of coordinating with global (proposed to occur through slower oscillations like theta and delta waves), and regional (thought to involve gamma waves) activities [3]. Resonating in unison has the important effect of enabling information transfer and so of regulating communication between brain domains [21]. On the other hand, oscillators must also disengage through desynchronization, where their frequencies are no longer aligned, to generate new combinations with functionally different outcomes. For example, both beta and mu basal ganglia rhythms show event-related desynchronization prior to movement in the basal ganglia, with sustained suppression during movement execution [22]. Desynchronization requires a discrete segregation of oscillator pairs to avoid functional overlap; that is, a qualitative bifurcation of the two that is fundamentally a nonlinear and dynamical event, for which several mechanisms are proposed [21], like phase resetting through pulsing, or noise-induced effects that entrain localized rhythms [20]. Phase shifting, or curve resetting, is a common mechanism for oscillatory control, one already implicated in Wilson Cowan excitatory inhibitory models. By means of spike timing-dependent plasticity, oscillatory phases can be advanced or delayed to adjust synchronization [20], a mechanism that could be evoked by neurostimulation.

Synchronization and desynchronization help the brain to maintain reliability as well as to achieve the flexibility needed for functional variance. Additionally, these "performance" needs must be contextualized in terms of global operation, which ultimately defines the sorts of mechanisms required for the "good" of the whole individual. Significantly, the resident oscillator field is not unimodal, but represents a broad distribution of oscillator attractors elicited by the network connectivity and determined by the physical parameters that give rise to them such as impedance resonance and anatomical configurations [3]. Neurostimulation may drive synchrony with a subset of oscillators but may do so only if the relative coupling between the source of neurostimulation and the neural oscillators is energetically preferred to other combinations, where local instabilities might otherwise disengage them [23].

Critically, for neurostimulation, rigid or full phase locking is rarely if ever achieved [21, 24], a natural physical feature permitting the separation of pair members with the corresponding potential to form new combinations. Due to the intrinsic tendency for oscillators to align (or disengage), influences of neurostimulation on neural oscillators can be expected to specifically impact the spectral power attained during DBS frequency output, including factors like the extent of phase alignment in the population [20], frequency modulation due to the phase dependency of the coupling constant [21], intermittency of alignment [23], and oscillator disruption that may be occasioned by excessive coupling strength [25]. The need for oscillators to recombine requires that synchronization be of only modest strength. This requirement has led to the current model for oscillator pairing, the Theory of Weakly Coupled Oscillators [3, 21], which is mathematically described by the Adler equation. (Weak here means that interactions lead to phase adjustments without strong perturbations of the oscillatory generative mechanisms.) The Adler equation, accordingly, includes terms for repulsion, termed detuning, and for coupling, both of which vary as a function of the frequency difference between pair members (**Figure 1**).

3.2 Weak associations and neurostimulation

Because perfect synchrony is not strictly attainable, the effect of increasing coupling strength is to increase synchronization residency within a preferred

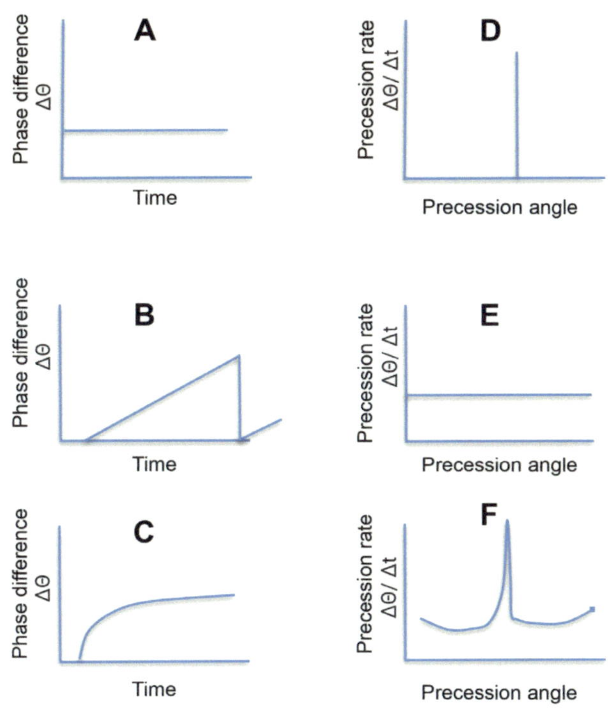

Figure 1.
Synchrony between two oscillators is governed by two factors, the difference between the intrinsic oscillator frequencies and the coupling strength between them. The individual phase evolution for each of two oscillators (A) and (B) is mathematically described: $d\Theta_A/dt = w_A(t)$ and $d\Theta_B/dt = w_B(t)$. From TWCO theory, the evolution of the phase precession angle, Θ_B, is: $d\Theta_P/dt = (w_A(t) - w_B(t)) + K\sin(\Theta_P(t)) + N_P$ (Adler equation). (A and D) Rigid phase locking occurs when the rate of precession equals 0 and the phase difference angle is a constant value. (B and E) The rate of precession is constant and oscillation precesses through all phase angles. (C and F) With coupling, the precession rate is variable and described by the sine of the phase precession angle. Slowing occurs when the phase difference angle is small, termed the phase overlap range, and speed increases when the phase difference is large, a phenomenon known as the Arnold tongue. Such frequency modulation effects result in information transfer in the region of phase overlap [21].

overlap range where oscillator frequency differences are minimal, mathematically described by the sine of the phase angle difference between oscillators. As a result, the oscillators continue to experience frequency modulation throughout the cycle, which is manifest in the continual change in their precession rates (**Figure 1**). (Frequency modulation is posited to lead to information transfer in the maximal overlap range).

Moreover, increasing coupling strength by neurostimulation for the purpose of improving synchronization with a neural oscillator is intrinsically limited and possesses an upper bound [25]. Neural oscillations exhibit stochastic behavior with intermittent synchronization, where neural signals go in and out of synchrony [23] revealing that synchronization (of weakly coupled oscillators) represents a statistical median where a predominant fraction of "micro" oscillating circuits determine the behavior of the population oscillator. Thus, the overall oscillatory distribution may be considered to have a certain phase variance range. Increases in coupling strength, accordingly, can be expected to shift only a proportion of the individual cycling circuits into a non-oscillatory range as increases in the strength of coupling progressively shift the population to a phase lock value near one (**Figure 2**).

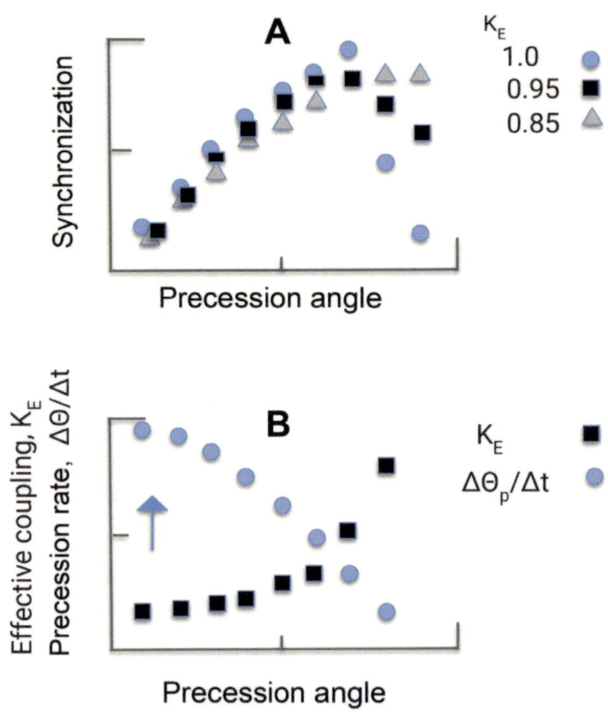

Figure 2.
Effects of varying coupling strength on oscillator attrition. Mathematically, synchronization can be defined in terms of the phase locking value at perfect constancy, that is, equal to 1, minus the influence due to phase precession and the loss of "micro" oscillators due to quenching. Normalized precession influences on synchronization are then described: $S(t) = 1 - d\Theta_P/dt\ (T - t)/d\Theta_P(T) - G((1 - d\Theta_P/dt\ (T - t)/d\Theta_P(T)))$, *where S(t) is the relative synchronization as a function t of the precession cycle (T). Ahn and Lubchinsky characterize an oscillating population microstructure [23] in terms of the frequency distribution of the phase differences present within the synchronized set. Using this variance, the proportion of oscillators entering a zone of attrition may then be described by a cumulative normal distribution. Thus only the optimally synchronized set will approach a phase lock value leading to quenching, which is expressed as a product of the cumulative normal distribution and the synchronized population, where G, the fraction entering attrition, can be obtained from the cumulative normal distribution, which is bounded, due to phase variance, at phase constancy.*
(A) Reduction in synchronization due to oscillator attrition. (B) Variation in the coupling strength constant as a function of the precession angle.

Taken together, the physical properties structuring brain oscillations define a set of parameters within which neurostimulatory intervention could modulate brain dysfunctions.

4. Epileptogenic spreading and neurostimulation affect higher order, global oscillations

Significantly, recent studies demonstrate that epileptic activity affects long-distance oscillatory associations in the brain, including those influencing higher order cognitive activity [26]. A key finding has been the detection of coupling between epileptic electrical activity and slow brain oscillations—posited to mediate interareal coordination of brain activity—in loci distant from seizure origins. Using a biomarker of experimental epileptogenesis, fast ripples (FRs) (high-frequency waveforms that can be induced by kainite injection) the study demonstrated the presence of nonrandom brain activity specifically associated with slow oscillations. Fast ripples were shown to couple with two bandwidths, a slow oscillation in the 3- to 5-Hz range and one involving interictal epileptic episodes in the 20- to 30-Hz range. Phase-amplitude coupling during these events aligned at 4.5 Hz frequency for phase and 27 Hz frequency for amplitude and was 2.1 times higher than during baseline. Domain-specific analyses additionally revealed that the frontal cortex and left and right hippocampi specifically increased in power at 3–5 Hz in all three regions indicating that the ripples were synchronized across these brain domains. Furthermore, the increase in synchronization converged toward a common value, revealing that distribution of phase differences tended to converge and to coincide with the slow oscillation. Additionally, frontal cortex synchronization was delayed with respect to the two hippocampi, demonstrating that functional connectivity was oriented from the hippocampi to the frontal cortices, a finding also confirmed by Grainger analysis. Altogether, the data revealed a strong influence of structured brain activity on epileptogenesis, with cross-frequency coupling between the slow oscillation and FRs shaping the latter's temporal pattern and directionality in the brain.

Critically, epileptic coupling with slow oscillations has been shown to modify memory consolidation, a higher order brain function [27]. Memory consolidation is known to require three patterns of network activity (and their corresponding physiological coupling): hippocampal ripples, neocortical slow oscillations, and neocortical sleep spindles. By selectively eliminating ripples, for instance, memory performance can be greatly impaired in laboratory animals. In normal functioning, the coupling of the three patterns between the hippocampi and prefrontal cortices during NREM sleep leads to consolidation. Experimentally, accordingly, these studies examined how epileptogenesis interfered with the temporal coupling between these events. Specifically, the introduction of experimentally induced, interictal episodes was used to reduce fast ripples. Multivariate correlations between experimentally induced IEDs and fast ripples and spindles then showed that the reduction in FR resulted in significant declines in task-related memory performance, demonstrating a direct effect between the epileptogenic event, the brain patterning, and the inability to recall learned tasks. Significantly, the experimentally induced IEDs modified structured, global activity involving slow oscillations. In all cases, the hippocampal IEDs induced a marked decrease in neuronal firing (relative to baseline firing) within 200 ms, a time window known to be correlated with neuronal hyperpolarization and reduced spiking during NREM sleep and anesthesia that corresponded to slow oscillation, delta waves.

4.1 Neurostimulation treatments

The effects of epilepsy on these higher order oscillatory structures suggest that neurostimulation could restore normal function by reversing these effects. Work in this area remains preliminary, but consistent with this hypothesis.

4.1.1 Vagal nerve stimulation

Therapeutic approaches using neurostimulation for epilepsy primarily involve vagal nerve stimulation (VNS), although other techniques such as deep brain stimulation and repetitive transcranial magnetic stimulation (rTMS) have seen limited use. Existing studies suggest that neurostimulation influences mechanisms of consciousness, which are altered during epilepsy [28]. For afferent vagal nerve fibers, the brainstem nucleus of the solitary tract (NST) is the main relay station. This nucleus has widespread projections to numerous areas in the forebrain, brainstem, thalamus, and areas involved in learning and memory formation (amygdala, hippocampus). Additionally, learning, memory encoding and recall are known to be modulated by arousal, an integral feature of consciousness. Consistent with the observations on the effect of epilepsy on memory consolidation, animal models of vagal nerve stimulation showed that it positively influenced hippocampal long-term potentiation (HLP). In humans, for instance, a chronic increased alertness is observed in VNS-implanted subjects with acute effects on memory consolidation.

4.1.2 DBS

DBS in epilepsy has been applied to a number of targets, including the thalamus (anterior and centromedian nuclei), cerebellum, and basal ganglia (subthalamic nucleus, caudate, substantia nigra pars reticulata). Via the brainstem and basal forebrain arousal systems, the thalamus is hypothesized to underpin consciousness through distributed mechanisms of arousal regulation. Of these, the anterior nucleus of the thalamus appears to underlie limbic seizures and to present in medically resistant seizure formation, whereas the centromedian nucleus of the thalamus is involved in the reticulothalamocortical system that is considered integral to the modulation of vigilance. Significantly, deep brain stimulation of the anterior nucleus of the thalamus has emerged as a promising therapy for drug resistant epilepsy, with recent findings indicating a key mechanistic role for brain oscillations. A study by Chang, for example, showed that desynchronization of the ipsilateral hippocampal background electrical activity over a broad frequency range influenced epileptic discharges, including interictal spikes and high-frequency oscillations [29]. Furthermore, high-frequency stimulation of the anterior nucleus of the thalamus appeared to decouple large-scale neural activity between the hippocampus and regionally distant cortical areas.

5. Summary and conclusion

Singer's discovery in the 1990s of patterned electrical activity for brain communication provided the conceptual basis for moving beyond temporal sequencing for encoded representations [30]. It also overcame the most significant theoretical limitation of Hubel and Wiesel's abstraction thesis for coding, which had been premised on their discovery of motion and edge detector cells in the occipital cortex. The use of rhythmic, typically oscillatory, activity for communication and the ordering of cognition has since been confirmed in a wide variety of studies. This understanding has enabled a sounder strategy for investigating the structure of brain operation and how the impairment of this structure might lead to brain dysfunction and disease. It has also opened a window to the new therapeutic modes of neuromodulation and neurostimulation. These recent forms of therapy, many described in this volume, are exploiting such understanding to yield the current profusion of medical applications now revolutionizing treatment for brain disease.

Author details

Denis Larrivee[1,2]

1 Loyola University Chicago, USA

2 Mind and Brain Institute, University of Navarra Medical School, Spain

*Address all correspondence to: sallar1@aol.com

References

[1] Udupa K, Chen R. The mechanisms of action of deep brain stimulation and ideas for the future development. Progress in Neurobiology. 2015;**133**:27-49

[2] Philip N et al. Low intensity transcranial current stimulation in psychiatry. The American Journal of Psychiatry. 2017;**174**(7):628-639

[3] Wang XJ. Neurophysiological and computational principles of cortical rhythms in cognition. Physiological Reviews. 2010;**90**:1195-1268

[4] Buzsaki G. Rhythms of the Brain. New York: Oxford University Press; 2006

[5] De Boer HM et al. The global burden and stigma of epilepsy. Epilepsy and Behavior. 2008;**12**(4):540-546

[6] Fisher RS et al. Epileptic seizures and epilepsy: Definitions proposed by the international league against epilepsy (ILAE) and the International Bureau for Epilepsy (IBE). Epilepsia. 2005;**46**(4):470-472

[7] Englot DJ et al. Regional and global connectivity disturbances in focal epilepsy, related neurocognitive sequelae, and potential mechanistic underpinnings. Epilepsia. 2016;**57**:1546-1557

[8] Rektor I et al. Association between the basal ganglia and large-scale brain networks in epilepsy. Brain Topography. 2013;**26**:355-362

[9] Benbadis SR et al. Putting it all together: Options for intractable epilepsy. An updated algorithm on the use of epilepsy surgery and neurostimulation. Epilepsy & Behavior. 2018;**88**:33-38

[10] Boison D et al. Homeostatic control of brain function—new approaches to understand epileptogenesis. Frontiers in Cellular Neuroscience. 2013;**7**(109):1-8

[11] Bazzigaluppi P et al. Hungry neurons: Metabolic insights on seizure dynamics. International Journal of Molecular Sciences. 2017;**18**(2269):1-14

[12] Renkawek K et al. Neonatal status convulsivus, spongiform encephalopathy, and low activity of Na+/K+-ATPase in the brain. Epilepsia. 1992;**33**:58-64

[13] During MJ, Spencer DD. Adenosine: A potential mediator of seizure arrest and postictal refractoriness. Annals of Neurology. 1992;**32**:618-624

[14] Brundege JM, Dunwiddie TV. Modulation of excitatory synaptic transmission by adenosine released from single hippocampal pyramidal neurons. The Journal of Neuroscience. 1966;**16**:5603-5612

[15] Wang X et al. Computational modelling of microseizures and focal seizure onset. In: Tetzlaff R, editor. Recent Advances in Predicting and Preventing Epileptic Seizures. Proceedings of the 5th International Workshop on Seizure Prediction. ProQuest EBook Central: World Scientific Publishing Co; 2014

[16] Allen PJ et al. Very high-frequency rhythmic activity during SEEG suppression in frontal lobe epilepsy. Electroencephalography and Clinical Neurophysiology. 1992;**82**:155

[17] Bartolomeia F, Naccache L. The global workspace (GW) theory of consciousness and epilepsy. Behavioural Neurology. 2011;**24**:67-74

[18] Guye M et al. The role of corticothalamic coupling in human temporal lobe epilepsy. Brain. 2006;**129**:1917-1928

[19] Deniau JM. Deep brain stimulation mechanisms: Beyond the concept of local functional inhibition. The European Journal of Neuroscience. 2010;**32**:1080-1091

[20] Canavier CC. Phase resetting as a tool of information transmission current opinions in. Neurobiology. 2015;**31**:206-213

[21] Lowet E et al. Quantifying neural oscillatory synchronization: A comparison between spectral coherence and phaselocking value approaches. PLoS One. 2015;**11**:e0146443

[22] Doesburg SM et al. From local inhibition to long-range integration: A functional dissociation of alpha-band synchronization across cortical scales in visuospatial attention. Brain Research. 2009;**1303**:97-110

[23] Ahn S, Rubchinsky LL. Short desynchronization episodes prevail in synchronous dynamics of human brain rhythms. Chaos. 2013;**23**:1-8

[24] Larrivee D. Global dynamics and local synchrony: Therapeutic prospects for implant learning devices. In: Internat Joint Conf Neural Networks. 2018. pp. 1-6

[25] Nandan M et al. Transition from amplitude to oscillation death in a network of oscillators. Chaos: An Interdisciplinary Journal of Nonlinear Science. 2014;**24**(4):1063

[26] Sheybani L et al. Large-scale 3-5 hz oscillation constrains the expression of neocortical fast ripples in a mouse model of mesial tem- poral lobe epileps. eNeuro. 2019;**6**(1):e0494-e0418

[27] Gelinas JN et al. Interictal epileptiform discharges induce hippocampal–cortical coupling in temporal lobe epilepsy. Nature Medicine. 2016;**22**(6):641-651

[28] Bagary M. Epilepsy, consciousness and neurostimulation. Behavioural Neurology. 2011;**24**:75-81

[29] Chang B. Deep brain stimulation works for drug-resistant epilepsy, but how? Epilepsy Currents. 2018;**18**(6):378-385

[30] Uhlhaas PJ, Singer W. High-frequency oscillations and the neurobiology of schizophrenia. Dialogues in Clinical Neuroscience. 2013;**15**(3):301-331

Chapter 2

Neuromodulation in the Age of Modern Neuroimaging Technologies

Mohammad Hossein Khosravi, Meysam Hoseinyazdi, Reza Jahankhah and Sara Haseli

Abstract

Most commonly used for the treatment of Parkinson's disease (PD), the deep brain stimulation (DBS) is a new neurosurgical method whose other applications are still under development. Neuroimaging has a variety of main roles in DBS including evaluating the final electrode contact position, localizing the target nucleus, and detecting complications. Despite being a neurosurgical method, successful DBS intervention is highly dependent on an appropriate neuroimaging technique. For achieving satisfying clinical results, DBS needs the presence of neuroradiologists. In this chapter, we have reviewed the role of neuroimaging in all stages of deep brain stimulation as well as the underlying mechanism in this domain.

Keywords: neuroimaging, neurostimulation, deep brain stimulation, functional neurosurgery

1. Introduction

Most commonly used for the treatment of Parkinson's disease (PD), the deep brain stimulation (DBS) is a new neurosurgical method which its other applications is still under development [1]. Neuroimaging has a variety of main roles in DBS including evaluating the final electrode contact position, localizing the target nucleus, and detecting complications.

Benabid et al. were the very first researchers who introduced the chronic high-frequency stimulation of the ventral intermediate nucleus (VIM) of the thalamus in early 1990s [2]. The authors used a subcutaneous pulse generator, which was implanted in the thoracic region, connected to chronic stimulating electrodes in the VIM for treatment of 6 patients with essential tremor and 26 patients with Parkinson's disease (PD). The patients maintained improvement up to 29 months. As the first clinical effort to introduce the chronic high-frequency stimulation of nuclei (deep brain stimulation), this study showed that this newly come up method could be used instead of common destructive surgeries such as thalamotomy.

Another similar technique, bilateral DBS of the subthalamic nucleus (STN), was then introduced by the Benabid team for the treatment of severe motor fluctuations and akinetic rigid Parkinson's disease [3]. In 2002, the USA food and drug administration (FDA) approved the treatment of Parkinson's disease by stimulation of bilateral STN and the stimulation of internal globus pallidus (GPi) was approved in 2003. Although advanced Parkinson's disease is the main indication for DBS, a number of different additional uses have been mentioned for DBS, such as Tourette syndrome, cluster headache, and dystonia as well as psychiatric indications such as major depression (MDD) and obsessive-compulsion disorders (OCDs).

Despite being a neurosurgical method, successful DBS intervention is highly dependent on an appropriate neuroimaging technique. For achieving satisfying clinical results, DBS needs the presence of neuroradiologists. In this chapter, we have reviewed the role of neuroimaging in all stages of deep brain stimulation.

2. Targets for DBS

A variety of indications and targets have been proposed for DBS since its starting era. Essential tremor and Parkinson's disease are among the most common and ancient indications of DBS, which are managed by stimulation of VIM nucleus [4–6]. On the other hand, STN and GPi are the most effective targets for Parkinson's disease DBS. It has also been reported that VIM DBS may relieve orthostatic tremor [6]. Tourette syndrome is another indication for DBS that is done through bilateral thalamic stimulation [7, 8].

Subthalamic nucleus (STN) stimulation by bilateral implantation of electrodes comprises a majority of DBS interventions for management of advanced Parkinson's disease [9, 10]. Intractable epilepsy is another described indication for STN DBS [11]. Recently, different psychologic disorders, such as OCD, have been discussed as possible indications for STN DBS [12]. Internal globus pallidus (GPi) is another target for DBS, which is more commonly indicated for managing dystonia and advanced Parkinson's disease [13–16]. Also, winter's cramp and Tourette syndrome have been managed by DBS of GPi [17–19]. Previous studies have shown that GPi DBS improves Yale Global Tic Severity Scale and reduces Tic in a range of 65–96%. An older reported indication for DBS is chronic pain for which a variety of targets have been proposed from internal capsule and periventricular gray matter to sensory thalamus [20, 21].

A variety of other targets have been come up for DBS in management of psychiatric disorders such as major depression or OCD [22–25]. On the other hand, cluster headache has been treated by hypothalamic DBS [26]. Also, seizures that are resistant to medical treatment have been managed by DBS of cerebellum, centromedian, or anterior nucleus of thalamus and hippocampus [26–28].

3. Pre-interventional imaging

Magnetic resonance imaging (MRI) is the most commonly used modality for pre-interventional brain assessment in Parkinson's disease patients who are candidates for DBS, whether STN DBS or bilateral GPi. Multiple lacunae, severe atrophy, or leukoencephalopathy are among the MRI abnormalities that contraindicate DBS surgery [29, 30]. Some features in MRI imaging are predictors of desired or non-appropriate postoperative results. For example, a normalized surface measure of mesencephalon is correlated with satisfying clinical effects of bilateral STN stimulation on motor disability in Parkinson's disease; while, a smaller surface of mesencephalon is more associated with non-desired results of stimulation [31]. Also, it has been mentioned that brain atrophy is not related to non-desired postoperative clinical results in patients who are candidates for bilateral STN stimulation. There is a supporting hypothesis for connecting these imaging features to post-interventional clinical results that believes that a small mesencephalic surface area is correlated with cognitive impairment and non-dopaminergic non-levodopa responsive axial motor symptoms that do not appropriately respond to STN stimulation.

Imaging modalities have an important role in targeting for DBS. Appropriate placement of electrodes is a sensitive and difficult neurosurgical technique, which involves highly skilled surgeons. In the first stage of DBS, anatomical landmarks are determined by MR imaging. Previously, invasive ventriculography was used to determine the anatomical landmarks for STN implantation; however, it is very uncommon these days [32]. MR imaging has two remarkable benefits: first of, it can be easily used for stereotactic targeting in DBS surgery and second, electrodes can be accurately implanted with no additional negative effects [33, 34]. Another option for targeting is MR imaging/CT fusion technique in which the data acquired from the two modalities are fused and MR imaging with stereotactic condition is not used anymore [35].

4. Imaging during intervention

Plain control radiographs are more commonly used by most of the neurosurgery teams during placement of implants to ensure that the electrodes are accurately following the predetermined pathway [36]. In addition, intraoperative use of MR imaging or CT scan has been recently developed for this purpose [37, 38].

Although it has remained a controversy, electrophysiological study of brain has been used intraoperatively for checking electrode placement in DBS surgery. Some neurosurgeons consider electrophysiologic mapping of the anatomic target during STN electrode implantation while others prefer not to apply it, as it prolongs the surgery and may be associated with risks and complications [39–41].

5. Postoperative imaging

In most of the cases, postoperative imaging is performed to detect the possible complications. CT scan is the most common modality that is used for this purpose. It seems that MR imaging has a higher sensitivity in comparison with CT scan for some complications; for example, electrode-related infections are more detected by MR imaging. Also, MR imaging correctly indicates the position of contact of implanted electrodes. MR imaging study provides a bunch of valuable data including the exact position of electrodes in case of clinical failure and also relationships between electrode and the target. Neurosurgeons more commonly register an atlas on postoperative MR imaging for checking the exact position of contact. Electrode heating is the most common complication of MR imaging, which is induced by electromagnetic waves [42, 43].

Post-interventional imaging has provided a remarkable source of data for discovering new therapeutic methods for many neurologic and psychiatric diseases. When undesired symptoms and manifestations are presented after DBS, researchers can assess the effect by imaging and this will lead to identification of new targets for managing a variety of disorders. It was found that bilateral hypothalamic DBS, which was used for treating morbid obesity, has evoked detailed autobiographic memories [44]. Also, the correlation of severe obsession and hyperactivity of caudate nucleus was found during intraoperative electrophysiologic study of caudate nucleus DBS in patients with OCD [45].

6. PET, fMRI, and DBS

Functional MRI (fMRI) is a neuroimaging modality with a wide range of application in both biomedical research and clinical studies. In addition to its high resolution for soft tissue imaging, MRI has the ability to assess physiological parameters including metabolites, diffusion, or hemodynamics [46]. Neuronal activity causes a secondary hemodynamic response, including a local vascular response, which can be measured by fMRI [47, 48]. fMRI has promoted our understanding about behavioral and translational neuroscience as it has provided human brain function maps in addition to conventional anatomical imaging.

When it comes to DBS, positron emission tomography (PET) scan is more preferred than fMRI as it provides a safer modality for studying patients during DBS intervention. PET is used for studying both mechanism and unexpected effects of DBS [49]. According to these facilities, PET has become a gold standard for imaging of in vivo neurochemistry.

Combination of fMRI and PET modalities has provided a terrific opportunity in research to understand the neurochemistry of brain and underlying biochemical nature of brain function.

7. Diffusion tensor imaging (DTI)

Diffusion tensor imaging is an emerging modality that enables us to characterize microstructure of white matter and this may help with further development of targeting methods and brain stimulation therapies [50]. The technology used behind the DTI is measuring three-dimensional movement of water molecules in biological tissue. DTI calculates diffusion of water in three dimensions by fitting a tensor to each voxel of a brain diffusion-weighted MR scan [51]. Three-dimensional visualization of brain white matter pathways can be provided by DTI-based tractography [52, 53]. This has resulted in better understanding of brain anatomical structure, which can be implied in neurosurgical procedures [54, 55].

Defining accurate position of targets is a key point in neurosurgical stimulation process. The role of DTI in detailed visualization of white matter becomes more important when the conventional imaging modalities cannot reliably show the putative target location [50]. Tractography-guided neuromodulation has been tried for DBS in patients with Parkinson's disease and dystonia. This will help surgeons with finding individual anatomic variations and so achieving better results.

8. Less invasive stimulation modalities

Neuromodulation carries a vast range of procedures from pharmacological interferences to the direct stimulation of brain with placed electrodes. Noninvasive brain stimulation (NIBS) devices work based on transferring electrical currents into the brain (usually cortex) through externally placed electrodes. These currents may be alternating or even created by magnetic fields [56]. In addition to its developed application in research, NIBS has dramatically entered to the clinical management of several neurologic/psychiatric disorders. Repeated trains of transcranial magnetic stimulation (rTMS) were first approved by FDA for management of major depressive disorders and obsessive-compulsive disorders, while migraine headaches are managed by single pulse TMS [56, 57].

A dynamic magnetic field is produced by TMS devices, which induces a consequent electric field through the skull and scalp. When this electric field is delivered to the motor cortex, neurons forming the corticospinal tract are depolarized at the junction of gray and white matter. In addition, axons in superficial layers of cortex including interneurons and thalamocortical afferents can be triggered by TMS pulses. TMS has effects on various brain neurotransmitter systems including their second messengers and receptors. Also, it promotes synaptic plasticity, which is a justification for TMS use in pain management. On the other hand, some previously published researches have indicated that TMS is effective in reducing frequency of epileptic attacks in patients with medically refractory epilepsy, without imposing any additional side effects. Another pilot study holds the belief that TMS in combination with EEG is an appropriate method for developing quantitative biomarkers of cortical hyperexcitability in patients with epilepsy [58].

A considerable problem with application of rTMS is its variable effects among different patients [59, 60]. This makes the research results' replication a problem and application of rTMS to clinical therapeutic setting a controversial issue. When we use rTMS in a precise cortical area, it will equally affect all the neuronal populations and consequent behaviors involving that area [61]. Therefore, combination of EEG and rTMS seems to be an appropriate method in order to specify the rTMS effects in patients through direct measurement of cortical responses to TMS pulses [62]. This helps with measurement of TMS-evoked potentials (TEPs) and the meantime effects of TMS on the recording EEG. Various TEPs' components are a reflection of activity in a precise area of cortical neurons. So, this may result in development of more selectively targeted forms of rTMS in non-motor areas of the cortex.

Transcranial direct current stimulation (tDCS) is another form of noninvasive brain stimulation techniques that is easily available and not extensive, while the exact mechanism of action has not been yet discovered [63, 64]. In this method, electrodes are placed on the scalp and they conduct weak prolonged (about 10–20 min) currents to brain tissues. Indeed, neuronal excitability is modulated in a polarity-specific manner by tDCS [65]. The modulatory effects of tDCS are the main role considered for this procedure as it shifts membrane polarity resulting to modifying the neuronal discharge. There are two subdivisions: anodal tDCS increases the rate of spontaneous neuronal firing by depolarizing resting membrane potential, while cathodal tDCS shifts the resting membrane potential to hyperpolarization, which leads into decreased cortical excitability [66]. tDCS has approved improving effects on patients with various types of anxiety disorders such as social anxiety disorders, generalized anxiety disorders, and anorexia nervosa as well as major depression and chronic pain [67–69].

Besides the proved applications of tDCS in previous studies, the effect of sham tDCS has not been yet completely assessed. Some previously conducted sham-controlled studies have reported inconsistent results with placebo response, which make this idea more important [70].

9. Neuroimaging and neurosurgical treatment of psychiatric disorders

Progresses in neuroimaging have resulted in developing a notable amount of new indications of DBS for psychiatric disorders. Discovering new functions and relationships for internal capsule, cingulate cortex and their networks is a result of modern neuroimaging techniques. In the major part of the situations, nodes of these networks are in the regions that are responsible for functional changes in psychiatric pathology that kind of confirms the benefits of conventional capsulotomy and cingulotomy [71].

These days, personalized medicine has become the most commonly mentioned subject in the modern medicine. All the medicine-related fields are trying to find ways that help with individualized treatment of the diseases, thus treating patients instead of diseases [72]. So, psychiatrists are following this trend and modern neuroimaging techniques may help them with finding proper treatment for each patient [73]. So far, neuroimaging was used only for checking the proper placement of electrodes and retrograde evaluation of interventional mechanisms; however, these modalities will be used for planning new treatment methods and targets for DBS in near future. Neuroimaging can provide lots of valuable data about connectivity and regional volume in each patient. Thus, it not only helps with choosing the most appropriate approach in psychiatric neurosurgery but also simplifies prediction of interventional outcomes [74–76].

Looking at the recent published studies around neuroimaging, we found out that developing neuroimaging techniques is leading to the age of "precision surgery." In this period of time, neuroimaging will change the face and approach to electrode implantation and patient selection as well as selection of surgical targets throughout individualized neuroanatomy extracted from modern neuroimaging modalities and technologies [74, 77, 78].

10. Conclusion

As the researches are getting more informative, more patients are going under DBS intervention especially for treating Parkinson's disease. In addition, as the modern technologies are developed, more new applications and targets are getting introduced for DBS. So, neuroimaging has a notable role in preoperative and postoperative sections as well as during DBS intervention. Further researches are required to discover more efficient imaging modalities that will lead to discovery of new targets and indications for DBS and functional neurosurgery.

Author details

Mohammad Hossein Khosravi[1]*, Meysam Hoseinyazdi[2], Reza Jahankhah[2] and Sara Haseli[3]

1 Department of Neurosurgery, School of Medicine, Iran University of Medical Sciences, Tehran, Iran

2 Medical Imaging Research Center, Shiraz University of Medical Sciences, Shiraz, Iran

3 Chronic Respiratory Diseases Research Center, National Research Institute of Tuberculosis and Lung Diseases (NRITLD), Shahid Beheshti University of Medical Sciences, Tehran, Iran

*Address all correspondence to: dr.mhkhosravi@gmail.com

References

[1] Dormont D, Seidenwurm D, Galanaud D, Cornu P, Yelnik J, Bardinet E. Neuroimaging and deep brain stimulation. American Journal of Neuroradiology. 2010;**31**(1):15-23

[2] Benabid AL, Pollak P, Hoffmann D, Gervason C, Hommel M, Perret J, et al. Long-term suppression of tremor by chronic stimulation of the ventral intermediate thalamic nucleus. The Lancet. 1991;**337**(8738):403-406

[3] Limousin P, Pollak P, Benazzouz A, Hoffmann D, Le Bas J-F, Perret J, et al. Effect on parkinsonian signs and symptoms of bilateral subthalamic nucleus stimulation. The Lancet. 1995;**345**(8942):91-95

[4] Lee JY, Kondziolka D. Thalamic deep brain stimulation for management of essential tremor. Journal of Neurosurgery. 2005;**103**(3):400-403

[5] Lyons KE, Pahwa R. Deep brain stimulation and essential tremor. Journal of Clinical Neurophysiology. 2004;**21**(1):2-5

[6] Guridi J, Rodriguez-Oroz MC, Arbizu J, Alegre M, Prieto E, Landecho I, et al. Successful thalamic deep brain stimulation for orthostatic tremor. Movement Disorders. 2008;**23**(13):1808-1811

[7] Maciunas RJ, Maddux BN, Riley DE, Whitney CM, Schoenberg MR, Ogrocki PJ, et al. Prospective randomized double-blind trial of bilateral thalamic deep brain stimulation in adults with Tourette syndrome. Journal of Neurosurgery. 2007;**107**(5):1004-1014

[8] Servello D, Porta M, Sassi M, Brambilla A, Robertson MM. Deep brain stimulation in 18 patients with severe Gilles de la Tourette syndrome refractory to treatment: The surgery and stimulation. Journal of Neurology, Neurosurgery, and Psychiatry. 2008;**79**(2):136-142

[9] Krack P, Limousin P, Benabid A, Pollak P. Chronic stimulation of subthalamic nucleus improves levodopa-induced dyskinesias in Parkinson's disease. The Lancet. 1997;**350**(9092):1676

[10] Moro E, Volkmann J, König I, Winkler S, Hiller A, Hassin-Baer S, et al. Bilateral subthalamic stimulation in Parkin and PINK1 parkinsonism. Neurology. 2008;**70**(14):1186-1191

[11] Theodore WH, Fisher RS. Brain stimulation for epilepsy. The Lancet Neurology. 2004;**3**(2):111-118

[12] Mallet L, Polosan M, Jaafari N, Baup N, Welter M-L, Fontaine D, et al. Subthalamic nucleus stimulation in severe obsessive–compulsive disorder. The New England Journal of Medicine. 2008;**359**(20):2121-2134

[13] Machado A, Rezai AR, Kopell BH, Gross RE, Sharan AD, Benabid AL. Deep brain stimulation for Parkinson's disease: Surgical technique and perioperative management. Movement Disorders: Official Journal of the Movement Disorder Society. 2006;**21**(S14):S247-SS58

[14] Yelnik J, Damier P, Bejjani B, Francois C, Gervais D, Dormont D, et al. Functional mapping of the human globus pallidus: Contrasting effect of stimulation in the internal and external pallidum in Parkinson's disease. Neuroscience. 2000;**101**(1):77-87

[15] Coubes P, Cif L, El Fertit H, Hemm S, Vayssiere N, Serrat S, et al. Electrical stimulation of the globus pallidus internus in patients with primary generalized dystonia: Long-term results. Journal of Neurosurgery. 2004;**101**(2):189-194

[16] Trottenberg T, Volkmann J, Deuschl G, Kühn A, Schneider G-H, Müller J, et al. Treatment of severe tardive dystonia with pallidal deep brain stimulation. Neurology. 2005;**64**(2):344-346

[17] Fukaya C, Katayama Y, Kano T, Nagaoka T, Kobayashi K, Oshima H, et al. Thalamic deep brain stimulation for writer's cramp. Journal of Neurosurgery. 2007;**107**(5):977-982

[18] Welter M-L, Mallet L, Houeto J-L, Karachi C, Czernecki V, Cornu P, et al. Internal pallidal and thalamic stimulation in patients with Tourette syndrome. Archives of Neurology. 2008;**65**(7):952-957

[19] Houeto J-L, Karachi C, Mallet L, Pillon B, Yelnik J, Mesnage V, et al. Tourette's syndrome and deep brain stimulation. Journal of Neurology, Neurosurgery, and Psychiatry. 2005;**76**(7):992-995

[20] Raslan AM. Deep Brain Stimulation for Chronic Pain: Can It Help? LWW; 2006

[21] Bittar RG, Kar-Purkayastha I, Owen SL, Bear RE, Green A, Wang S, et al. Deep brain stimulation for pain relief: A meta-analysis. Journal of Clinical Neuroscience. 2005;**12**(5):515-519

[22] Rauch SL, Dougherty DD, Malone D, Rezai A, Friehs G, Fischman AJ, et al. A functional neuroimaging investigation of deep brain stimulation in patients with obsessive–compulsive disorder. Journal of Neurosurgery. 2006;**104**(4):558-565

[23] Aouizerate B, Martin-Guehl C, Cuny E, Guehl D, Amieva H, Benazzouz A, et al. Deep brain stimulation for OCD and major depression. The American Journal of Psychiatry. 2005;**162**(11):2192

[24] Holtzheimer IIIPE, Nemeroff CB. Advances in the treatment of depression. NeuroRx. 2006;**3**(1):42-56

[25] Mayberg HS, Lozano AM, Voon V, McNeely HE, Seminowicz D, Hamani C, et al. Deep brain stimulation for treatment-resistant depression. Neuron. 2005;**45**(5):651-660

[26] Schoenen J, Di Clemente L, Vandenheede M, Fumal A, De Pasqua V, Mouchamps M, et al. Hypothalamic stimulation in chronic cluster headache: A pilot study of efficacy and mode of action. Brain. 2005;**128**(4):940-947

[27] Velasco F, Carrillo-Ruiz JD, Brito F, Velasco M, Velasco AL, Marquez I, et al. Double-blind, randomized controlled pilot study of bilateral cerebellar stimulation for treatment of intractable motor seizures. Epilepsia. 2005;**46**(7):1071-1081

[28] Andrade D, Zumsteg D, Hamani C, Hodaie M, Sarkissian S, Lozano A, et al. Long-term follow-up of patients with thalamic deep brain stimulation for epilepsy. Neurology. 2006;**66**(10):1571-1573

[29] Landi A, Parolin M, Piolti R, Antonini A, Grimaldi M, Crespi M, et al. Deep brain stimulation for the treatment of Parkinson's disease: The experience of the Neurosurgical Department in Monza. Neurological Sciences. 2003;**24**(1):s43-ss4

[30] Welter M, Houeto J, Tezenas du Montcel S, Mesnage V, Bonnet A, Pillon B, et al. Clinical predictive factors of subthalamic stimulation in Parkinson's disease. Brain. 2002;**125**(3):575-583

[31] Bonneville F, Welter M, Elie C, du Montcel ST, Hasboun D, Menuel C, et al. Parkinson disease, brain volumes, and subthalamic nucleus stimulation. Neurology. 2005;**64**(9):1598-1604

[32] Breit S, LeBas J-F, Koudsie A, Schulz J, Benazzouz A, Pollak P, et al. Technique applications—Pretargeting for the implantation of stimulation electrodes into the subthalamic nucleus: A comparative study of magnetic resonance imaging and ventriculography. Neurosurgery-Hagerstown. 2006;**58**(2):83-95

[33] Simon SL, Douglas P, Baltuch GH, Jaggi JL. Error analysis of MRI and Leksell stereotactic frame target localization in deep brain stimulation surgery. Stereotactic and Functional Neurosurgery. 2005;**83**(1):1-5

[34] Menuel C, Garnero L, Bardinet E, Poupon F, Phalippou D, Dormont D. Characterization and correction of distortions in stereotactic magnetic resonance imaging for bilateral subthalamic stimulation in Parkinson disease. Journal of Neurosurgery. 2005;**103**(2):256-266

[35] Liu X, Rowe J, Nandi D, Hayward G, Parkin S, Stein J, et al. Localisation of the subthalamic nucleus using Radionics Image Fusion™ and Stereoplan™ combined with field potential recording. Stereotactic and Functional Neurosurgery. 2001;**76**(2):63-73

[36] Dormont D, Cornu P, Pidoux B, Bonnet A-M, Biondi A, Oppenheim C, et al. Chronic thalamic stimulation with three-dimensional MR stereotactic guidance. American Journal of Neuroradiology. 1997;**18**(6):1093-1107

[37] Martin AJ, Larson PS, Ostrem JL, Keith Sootsman W, Talke P, Weber OM, et al. Placement of deep brain stimulator electrodes using real-time high-field interventional magnetic resonance imaging. Magnetic Resonance in Medicine: An Official Journal of the International Society for Magnetic Resonance in Medicine. 2005;**54**(5):1107-1114

[38] Fiegele T, Feuchtner G, Sohm F, Bauer R, Anton JV, Gotwald T, et al. Accuracy of stereotactic electrode placement in deep brain stimulation by intraoperative computed tomography. Parkinsonism & Related Disorders. 2008;**14**(8):595-599

[39] Bejjani B-P, Dormont D, Pidoux B, Yelnik J, Damier P, Arnulf I, et al. Bilateral subthalamic stimulation for Parkinson's disease by using three-dimensional stereotactic magnetic resonance imaging and electrophysiological guidance. Journal of Neurosurgery. 2000;**92**(4):615-625

[40] Koike Y, Shima F, Nakamizo A, Miyagi Y. Direct localization of subthalamic nucleus supplemented by single-track electrophysiological guidance in deep brain stimulation lead implantation: Techniques and clinical results. Stereotactic and Functional Neurosurgery. 2008;**86**(3):173-178

[41] Tabbal SD, Revilla FJ, Mink JW, Schneider-Gibson P, Wernle AR, De Erausquin GA, et al. Safety and efficacy of subthalamic nucleus deep brain stimulation performed with limited intraoperative mapping for treatment of Parkinson's disease. Operative Neurosurgery. 2007;**61**(Suppl_3) ONS-119-ONS-29

[42] Rezai AR, Baker KB, Tkach JA, Phillips M, Hrdlicka G, Sharan AD, et al. Is magnetic resonance imaging safe for patients with neurostimulation systems used for deep brain stimulation? Neurosurgery. 2005;**57**(5):1056-1062

[43] Rezai AR, Phillips M, Baker KB, Sharan AD, Nyenhuis J, Tkach J, et al. Neurostimulation system used for deep brain stimulation (DBS): MR safety issues and implications of failing to follow safety recommendations. Investigative Radiology. 2004;**39**(5):300-303

[44] Hamani C, McAndrews MP, Cohn M, Oh M, Zumsteg D, Shapiro CM, et al. Memory

enhancement induced by hypothalamic/fornix deep brain stimulation. Annals of Neurology: Official Journal of the American Neurological Association and the Child Neurology Society. 2008;**63**(1):119-123

[45] Guehl D, Benazzouz A, Aouizerate B, Cuny E, Rotgé J-Y, Rougier A, et al. Neuronal correlates of obsessions in the caudate nucleus. Biological Psychiatry. 2008;**63**(6):557-562

[46] Sander CY, Hesse S. News and views on in vivo imaging of neurotransmission using PET and MRI. The Quarterly Journal of Nuclear Medicine and Molecular Imaging. 2017;**61**(4):414

[47] Fox PT. The coupling controversy. NeuroImage. 2012;**62**(2):594-601

[48] Devor A, Dunn AK, Andermann ML, Ulbert I, Boas DA, Dale AM. Coupling of total hemoglobin concentration, oxygenation, and neural activity in rat somatosensory cortex. Neuron. 2003;**39**(2):353-359

[49] Trošt M, Su S, Su P, Yen R-F, Tseng H-M, Barnes A, et al. Network modulation by the subthalamic nucleus in the treatment of Parkinson's disease. NeuroImage. 2006;**31**(1):301-307

[50] Tohyama S, Walker MR, Sammartino F, Krishna V, Hodaie M. The utility of diffusion tensor imaging in neuromodulation: Moving beyond conventional magnetic resonance imaging. Neuromodulation: Technology at the Neural Interface. 2020

[51] Alexander AL, Lee JE, Lazar M, Field AS. Diffusion tensor imaging of the brain. Neurotherapeutics. 2007;**4**(3):316-329

[52] Basser PJ, Pajevic S, Pierpaoli C, Duda J, Aldroubi A. In vivo fiber tractography using DT-MRI data. Magnetic Resonance in Medicine. 2000;**44**(4):625-632

[53] Hagmann P, Kurant M, Gigandet X, Thiran P, Wedeen VJ, Meuli R, et al. Mapping human whole-brain structural networks with diffusion MRI. PLoS One. 2007;**2**(7):e597

[54] Lerner A, Mogensen MA, Kim PE, Shiroishi MS, Hwang DH, Law M. Clinical applications of diffusion tensor imaging. World Neurosurgery. 2014;**82**(1-2):96-109

[55] Sundgren P, Dong Q, Gomez-Hassan D, Mukherji S, Maly P, Welsh R. Diffusion tensor imaging of the brain: Review of clinical applications. Neuroradiology. 2004;**46**(5):339-350

[56] Hallett M. Transcranial magnetic stimulation: A primer. Neuron. 2007;**55**:187-199

[57] Leung A, Shirvalkar P, Chen R, Kuluva J, Vaninetti M, Bermudes R, et al. Transcranial magnetic stimulation for pain, headache, and comorbid depression: INS-NANS Expert Consensus Panel Review and Recommendation. Neuromodulation: Technology at the Neural Interface. 2020

[58] Van Haerents S, Chang BS, Rotenberg A, Pascual-Leone A, Shafi MM. Noninvasive brain stimulation in epilepsy. Journal of Clinical Neurophysiology. 2020;**37**(2):118-130

[59] Simeoni S, Hannah R, Sato D, Kawakami M, Rothwell J, Gigli GL. Effects of quadripulse stimulation on human motor cortex excitability: A replication study. Brain Stimulation: Basic, Translational, and Clinical Research in Neuromodulation. 2016;**9**(1):148-150

[60] Vallence A-M, Goldsworthy MR, Hodyl NA, Semmler JG, Pitcher JB, Ridding MC. Inter-and intra-subject variability of motor cortex plasticity following continuous

theta-burst stimulation. Neuroscience. 2015;**304**:266-278

[61] Hannah R, Rocchi L, Tremblay S, Rothwell JC. Controllable pulse parameter TMS and TMS-EEG as novel approaches to improve neural targeting with rTMS in human cerebral cortex. Frontiers in Neural Circuits. 2016;**10**:97

[62] Ilmoniemi RJ, Kičić D. Methodology for combined TMS and EEG. Brain Topography. 2010;**22**(4):233

[63] Nitsche MA, Cohen LG, Wassermann EM, et al. Transcranial direct current stimu-lation: State of the art 2008. Brain Stimulation. 2008;**1**:206-223

[64] Benussi A, Pascual-Leone A, Borroni B. Non-invasive cerebellar stimulation in neurodegenerative ataxia: A literature review. International Journal of Molecular Sciences. 1948;**2020**(21):6

[65] Pellicciari MC, Miniussi C. Transcranial direct current stimulation in neurodegenerative disorders. The Journal of ECT. 2018;**34**(3):193-202

[66] Nitsche MA, Paulus W. Excitability changes induced in the human motor cortex by weak transcranial direct current stimulation. The Journal of Physiology. 2000;**527**(3):633-639

[67] Stein DJ, Medeiros LF, Caumo W, Torres IL. Transcranial direct current stimulation in patients with anxiety: Current perspectives. Neuropsychiatric Disease and Treatment. 2020;**16**:161

[68] Lin Y, Zhang C, Wang Y. A randomized controlled study of transcranial direct current stimulation in treatment of generalized anxiety disorder. Brain Stimulation: Basic, Translational, and Clinical Research in Neuromodulation. 2019;**12**(2):403

[69] Heeren A, Billieux J, Philippot P, De Raedt R, Baeken C, de Timary P, et al. Impact of transcranial direct current stimulation on attentional bias for threat: A proof-of-concept study among individuals with social anxiety disorder. Social Cognitive and Affective Neuroscience. 2017;**12**(2):251-260

[70] Horvath JC, Forte JD, Carter O. Evidence that transcranial direct current stimulation (tDCS) generates little-to-no reliable neurophysiologic effect beyond MEP amplitude modulation in healthy human subjects: A systematic review. Neuropsychologia. 2015;**66**:213-236

[71] Dyster TG, Mikell CB, Sheth SA. The co-evolution of neuroimaging and psychiatric neurosurgery. Frontiers in Neuroanatomy. 2016;**10**:68

[72] Mirnezami R, Nicholson J, Darzi A. Preparing for precision medicine. The New England Journal of Medicine. 2012;**366**(6):489-491

[73] Costa e Silva JA. Personalized medicine in psychiatry: New technologies and approaches. Metabolism. 2013;**62**:S40-SS4

[74] Banks GP, Mikell CB, Youngerman BE, Henriques B, Kelly KM, Chan AK, et al. Neuroanatomical characteristics associated with response to dorsal anterior cingulotomy for obsessive-compulsive disorder. JAMA Psychiatry. 2015;**72**(2):127-135

[75] Mayberg HS, Liotti M, Brannan SK, McGinnis S, Mahurin RK, Jerabek PA, et al. Reciprocal limbic-cortical function and negative mood: Converging PET findings in depression and normal sadness. The American Journal of Psychiatry. 1999;**156**(5):675-682

[76] Seminowicz D, Mayberg H, McIntosh A, Goldapple K, Kennedy S, Segal Z, et al. Limbic–frontal circuitry in major depression: A path modeling metanalysis. NeuroImage. 2004;**22**(1):409-418

[77] Rück C, Karlsson A, Steele JD, Edman G, Meyerson BA, Ericson K, et al. Capsulotomy for obsessive-compulsive disorder: Long-term follow-up of 25 patients. Archives of General Psychiatry. 2008;**65**(8):914-921

[78] Riva-Posse P, Choi KS, Holtzheimer PE, McIntyre CC, Gross RE, Chaturvedi A, et al. Defining critical white matter pathways mediating successful subcallosal cingulate deep brain stimulation for treatment-resistant depression. Biological Psychiatry. 2014;**76**(12):963-969

Chapter 3

Deep Brain Stimulation Approach in Neurological Diseases

Dev Priya and Pathak Abhishek

Abstract

The technique was emanated in early 1960s; nowadays, deep brain stimulation (DBS) has become a huge practice in treatment of various movement disorders along with some psychiatric disorders. The advancement of DBS in different neurodegenerative diseases and managing patients with refractory brain disorders are closely related to the developments in technology. This development in regard with the device advancement along with the safe coupling of DBS to high-resolution imaging can help us to shape our knowledge in brain-wide networks and circuits linked with clinical aspects. DBS is found to be useful in learning and memory. On the contrary, traditional epilepsy surgeries are more complicated and technologically DBS is easier and more feasible. There are mild adverse effects of this DBS treatment, but a number of studies have shown positive treatment outcome with movement disorders and many kinds of psychiatric disorders too.

Keywords: deep brain stimulation, neuromodulation, brain, movement disorder, neurodegenerative disease, psychiatric disorder

1. Introduction

Neuromodulation is an increasingly rising field in the successful treatment of neurological disorders [1, 2]. Neurostimulation allows highly flexible alteration of disease symptoms. A number of medications fail due to severe side effects that outweigh the medication benefit, but neurostimulation has been so long to be potentially used as a treatment option for several movement disorders [2], with mild side effects with unknown mechanism of action in other disorders [3].

2. Types of Neuromodulation techniques

1. Deep brain stimulation (DBS) is an approved option for the treatment of intractable forms of various diseases. It involves inflecting the dysfunctional neuronal networks by long-term electrical stimulation, which utilizes implanting electrodes placed in the target neurological site that excites the neuronal circuits [4]. In recent years, evolution of DBS has revolutionized the treatment few neurological diseases especially in the treatment of movement disorders [5].

2. Vagal nerve stimulation (VNS) uses a device to stimulate the vagus nerve via electrical impulses. VNS is very helpful for people who have not responded to

intensive antiepileptic drug treatment and suffers from their adverse effects. FDA has approved VNS in 1997 for the treatment of epilepsy, depression, and various other disorders.

3. Transcranial magnetic stimulation (TMS) is a noninvasive brain stimulation by producing electrical impulses at a specific area of the brain through electromagnetic induction or by changing magnetic field [6].

4. Spinal cord stimulation (SCS) is useful in the treatment of long-lasting pain, which utilizes a stimulator that gives an electrical stimulus to the spinal cord.

5. Epidural motor cortex stimulation technique is highly useful in the treatment of intractable long-term neuropathic pain.

6. rTMS is useful in the treatment of experimental pain, neuropathic pain, and nonneuropathic chronic conditions.

7. Transcranial direct current stimulation is a highly used noninvasive technique altering neuronal plasticity. It is moderately used in treating neuropathic pain and fibromyalgia [7].

3. Deep brain stimulation (DBS)

DBS is an electrode implantation method using stereotactic techniques into the deep regions of brain for modulating neuronal function. An implantable pulse generator (IPG) is attached below the clavicle region, with an intention to treat neurological and psychiatric conditions. This attached IPG works on battery and delivers electrical stimulation, which is regulated externally by patients with the help of the remote. The electronic components like frequency, pulse, voltage, and other parameters can be altered to attain maximum efficacy of the treatment. It is believed that it works on excitation and inhibition of neurons present nearby the electrodes, but the exact mechanism is still unknown.

Low-frequency stimulation seems to excite nearby neurons, while high-frequency stimulation may decrease local activity leading to rescindable functional lesion. This simple-minded opinion for the mechanistic action has been a challenge in recent years, and more comprehensive knowledge may promote enhanced DBS treatments [8].

4. Brief chronicle of DBS

4.1 Early history

During the early 1900s' experiments, first stereotactic frame was designed that allowed stimulation of deeper regions of brain. In 1947, X-ray pneumoencephalography was developed that enabled surgeons to locate the target with the help of detailed stereotactic atlas that was developed later on. In 1950, stereotactic techniques were used for the tremor treatment. Later, in 1963, Albe Fessard reported high-frequency (~100–200 Hz) electrical stimulation for the first time in the ventral intermediate thalamic nucleus that could substantially alleviate Parkinsonian tremor [9].

4.2 The last 50 years

In 1960, levodopa treatment development was highly effective for Parkinsonian symptoms with lesser risk and expense compared to DBS implantation and this led the curtailing of early forms of DBS research.

Inspite of the drawbacks, the research for use of DBSnever stopped. DBS continued to observe restricted use in intractable chronic treatment, with Medtronic Inc. (Minneapolis, MN, USA) and released the first fully implanted DBS systems commercially accessible for this purpose in the mid-1970s [10].

Other study groups investigated the use of thalamic DBS to treat consciousness diseases and reported few benefits. By the end of 1980s, it was evident that using levodopa would not hold the promising effects, after years of therapy, and patients developed wearing off along with the side effects like dyskinesias. Meanwhile, the technology of implantable medical devices had improved to the stage that it was routinely used for chronically implanted devices like cardiac pacemakers and spinal cord stimulators. The animal model study eventually got translated into clinical practices, and the first subthalamic nucleus (STN) DBS study got published [11]. By the beginning of the century, clinical use of DBS in Parkinsonian disorders has begun to become common [8].

5. Rationale and mechanisms of action

Although the exact mechanisms of action of DBS are still elusive in spite of extensive research, several theories have been put forward. These proposed mechanisms can be divided according to the latency of onset of the effects from the time of stimulation into acute (seconds to hours) and chronic (days to months). The two major proposed mechanisms are as follows:

1. Electrophysiological and neurotransmitter modulation 395 likely explain the acute effects.

2. Plasticity and neurogenesis may explain the chronic effects [12].

However, there is a considerable overlap among the proposed mechanisms and one group of mechanisms has effects over the other, as described in detail in the following sections. Furthermore, depending on the methods used to investigate the mechanisms of action, different aspects of stimulation effects are tested. With an integrative approach combining investigations employing different modalities, one can understand the general effects of DBS.

5.1 Modalities used to study the mechanisms of DBS

Different methods have been used to quantify the changes produced by the DBS at the cellular, tissue and system levels to study the mechanisms of action of DBS. These modalities can be broadly classified into electrophysiological, imaging, biochemical, and molecular methods. Imaging techniques such as positron emission tomography (PET) and functional MRI (fMRI) provide information on both local- and system-level changes. These are complementary methods: functional imaging studies have high spatial resolution, whereas electrophysiological methods have high temporal resolution. Moreover, electrophysiological methods directly measure neuronal activities rather than indirect measures of neural activities using blood-flow changes measured by imaging methods [13].

There are several hypotheses proposed by different schools of thought, to explain the processes by which DBS works. Accepted and popular hypothesis relied on the alteration of pathological brain circuit activity induced by stimulation [12, 14]. The stimulating impacts that are accountable for this disturbance occur at protein, ionic, cellular, and network levels to produce symptom improvements [15]. While it is presently unclear that which of the DBS' wide-ranging impacts are needed and adequate to generate therapeutic results, it is evident that high-frequency (~100 Hz) pulse stations (~0.1 ms) produce network reactions that are essentially distinct from low-frequency (~10 Hz) stimulation. The electrodes implanted into the brain redistribute the charged particles (such as Na+ and Cl−ions) throughout the extracellular space, which generates electric field and ultimately leads to the manipulation of sodium channel protein's voltage sensor embedded in the neuron membrane [16]. The opening of sodium channels at the cellular level may generate a potential action for initiation of axons and can propagate in both orthodromic and antidromic directions. DBS causes, activated axons are able to follow very high fidelity stimulus rates at ~100 Hz, but these high-frequency synaptic transmissions are less robust and much complex than that of axonal transmission [17, 18].

Under such high-frequency activity, postsynaptic receptors can be depressed and axon terminals can exhaust their released pool of neurotransmitters [19, 20]. Even though these synapses appear to be active in DBS, theories of information processing suggest that they could become low-pass filters that can block low-frequency signal transmission [21]. This general mechanism, defined as "synaptic filtering," may play a crucial role in DBS, hampering the transmission of oscillatory activity patterns throughout the related networks of brain via neurons [22].

DBS' simple biophysical consequences offers a background where the patterns of network activity observed in patients can begin to be interpreted. The oscillation frequency of the stimulation signal is virtually zero as stimulation intensity remains unchanged during DBS, which could produce what is known as an "information lesion" in stimulated neurons [23]. According to this theory, action potential induced by DBS essentially bypasses some endogenous activity directly within the stimulated nerves and therefore slows down the transmission of oscillatory activity via the network. Nonetheless, not too many researches support the statement that high-frequency DBS causes lesion. Research with asleep and behavioral primates indicates how DBS can serve as a filter, which allows certain sensorimotor-related regulation of neuronal activity in the activated area, whereas specifically suppressing pathological low-frequency oscillation propagation [24, 25]. Certain basal ganglia activities, like those of reward-based decision-making or motor sequence learning, can often be retained during STN DBS or globus pallidus [26].

Certain factors may also have significant roles in treatment mechanism of DBS for PD like high-frequency DBS could provide an appropriate information lesion that inhibits the propagation of low-frequency oscillations, unlike low-frequency synchronization, could have no impact on broader network function [27, 28]. One of the advantages of this system is that high-frequency DBS is a standard device that can overcome various forms of clinical low-frequency excitations, like mobile tremor, dystonia, and akinesia rigidity [29].

The above proposed mechanism of DBS goes some way to explain only the acute effects of DBS in movement disorders, but this would not explain long-latency, chronic-adaptive alterations, which arise in individuals with dystonia following DBS and it may describe the psychological response to DBS. There might be possibility that low oscillating frequencies are strongly enhanced by long-term potentiation, while stimulation of high-frequency seems to have smaller plasticity effect. Therefore, replacing low-frequency patterns with high frequency can reverse those symptoms associated with chronic disease [30]. DBS often takes months to get maximum benefit in various disorders, such as dystonia, depression, and epilepsy [31].

5.2 Open- vs. close-loop stimulation system

Nowadays, the open-loop system is embedded in many cases for DBS in which related parameters such as frequency, amplitude, and duty cycle can be adjusted by trained physicians. Stimulation, in this method, is fixed for initial months of treatment, then later can be adjusted based on patient's symptoms and overall conditions.

A closed-loop system receives continuous feedback from the patient's neuronal circuits of brain by a present and programmed algorithm and thus appears to be an effective stimulation, and the parameters are adjusted real time. The implanted device causes physiological changes, both over long and short term, via automatic therapeutic parameter delivery with the ability to sense brain signals. Though there are no randomized controlled trials, comparing the therapeutic effect of open- vs. closed-loop system, few researchers opine that closed-loop method are more effective than the open-loop system. Through their novel closed-loop method, to compare the effectiveness of open-loop systems using two neurons, they demonstrated that closed-loop system with implantable electrodes in GPi region has better results on the disease motor symptoms in PD patients than the open-loop and high-frequency systems [32, 33].

6. DBS in different neurodegenerative diseases

The common form of dementia, AD, treated with lesser efficiency of success in treatment via this technique has been used to modulate nonfunctional neuronal circuits with abnormalities seen in cortical and subcortical areas of the brain. Treatment helps in altering cholinesterase inhibitors and NMDA receptor antagonist [31]. DBS is a significant option for treatment of movement disorders that are intractable to drugs namely Parkinson's disease, essential tremors, dystonia, and have recently shown to be effective against treatment of OCDs, depression, and Tourette syndrome [5, 31].

7. DBS in movement disorders

DBS became the standard therapy refractory over the last 25 years for individuals with motor circuit disabilities, most notably PD, dystonia, and essential tremor. DBS use has now been confined to high-income and developing countries [34]. Hospital-discharge-based studies of US database has showed that >30,000 DBS surgeries were performed during 2002 and 2011, and the publications on DBS have also risen over the same period of time [35].

7.1 Parkinson's disease

Over the last 10 years, STN is used as a target for DBS in PD [36]. GPi is also used as a target, but the choice between STN and GPi is often guided by the biomedical group based on the medical context of the patient.

Multiple studies have already shown that STN DBS produces continuous symptom relief even after 5–10 years of treatment, although with cognition and gait regression due to the unremitting development of the underlying degenerative disorder [37]. In PD diagnosis, DBS is called the "second honeymoon" (dopaminergic therapy is the first). Instability in posture and freezing can be improved by DBS at pedunculopontine nucleus region of the brain [38].

Based on previous studies, there is a general concept of DBS that it can improve PD patients with advance kind of symptoms like motor fluctuation, dyskinesias secondary to chronic levodopa as well as those with refractory and marked tremor. But based on studies of EARLYSTIM findings, DBS can also improve early stages of PD [39]. Due to these advantages of DBS, it is now been under clinical trials for those patients who are eliminated from surgery due to age factor, along with those patients with motor fluctuations in whom medication is effective. Due to the inherent risk of DBS like hemorrhage and infection, such trials face ethical issues [40].

7.2 Epilepsy

Earlier it was thought that DBS can switch open resective surgery in epilepsy, but after studies on DBS of the anterior nucleus of the thalamus (ANT), it was stifled. These researches imposed well on the efficacy of DBS but simultaneously also demonstrated that many patients did not attain seizure freedom after the DBS treatment [41, 42]. Closed-loop stimulation is a hopeful technology in epilepsy that can sense seizure activity with electrode and also can send electrical stimulations to brain to thwart propagation of seizure [43].

7.3 Essential tremor

After various studies, DBS was recommended by FDA in 1997 for the initial tremor symptoms of the movement disorder [44]. Along with DBS, other therapies such as lesional surgery have also been used for the treatment of essential tremors. DBS is a better choice due to its safety as well as adjustability of the stimulation, which is not provided by the lesional therapy [45]. Thalamic DBS is used in tremors of multiple sclerosis patients [46].

7.4 Dystonia

DBS had played a crucial role in dystonia treatment [47, 48]. Pallidal DBS, for instance, is the first-line treatment in childhood generalized dystonic disease. The most significant determinant of results was age at which surgery was performed and the duration of disorder [49–51]. Genetic makeup of patients has also been important in evaluating the outcome, as individual with DYT1 dystonia are benefited more than the DYT6 dystonia [52]. Therefore, genetic testing of patients undergoing DBS treatment would suggest which candidate is going to be benefited more [53]. The posteroventral lateral GPi in dystonia is the utmost recognized target for DBS [54]. GPi stimulation offers significant recovery in dystonic patients with adversarial effects on low frequency. The STN and the thalamus are two other targets for DBS. Despite of positive outcomes of STN DBS, the therapeutic use is still restricted [55]. An additional important target is sensorimotor thalamus, which in the age of radiofrequency lesioning, was considered as standard target [56, 57]. The mode of action of DBS in clinical improvement is quite intricate because of delayed and progressive effect exhibited over a period of months. The underlying mechanism for this was hypothesized as the alteration of maladaptive plasticity, progressive motor learning, and modification in pathological oscillatory activity in basal ganglia circuitry [58]. Dystonia can recur within minutes to hours after discontinuation of stimulation during the initial postoperative period; the advantages from stimulation that has been administered for several years can persist for days and weeks after discontinuation [59, 60]. Therefore, DBS acts as a true treatment in case of dystonia where progressive treatments are absent or poorly successful. This rationale has contributed an EARLYSTIM study in dystonia [61].

7.5 Alzheimer disease (AD)

AD is perhaps the most prevailing neurodegenerative disease but is characterized with years of gradual reduction in neurocognitive parameters. Many DBS strategies have been identified for AD, including areas anterior to the fornix, entorhinal cortex, and the nucleus basalis of Meynert (NBM). Several studies suggest that DBS can affect cognitive function in AD. Nonetheless, outcome influencing factors such as baseline neuroanatomical substrates, surgical technique, placement of lead, and target population choice are the challenges for DBS [62].

8. DBS in psychiatric disorders

Psychiatric disorders are assorted conditions affecting multiple pathways with overlap. Such disorders have few (if any) biochemical markers that support treatment and outcomes, and there is a lack of data for its outcome assessment in patients. Thus, this affects the designing of clinical trial studies. In addition, the quality of surgical trials is also hindered due to significant selection barriers [63]. In an attempt to alleviate refractory psychiatric symptoms, numerous prospective studies have been done to evaluate if focal disruption at specific anatomic targets can impact circuit-wide or network-wide changes. Though the strategy is enticing, there are still some challenges.

8.1 Tourette syndrome

Due to the behavioral and cognitive issues in these patients, less than 300 patients have endured DBS treatment across the world. Patients with chronic symptoms are improved less than those with mild symptoms as per a meta-analysis [64]. A randomized controlled trial in 2017 did not report any significant improvement of tics in Tourette syndrome patients treated with anteromedial GPi stimulation during the initial blinded phase of the study; however, tics improvement was documented during the study's transparent period [65]. There is need of more randomized control trials for further development of DBS treatment in these patients.

8.2 Major depression

Major depression is a serious disorder that can impact quality of life day-to-day working and, eventually, life expectancy significantly [66, 67]. As a result of advancement of imaging techniques, there is a suggestion that depression occurs due to alteration in mood-related circuits, which can be reversed with neuromodulation along with other antidepressant therapies.

8.3 Bipolar disorder

Bipolar disorders are associated with acute and strong emotive condition, which are episodic and known as mood episodes; these disorders are less common than major depression but are linked with increased risk of suicide. Effective targets in bipolar disorders for DBS are thought to be SCC, the nucleus accumbens, and slMFB, but studies are less [68].

8.4 Obsessive: compulsive disorder

Obsessive–compulsive disorder (OCD) is a debilitating psychological condition, which is characterized by obsessions combined with time-consuming and subjectively anxiolytic behaviors. Several targets were proposed for OCD treatment, but STN DBS was found to be the most effective with significant reduction in OCD symptoms [69].

8.5 Anorexia nervosa

Anorexia nervosa is a severe, prevalent, and has one of the highest mortalities among any psychiatric disorder. The limbic and emotional circuits are involved activating and upholding the disorder. The limited availability of treatment in refractory anorexia nervosa and positive outcomes of DBS in mood-related circuits have led the curiosity for DBS targets availability in anorexia nervosa condition. Several research articles are published on SCC DBS target with significant reduction in depression and anxiety [70]. However, further studies are needed for convincing target for DBS.

9. Pain

For patients with pain, the analysis of DBS outcome is more challenging than in motor movement disorders due to rationality of pain self-assessment. Though nociceptive pain can usually be kept in check with opiate medication, DBS targets in the thalamus or cingulum are considered for patients with severe refractory neuropathic pain [30, 71, 72].

10. Positive influence of the DBS treatment

There are a number of side effects via medication that is highly reduced by neuromodulation technique. Seizure frequencies and mortality were decreased, but the results were not evaluated. Successful results of DBS on movement disorder and vagal nerve stimulation for epilepsy [73, 74]. DBS is a best way to treat extrapyramidal motor disorder namely dyskinesia, tremors, rigidity, and dystonia [75–77]. GPi-DBS, in primary generalized dystonia, was proved to be very successful, and it can be used as an effective treatment option [78]. Although with mild treatment side effects, a number of studies have shown positive treatment outcome in chronic disorders of consciousness with unknown mechanism of action [79]. DBS is found to beneficial in enhancing altered learning and memory. In rodents' model of dementia, mesial temporal DBS has shown positive results. Improvement in visual memory is seen in patients who underwent unilateral amygdalohippocampal DBS [80]. DBS helps in regaining of learning, memory, and altered communication skills in patients of postbrain injury with disorders of consciousness [81].

11. Negative influence of the treatment

Severe harmful effects of DBS are seen on dominant side of hippocampal region. Bilateral hippocampal DBS may cause memory dysfunction in epilepsy patients. Though DBS, is supposed to be safe, the adverse events can be seen in 7.5–8.5% of patients. The major adverse effects being, infections, intraoperative seizures and other complications [7].

12. Evolution in DBS technologies

Evolutions in technologies have led to the advancement in pain management in DBS. Several technologies related to spinal cord stimulation like Expanded MRI labeling, pulse modifier (generator as well as shrinker), dorsal root ganglia stimulating leads, and so on have benefited a lot due to high-frequency and high-density strategies of software [82–85]. The major problem in DBS is the inappropriate dose, for which no new technology has been developed for the past two decades; therefore, there is lack of competitiveness in DBS technology [30].

13. Summary

DBS is a neurosurgical procedure that utilizes lead-implanted electrodes that is placed chronically in the target areas of the brain well connected to pulse generator, which excites the neuronal circuits [1, 4, 5]. It is an invasive neuromodulation technique that was emanated in early 1960s [1]. Recently, DBS has become a huge practice in treatment of various movement disorders along with some psychiatric disorders [4, 5]. As compared to other neurosurgical options, lower chances of complications are seen with this technique [5]. Although with mild treatment side effects, a number of studies have shown positive treatment outcome in chronic disorders of consciousness with unknown mechanism of action [79]. Growth in DBS in respect to pathway and its impact on neuronal circuit has been mainly propelled by preclinical, neurophysiological, and computational research. Significant needs and prospect have evolved innovative techniques and technologies that have improved tolerability as well as research design, but DBS is still growing in many areas to manage cerebral diseases safely and efficiently.

Acknowledgements

I would like to thank Dr. D Joshi, Dr. R N Chaurasia, Dr. V N Mishra, and Institute of Medical Sciences for their support and encouragement. There was no funding provided for this study.

Conflict of interest

The authors have no conflict of interest.

Abbreviations

DBS	deep brain stimulation
VNS	vagal nerve stimulation
TMS	transcranial magnetic stimulation
SCS	spinal cord stimulation
rTMS	repetitive transcranial magnetic stimulation
AD	Alzheimer's disease
NMDA	N-methyl-d-aspartate
GPi-DBS	globus pallidus internus deep brain stimulation

Author details

Dev Priya and Pathak Abhishek*
Department of Neurology, Institute of Medical Sciences, Banaras Hindu University, India

*Address all correspondence to: abhishekpathakaiims@gmail.com

References

[1] Doruk Camsari D, Kirkovski M, Croarkin PE. Therapeutic applications of invasive neuromodulation in children and adolescents. The Psychiatric Clinics of North America. 2018;**41**(3):479-483

[2] Fisher RS, Velasco AL. Electrical brain stimulation for epilepsy. Nature Reviews. Neurology. 2014;**10**(5):261-270

[3] Oliveira L, Fregni F. Pharmacological and electrical stimulation in chronic disorders of consciousness: New insights and future directions. Brain Injury. 2011;**25**(4):315-327

[4] Lemaire JJ, Sontheimer A, Nezzar H, Pontier B, Luauté J, Roche B, et al. Electrical modulation of neuronal networks in brain-injured patients with disorders of consciousness: A systematic review. Annales Françaises d'Anesthèsie et de Rèanimation. 2014;**33**(2):88-97

[5] Falowski SM, Ooi YC, Bakay RA. Long-term evaluation of changes in operative technique and hardware-related complications with deep brain stimulation. Neuromodulation. 2015;**18**(8):670-677

[6] Albert GC, Cook CM, Prato FS, Thomas AW. Deep brain stimulation, vagal nerve stimulation and transcranial stimulation: An overview of stimulation parameters and neurotransmitter release. Neuroscience and Biobehavioral Reviews. 2009;**33**(7):1042-1060

[7] Cruccu G, Garcia-Larrea L, Hansson P, Keindl M, Lefaucheur JP, Paulus W, et al. EAN guidelines on central neurostimulation therapy in chronic pain conditions. European Journal of Neurology. 2016;**23**(10):1489-1499

[8] Pycroft L, Stein J, Aziz T. Deep brain stimulation: An overview of history, methods, and future developments. Brain and Neuroscience Advances. 2018;**2**:1-6

[9] Albe Fessard D, Arfel G, Guiot G, et al. Characteristic electric activities of some cerebral structures in man. Annales de Chirurgie. 1963;**17**:1185-1214

[10] Hosobuchi Y, Adams JE, Rutkin B. Chronic thalamic stimulation for the control of facial anesthesia dolorosa. Archives of Neurology. 1973;**29**(3):158-161

[11] Pollak P, Benabid AL, Gross C, et al. Effects of the stimulation of the subthalamic nucleus in Parkinson disease. Revista de Neurologia. 1993;**149**(3):175-176

[12] Lozano AM, Lipsman N. Probing and regulating dysfunctional circuits using deep brain stimulation. Neuron. 2013;**77**:406-424

[13] Udupa K, Chen R. The mechanisms of action of deep brain stimulation and ideas for the future development. Progress in Neurobiology. 2015;**1386**:1-23

[14] Ashkan K, Rogers P, Bergman H, Ughratdar I. Insights into the mechanisms of deep brain stimulation. Nature Reviews. Neurology. 2017;**13**:548-554

[15] McIntyre CC, Anderson RW. Deep brain stimulation mechanisms: The control of network activity via neurochemistry modulation. Journal of Neurochemistry. 2016;**139**(Suppl 1): 338-345

[16] Groome JR. The voltage sensor module in sodium channels. Handbook of Experimental Pharmacology. 2014;**221**:7-31

[17] Bucher D, Goaillard JM. Beyond faithful conduction: Short-term dynamics, neuromodulation, and long-term regulation of spike propagation

in the axon. Progress in Neurobiology. 2011;**94**:307-346

[18] Miocinovic S et al. Computational analysis of subthalamic nucleus and lenticular fasciculus activation during therapeutic deep brain stimulation. Journal of Neurophysiology. 2006;**96**:1569-1580

[19] Llinas RR, Leznik E, Urbano FJ. Temporal binding via cortical coincidence detection of specific and nonspecific thalamocortical inputs: A voltage-dependent dye-imaging study in mouse brain slices. Proceedings of the National Academy of Sciences of the United States of America. 2002;**99**:449-454

[20] Rosenbaum R et al. Axonal and synaptic failure suppress the transfer of firing rate oscillations, synchrony and information during high frequency deep brain stimulation. Neurobiology of Disease. 2014;**62**:86-99

[21] Lindner B, Gangloff D, Longtin A, Lewis JE. Broadband coding with dynamic synapses. The Journal of Neuroscience. 2009;**29**:2076-2088

[22] Montgomery EB Jr, Baker KB. Mechanisms of deep brain stimulation and future technical developments. Neurological Research. 2000;**22**:259-266

[23] Grill WM, Snyder AN, Miocinovic S. Deep brain stimulation creates an informational lesion of the stimulated nucleus. Neuroreport. 2004;**15**:1137-1140

[24] Agnesi F, Johnson MD, Vitek JL. Deep brain stimulation: How does it work? Handbook of Clinical Neurology. 2013;**116**:39-54

[25] Zimnik AJ, Nora GJ, Desmurget M, Turner RS. Movement-related discharge in the macaque globus pallidus during high-frequency stimulation of the subthalamic nucleus. The Journal of Neuroscience. 2015;**35**:3978-3989

[26] Wichmann T, DeLong MR. Deep brain stimulation for movement disorders of basal ganglia origin: Restoring function or functionality? Neurotherapeutics. 2016;**13**:264-283

[27] Moran A, Stein E, Tischler H, Bar-Gad I. Decoupling neuronal oscillations during subthalamic nucleus stimulation in the parkinsonian primate. Neurobiology of Disease. 2012;**45**:583-590

[28] Wilson CJ, Beverlin B II, Netoff T. Chaotic desynchronization as the therapeutic mechanism of deep brain stimulation. Frontiers in Systems Neuroscience. 2011;**5**:50

[29] Guridi J, Alegre M. Oscillatory activity in the basal ganglia and deep brain stimulation. Movement Disorders. 2017;**32**:64-69

[30] Tass PA, Majtanik M. Long-term anti-kindling effects of desynchronizing brain stimulation: A theoretical study. Biological Cybernetics. 2006;**94**:58-66

[31] Lozano AM, Lipsman N, Bergman H, Brown P, Chabardes S, et al. Deep brain stimulation: Current challenges and future directions. Nature Reviews. Neurology. 2019;**15**(3):148-160

[32] Rosin B, Slovik M, Mitelman R, Rivlin-Etzion M, Haber SN, Israel Z, et al. Closed-loop deep brain stimulation is superior in ameliorating parkinsonism. Neuron. 2011;**72**:370-384

[33] Ghasemi P, Sahraee T, Mohammadi A. Closed- and open-loop deep brain stimulation: Methods, challenges, current and future aspects. Journal of Biomedical Physics and Engineering. 2018;**8**(2):209-216

[34] Bick SKB, Eskandar EN. Neuromodulation for restoring memory. Neurosurgical Focus. 2016;**40**(5):E5

[35] Jourdain VA, Schechtmann G. Health economics and surgical treatment for Parkinson's disease in a world perspective: Results from an international survey. Stereotactic and Functional Neurosurgery. 2014;**92**:71-79

[36] Schnurman Z, Kondziolka D. Evaluating innovation. Part 1: The concept of progressive scholarly acceptance. Journal of Neurosurgery. 2016;**124**:207-211

[37] Deuschl G et al. Stimulation of the subthalamic nucleus at an earlier disease stage of Parkinson's disease: Concept and standards of the EARLYSTIM-study. Parkinsonism & Related Disorders. 2013;**19**:56-61

[38] Rizzone MG et al. Long-term outcome of subthalamic nucleus DBS in Parkinson's disease: From the advanced phase towards the late stage of the disease? Parkinsonism & Related Disorders. 2014;**20**:376-381

[39] Hamani C et al. Pedunculopontine nucleus region deep brain stimulation in Parkinson disease: Surgical anatomy and terminology. Stereotactic and Functional Neurosurgery. 2016;**94**:298-306

[40] Schuepbach WM et al. Neurostimulation for Parkinson's disease with early motor complications. The New England Journal of Medicine. 2013;**368**:610-622

[41] DeLong MR et al. Effect of advancing age on outcomes of deep brain stimulation for Parkinson disease. JAMA Neurology. 2014;**71**:1290-1295

[42] Fisher R et al. Electrical stimulation of the anterior nucleus of thalamus for treatment of refractory epilepsy. Epilepsia. 2010;**51**:899-908

[43] Salanova V et al. Long-term efficacy and safety of thalamic stimulation for drug-resistant partial epilepsy. Neurology. 2015;**84**:1017-1025

[44] Jobst BC et al. Brain-responsive neurostimulation in patients with medically intractable seizures arising from eloquent and other neocortical areas. Epilepsia. 2017;**58**:1005-1014

[45] Hariz MI et al. Multicentre European study of thalamic stimulation for parkinsonian tremor: A 6 year follow-up. Journal of Neurology, Neurosurgery, and Psychiatry. 2008;**79**:694-699

[46] Elias WJ et al. A randomized trial of focused ultrasound thalamotomy for essential tremor. The New England Journal of Medicine. 2016;**375**:730-739

[47] Oliveria SF et al. Safety and efficacy of dual-lead thalamic deep brain stimulation for patients with treatment-refractory multiple sclerosis tremor: A single-Centre, randomised, single-blind, pilot trial. Lancet Neurology. 2017;**16**:691-700

[48] Volkmann J et al. Pallidal neurostimulation in patients with medication-refractory cervical dystonia: A randomised, sham-controlled trial. Lancet Neurology. 2014;**13**:875-884

[49] Kupsch A et al. Pallidal deep-brain stimulation in primary generalized or segmental dystonia. The New England Journal of Medicine. 2006;**355**:1978-1990

[50] Andrews C, Aviles-Olmos I, Hariz M, Foltynie T. Which patients with dystonia benefit from deep brain stimulation? A metaregression of individual patient outcomes. Journal of Neurology, Neurosurgery, and Psychiatry. 2010;**81**:1383-1389

[51] Isaias IU et al. Factors predicting protracted improvement after pallidal DBS for primary dystonia: The role of age and disease duration. Journal of Neurology. 2011;**258**:1469-1476

[52] Lumsden DE et al. Proportion of life lived with dystonia inversely

correlates with response to pallidal deep brain stimulation in both primary and secondary childhood dystonia. Developmental Medicine and Child Neurology. 2013;**55**:567-574

[53] Panov F et al. Pallidal deep brain stimulation for DYT6 dystonia. Journal of Neurology, Neurosurgery, and Psychiatry. 2012;**83**:182-187

[54] Jinnah HA et al. Deep brain stimulation for dystonia: A novel perspective on the value of genetic testing. Journal of Neural Transmission (Vienna). 2017;**124**:417-430

[55] Moro E et al. Efficacy of pallidal stimulation in isolated dystonia: A systematic review and meta-analysis. European Journal of Neurology. 2017;**24**:552-560

[56] Ostrem JL et al. Subthalamic nucleus deep brain stimulation in primary cervical dystonia. Neurology. 2011;**76**:870-878

[57] Loher TJ, Pohle T, Krauss JK. Functional stereotactic surgery for treatment of cervical dystonia: Review of the experience from the lesional era. Stereotactic and Functional Neurosurgery. 2004;**82**:1-13

[58] Pauls KA et al. Deep brain stimulation in the ventrolateral thalamus/subthalamic area in dystonia with head tremor. Movement Disorders. 2014;**29**:953-959

[59] Ruge D et al. Deep brain stimulation effects in dystonia: Time course of electrophysiological changes in early treatment. Movement Disorders. 2011;**26**:1913-1921

[60] Grips E et al. Patterns of reoccurrence of segmental dystonia after discontinuation of deep brain stimulation. Journal of Neurology, Neurosurgery, and Psychiatry. 2007;**78**:318-320

[61] Cif L et al. The influence of deep brain stimulation intensity and duration on symptoms evolution in an OFF stimulation dystonia study. Brain Stimulation. 2013;**6**:500-505

[62] Vidailhet M, Grabli D, Roze E. Pathophysiology of dystonia. Current Opinion in Neurology. 2009;**22**:406-413

[63] Lozano AM et al. A phase II study of fornix deep brain stimulation in mild Alzheimer's disease. Journal of Alzheimer's Disease. 2016;**54**:777-787

[64] Eitan R et al. One year double blind study of high versus low frequency subcallosal cingulate stimulation for depression. Journal of Psychiatric Research. 2018;**96**:124-134

[65] Baldermann JC et al. Deep brain stimulation for Tourette-syndrome: A systematic review and meta-analysis. Brain Stimulation. 2016;**9**:296-304

[66] Welter ML et al. Anterior pallidal deep brain stimulation for Tourette's syndrome: A randomised, double-blind, controlled trial. Lancet Neurology. 2017;**16**:610-619

[67] Blair-West GW, Cantor CH, Mellsop GW, Eyeson-Annan ML. Lifetime suicide risk in major depression: Sex and age determinants. Journal of Affective Disorders. 1999;**55**:171-178

[68] Whiteford HA et al. Estimating remission from untreated major depression: A systematic review and meta-analysis. Psychological Medicine. 2013;**43**:1569-1585

[69] Gippert SM et al. Deep brain stimulation for bipolar disorder-review and outlook. CNS Spectrums. 2017;**22**:254-257

[70] Mallet L et al. Subthalamic nucleus stimulation in severe obsessive-compulsive disorder. The

New England Journal of Medicine. 2008;**359**:2121-2134

[71] Lipsman N et al. Deep brain stimulation of the subcallosal cingulate for treatment-refractory anorexia nervosa: 1 year follow-up of an open-label trial. Lancet Psychiatry. 2017;**4**:285-294

[72] Boccard SG, Pereira EA, Moir L, Aziz TZ, Green AL. Long-term outcomes of deep brain stimulation for neuropathic pain. Neurosurgery. 2013;**72**:221-230

[73] Boccard SGJ et al. Long-term results of deep brain stimulation of the anterior cingulate cortex for neuropathic pain. World Neurosurgery. 2017;**106**:625-637

[74] Limousin P et al. Effect of parkinsonian signs and symptoms of bilateral subthalamic nucleus stimulation. Lancet. 1995;**345**:91-95

[75] Morris GL 3rd, Mueller WM. Long-term treatment with vagus nerve stimulation in patients with refractory epilepsy. The Vagus nerve stimulation study group E01–E05. Neurology. 1999;**53**:1731-1735

[76] Coubes P, Cif L, El Fertit H, et al. Electrical stimulation of the globus pallidus internus in patients with primary generalized dystonia: Long-term results. Journal of Neurosurgery. 2004;**101**:189-194

[77] Castrioto A, Lozano AM, Poon YY, Lang AE, Fallis M, Moro E. Ten-year outcome of subthalamic stimulation in Parkinson disease: A blinded evaluation. Archives of Neurology. 2011;**68**(12):1550-1556

[78] Zhang K, Bhatia S, Oh MY, Cohen D, Angle C, Whiting D. Long-term results of thalamic deep brain stimulation for essential tremor. Journal of Neurosurgery. 2010;**112**:1271-1276

[79] Mills KA, Starr PA, Ostrem JL. Neuromodulation for dystonia: Target and patient selection. Neurosurgery Clinics of North America. 2014;**25**(1):59-75

[80] Leone M, Franzini A, Bussone G. Stereotactic stimulation of posterior hypothalamic gray matter in a patient with intractable cluster headache. The New England Journal of Medicine. 2001;**345**:1428-1429

[81] Leone M, Franzini A, Proietti Cecchini A, et al. Success, failure and putative mechanisms in hypothalamic stimulation for drug-resistant chronic cluster headache. Pain. 2013;**154**:89-94

[82] Leone M, Proietti CA. Deep brain stimulation in headache. Cephalalgia. 2016;**36**(12):1143-1148

[83] Pilitsis JG et al. 124 low-back pain relief with a new 32-contact surgical lead and neural targeting algorithm. Neurosurgery. 2016;**63**(Suppl 1):151

[84] Sun FT, Morrell MJ. Closed-loop neurostimulation: The clinical experience. Neurotherapeutics. 2014;**11**:553-563

[85] Deer T et al. Prospective, multicenter, randomized, double-blinded, partial crossover study to assess the safety and efficacy of the novel neuromodulation system in the treatment of patients with chronic pain of peripheral nerve origin. Neuromodulation. 2016;**19**:91-100

Section 2

Neurostimulation in the Medical Management of Spasticity

Chapter 4

Spasticity: Diagnosis and Treatment

Alexander Kovalenko, Viktor Misikov, Konstantin Sinelnikov, Valeriy Shamigulov, Dmitrii Iskra, Svetlana E. Khatkova and Denis V. Kovlen

Abstract

This chapter presents the technology of spasticity treatment—from diagnosis and treatment to quality control of treatment and rehabilitation. The diagnosis is based on methods of manual testing and differential diagnosis of spastic muscles, methods of quantitative assessment of spasticity on the basis of the Tardieu scale. The methodical development of the Tardieu scale with variants of its full and reduced use is presented. The basic patterns of spasticity of the upper and lower limbs are given. Schemes of management of patients with spasticity with indication of control points for application of methods of an assessment that shows efficiency of treatment and rehabilitation are presented. The methodology of spasticity treatment using botulinum neurotoxin (BoNT), including ultrasonic navigation, orientation of intramuscular motor endpoint of muscles (IME), is described. IME location diagrams and ultrasound picture of muscles are presented. Scales are proposed to assess the effect of spasticity on the functions of the upper and lower limbs. In conclusion, a variant of complex treatment of spasticity and original patient models are proposed, the use of which makes it possible to calculate the cost of BoNT.

Keywords: spasticity, patterns of spasticity, testing of spastic muscles, modified Tardieu scale (MTS), botulinum neurotoxin (BoNT), ultrasonic navigation, intramuscular motor endpoint (IME), rehabilitation

1. Introduction

Spasticity as the most important component of the defeat syndrome of the upper motor neuron is a motor disorder characterized by a speed-dependent increase in tonic stretching reflexes (muscle tone) with increased tendon reflexes, due to hyperexcitability of the stretching reflex, as one of the components of the syndrome [1]. It is detected in more than 12 million people in the world and is the cause of disability in 12–27% of them [2, 3]. The list of nosological forms in which the structure of the injury syndrome in the *upper motor neuron lesion* (UMNL) observed spastic hypertonicity is significant. It is determined in approximately 20–40% of stroke survivors, 14% of traumatic brain injury survivors, 65–78% of patients with spinal cord lesions, and 85% of patients with multiple sclerosis [4, 5].

Spasticity is a major obstacle to the recovery of the patients who have suffered brain damage. The work of restoring movement becomes impossible with the unresolved issue of spasticity, the treatment of which expands the frame of "the rehabilitation window" and defines the rehabilitation terms. In addition, in the absence of spasticity treatment, the risk of paresis complications increases: contractures, bedsores, limb deformities, pain, muscle spasms, etc. [6].

The development of spasticity is directly related to the initial stages of recovery of movement in paretic limbs. In 1–3 weeks after UMNL, the connections of the cerebral cortex with the structures of the extrapyramidal system (EPS) begin to recover. Recovery time varies depending on the degree of damage: from 2 weeks to 3 months [7].

During this period, the initiation of movements, in accordance with their image in the associative cortex, is able to be realized through intact EPS pathways. This efferent flow, reaching α-small motor neurons (MN), increases the tone in the muscles innervated by them (1st movement phase) for subsequent implementation of the dynamic phase (2-phase motion). However, the latter does not receive a sufficiently powerful efferentation due to the continuing defective functioning of the pyramid path. The result of this is the lack of inclusion of a sufficient number of inhibitory cells (Renshaw), which could inhibit α-small MN and lower muscle tone [7, 8].

Spasticity in strokes is usually formed in the first 3 months after the vascular accident. Its first signs usually begin to appear by the beginning of the 3rd week. The process of spasticity development is quite dynamic and variable. The terms of spasticity development from the first signs of tonus increase to the formed pattern in 2–5 weeks [9–11].

The development of spastic syndrome depends on many reasons: pain, stress, violation of proprioception, violation of the image of the body scheme and balance, tension and phobias with instability in a sitting or walking position.

Pain syndrome has a special place in the development of spasticity. For example, pain in the shoulder joint is directly associated with the development of spasticity. The absence of pain or its temporary relief in 83% of cases reduces the severity of spasticity.

Instability and uncertainty when walking, as well as stress, significantly affect the development of spasticity in the upper limb. So, spasticity in the hand, often develops in patients with severe weakness of the lower limb who retained the ability to move. During the period of yet unformed pattern of spasticity, these patients begin to strain, bend, and bring paretic arm to maintain balance while walking, which in 3–4 weeks causes the formed pattern of spasticity of the upper limb [12–14].

An important role in the development of spasticity plays the violation of proprioception, which leads to the violation of the image of the body scheme. Lack of afferentation triggers mechanisms that should increase the power of information from the tendons and joints receptors. In the case of spasticity, when dynamic muscle contraction is impossible due to paresis, it leads to activation of spinal and supraspinal mechanisms of tonus enhancement [15, 16].

Thus, the main directions in the rehabilitation of the consequences injury to the upper motor neuron and in the treatment of spasticity are:

- creating conditions precluding the need for the injury. For this purpose, analgesics, anxiolytics, as well as special styling, exercise therapy and hardware techniques are used, which activate proprioception, forming an associative image of the body scheme;

- the start of the physiological mechanisms of spasticity by activating muscle antagonists (taping, magnetic, electric stimulation, etc.) and initiating the mechanism of reciprocal interaction (kinesitherapy and other techniques);
- the use of methods that enable balancing the activity phases of the movement by reducing the activity in the 1st phase, up to severity 2nd (BoNT injections, stretching).

The most common complications of spasticity are contractures. They, together with spasticity, serve as the main obstacle to rehabilitation measures. The most common are the contractures of the shoulder (86%) and ankle (19%) joints. Adaptogenes of these contractures is different. Ankle contracture occurs among patients with late motor activity, severe paresis (70%), low motivation (81%), and incorrect treatment (23%). In contrast, shoulder contracture in 71% of cases is caused by the activity and verticalization of the patient in the first 14 days after the stroke. The shoulder joint, having the largest volume of movements, completely assumes all weight of the upper limb. With paresis and initial hypotension, often occurring after a stroke, the entire weight of the arm (4–7 kg) falls on the ligamentous apparatus of the joint, its articular bag, causing their trauma and pain. This, in turn, leads to the progressing severity of spasticity, as well as periarticular and articular changes [13].

By 6 months after the stroke, 90% of cases of spasticity, 36% of joint contractures, and 57% of tendon-muscle contractures (internal spasticity) are formed. At the same time, of all cases of spasticity, the manifestation of its signs in 77.3% of patients falls on the first 2–3 weeks. As a rule, the severity of spasticity in the first 2 weeks does not exceed 1–2 points on the Modified Ashworth scale (MAS). Increased spasticity by 1-point MAS increases the consumption of botulinum neurotoxin (BoNT) by 100–200 Units, which significantly increases the cost of treatment. Thus, early detection and treatment of spasticity reduces the cost of therapeutic rehabilitation measures [13, 14].

In the muscles involved in the spasticity pattern, diffuse muscle changes (DMC) develop over time in a form of connecting tissue substitution. There are no clear time criteria for the development of DMC. Among many patients with a disease duration of more than 4 years, the muscle structure is preserved. Some DMC develop within 6 months. Clinical signs of DMC are the following: low tissue turgor, decreased muscle volume, and significant restriction of movement, up to its total absence. While ultrasounding such muscles, in addition to reducing the volume, a hyperechogenic signal is registered (**Figure 1**) [17].

Currently, a classification has been adopted in which generalized, regional, and focal forms of spasticity are distinguished. There are also patterns of spasticity characteristic of different joints and muscles of the upper and lower limbs. Depending on the form and pattern of spasticity, the strategy and tactics of its treatment are determined [10]:

- generalized spasticity with pain—central muscle relaxants;
- focal and segmental spasticity—drugs BoNT;
- spasticity with marked para- or tetraparesis—intrathecal baclofen [15].

For effective treatment of spasticity with BoNT drugs, it is necessary to determine the spasticity pattern with verification of the muscles that form it; and then their correct introduction into the target muscle.

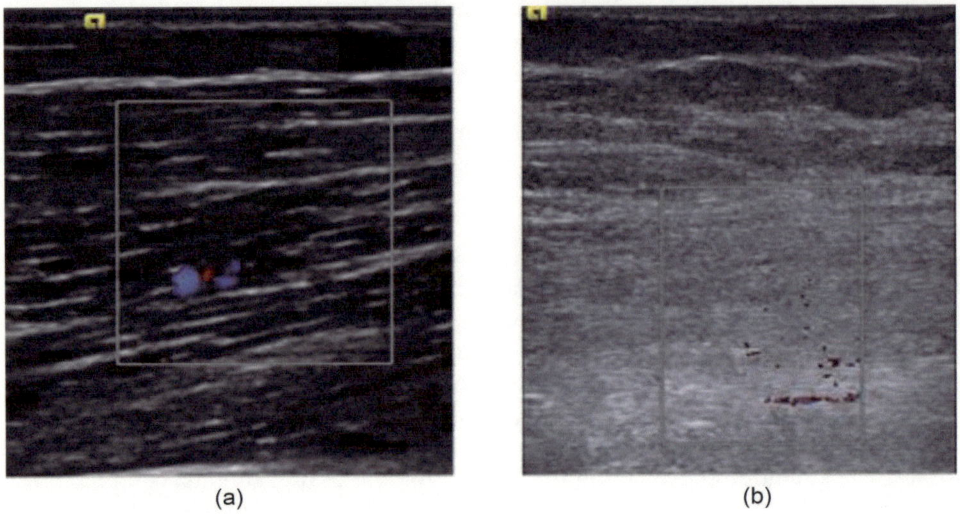

Figure 1.
Ultrasound picture of normal muscle tissue (a) and muscles with hyperechogenic ultrasonic signal due to DMC (b).

Twelve main clinical patterns of spasticity for the upper (5) and lower (7) limbs have been identified. Spasticity patterns for the hands include various, mainly flexor, variants of flexion in the joints: retracting the shoulder, elbow flexion, forearm pronation, wrist flexion, and finger flexion [18]. Spasticity patterns for the leg consist of hip reduction, knee flexion, knee extension, plantar flexion of the foot, equinovarus positioning of the foot, flexion of the fingers, and extension of the thumb [19].

2. Clinical diagnostic of spasticity

2.1 Manual testing of muscles for spasticity

Muscle testing is required to identify specific muscles involved in the spasticity pattern. All spastic muscle testing methods are based on two principles:

1. Identification and activation of exclusive and additional functions of the studied muscle.

2. Differentiation of movements for muscles with the same function, but passing through a different number of joints.

For spasticity patterns in the arm, an anatomical description is used with a representation of all the muscles that could perform a given movement in the joints (**Figure 2**). For differentiation of compensatory inclusions of muscles, it is necessary after definition of type of a pattern of spasticity in a hand to carry out manual testing.

2.1.1 Upper limb muscle testing

Bringing and pronation of the shoulder. At the heart of the restriction of movements in the shoulder with spasticity are problems with the withdrawal,

DOI: http://dx.doi.org/10.5772/intechopen.91046

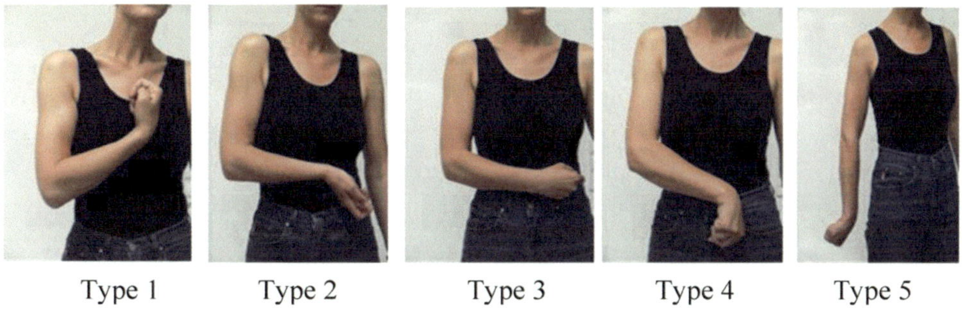

Figure 2.
Types of upper limb spasticity patterns [16].

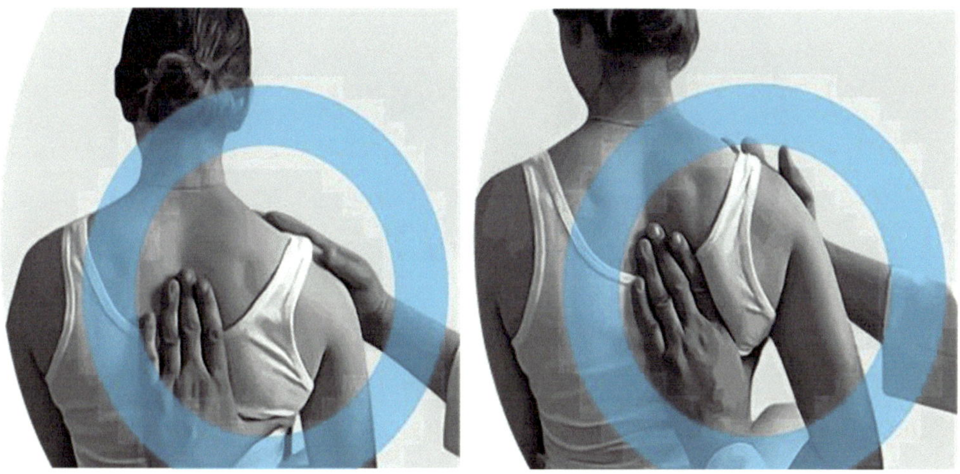

Figure 3.
M. Subscapularis spasticity testing.

lifting of the shoulder, and its supination. Almost all the muscles of the shoulder girdle can influence these movement vectors, but most often it is done by the following: *m. Pectoralis* major (PM) (90%), *m. Subscapularis* (S/s) (20%), and *m. Laissimus dorsi* (LD) (5%).

Spasticity PM and LD is diagnosed when the shoulder is raised and withdrawn with the express tension of their lateral edge (the anterior and posterior walls of the axillary cavity, respectively). Diagnosis is done visually and by palpation.

S/s retracts the shoulder and rotates it inward. Spasticity is diagnosed by lifting, retraction and supination of the shoulder by visual and palpatory control of the lower angle and medial edge of the scapula. Normally, the shoulder is withdrawn without moving the blade to the horizontal level (80–90°). Thus, if the movement of the blade begins before reaching this level, there is an increase in tone in S/s. There is individual variability, so it is necessary to compare this movement with the intact hand (**Figure 3**).

Elbow flexors. The main muscles flexing the elbow are mm. Brachioradialis (BR), Brachialis (Br), and Biceps brachii (BB) (muscles are listed by importance in the spasticity pattern). BB is also a powerful arch support of the forearm. The muscles are tested when provoking a stretch reflex (muscle stretching reflex, mitotic reflex) at different rates of extension in the elbow joint. The reaction of BR and BB is evaluated visually and by palpation (**Figures 4** and **5**). The reaction of Br can only be assessed by palpation, gripping, with your own fingers upon humerus

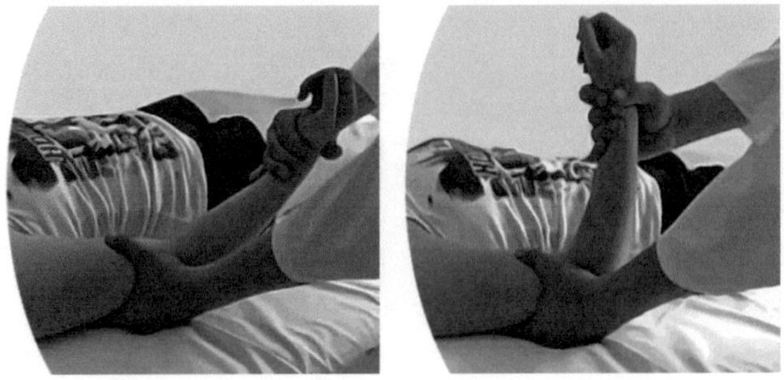

Figure 4.
M. Biceps brachii spasticity testing.

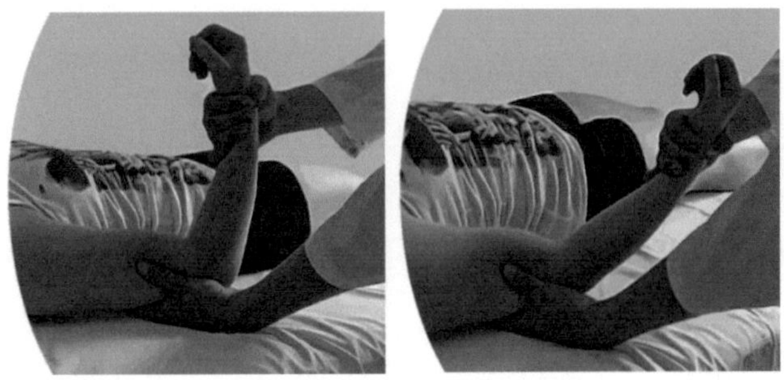

Figure 5.
M. Brachialis spasticity testing.

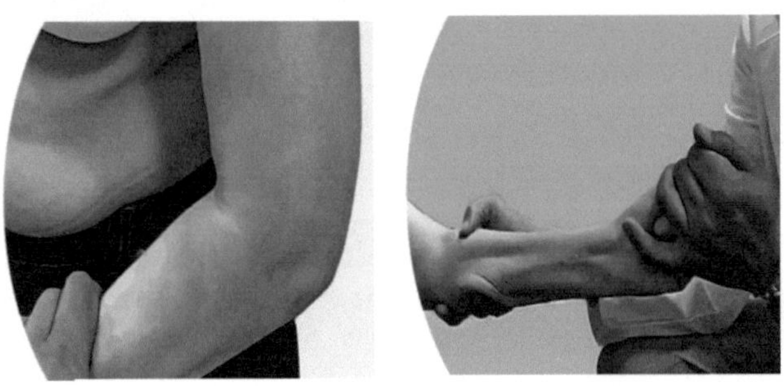

Figure 6.
M. Brachioradialis spasticity testing.

from below (rear). Win case of spasticity in response to a sharp extension in the elbow joint under the fingertips you feel tension (**Figure 6**).

Forearm pronators. Forearm pronates three muscles: mm. Pronator teres (PT) and Pronator quadratus (PQ) and m. Flexor carpi radialis (FCR). PT and FCR in pronation act as a single functional unit. In some cases, with ultrasound of these muscles, you can find the lack of a clear boundary between them, which once again confirms the generality of their function. Testing these two muscles is based on provoking the stretch reflex in response to rapid supination. The presence of spasticity in FCR is manifested visually and confirmed by palpation. Spasticity in PT can be determined only by palpation, putting your fingers on the middle line of the forearm 2–4 cm below the elbow bend and producing supination. Sometimes when assessing pronator spasticity, FCR is more stressful than PT.

Flexors of the hand and fingers. Testing is performed by back flexion in the wrist joint. If no significant resistance is felt during this movement, and the fingers are progressively flexed as the hand is extended, this means that neither of the two flexors of the hand (m. Flexor carpi radialis and m. Flexor carpi ulnaris) participates in its flexion. Pathological flexion of the hand in this case is due to spasticity m. Flexor digitorum profundus (FDP) and m. Flexor digitorum superficialis (FDS) (**Figure 7**).

In order to distinguish spasticity in FDS and FDP, you can extend the wrist joint. In this movement, it is necessary to pay attention to the proximal and distal interphalangeal joints of the fingers. If it is found that the distal interphalangeal joints are bent to a greater extent, this indicates the spasticity of the deep flexor of the fingers. If the proximal interphalangeal joints-superficial flexor fingers (**Figure 8**). If this bends the distal phalanx of the thumb—this indicates spasticity m. Flexor pollicis longus (**Figure 9**).

If manipulations in the wrist joint did not have any effect on the position of the thumb, it means that the muscles of the hand are responsible for its position: mm. Flexor pollicis brevis, Opponens pollicis Adductor pollicis (**Figure 10**).

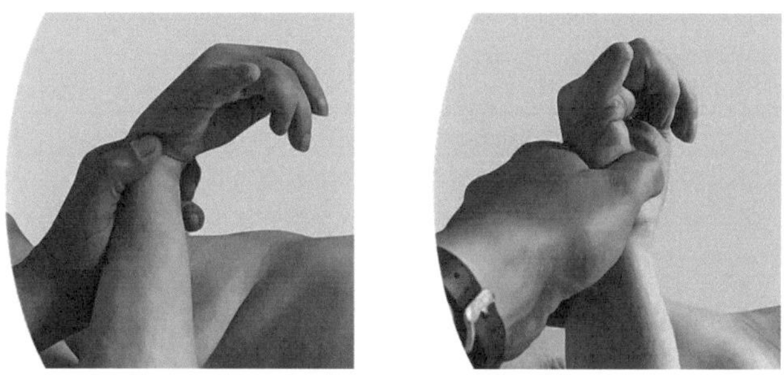

Figure 7.
M. Flexor digitorum profundus u m. Flexor digitorum superficialis spasticity testing.

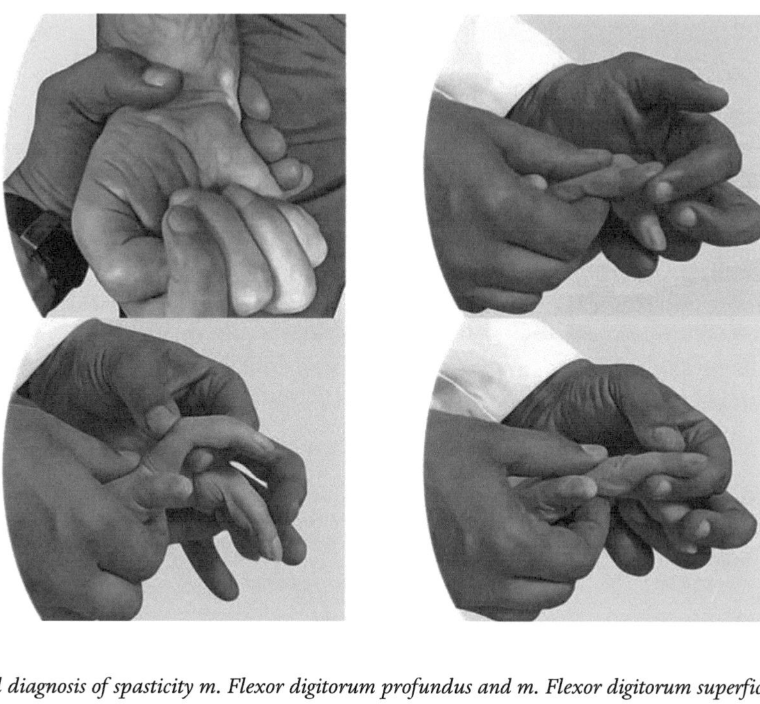

Figure 8.
Differential diagnosis of spasticity m. Flexor digitorum profundus and m. Flexor digitorum superficialis.

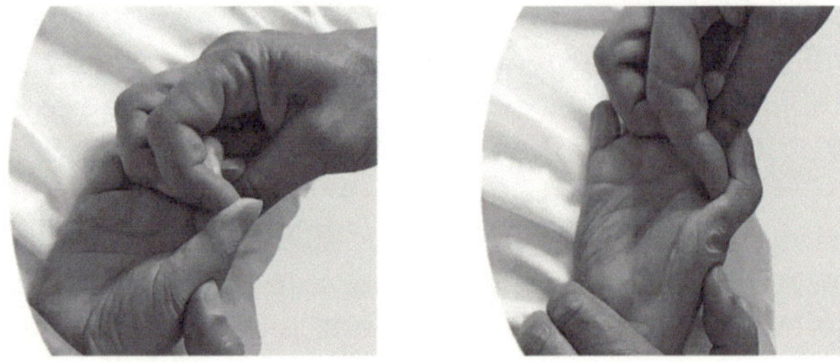

Figure 9.
M. Flexor pollicis longus spasticity testing.

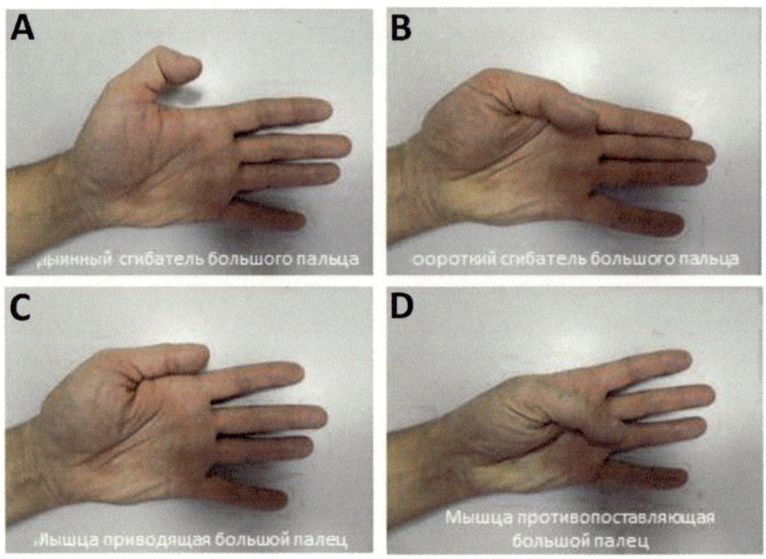

Figure 10.
Patterns in spasticity of the muscles of the hand. (A) m. Flexor pollicis longus, (B) m. Flexor pollicis brevis, (C) m. Adductor pollicis, and (D) m. Opponens pollicis.

2.1.2 Lower limb muscle testing

While a professional consensus has been formed on the upper limb spasticity patterns based on the work of H. Hefter, a consolidated opinion on the lower limb spasticity patterns has not been developed, and the question of determining target muscles and BoNT dosages still remains open [11].

The peculiarity of the lower limb patterns is the ambiguity of their distribution among clinical nosological forms. This fact and the remaining unclear features of the pathogenesis of spasticity is that it does not allow you to choose and apply to the patterns of the lower limb a single classification principle. We can only say about the predominant frequency of occurrence of a particular pattern in any nosology.

Thus, we can distinguish:

1. Spasticity patterns in cerebral palsy.

    - Flexion of hip and knee joints.

    - Internal rotation and the tibia adducci.

    - equinus.

- Valgus or varus.
- Exterior turn stop.
- Adduction.

2. Patterns of spasticity in multiple sclerosis.
   - Adduction.
   - Flexion or extension of the hip.
   - Of equinus.
   - Flexion or extension of the knee.
3. Spasticity patterns in severe brain injury, encephalitis, and spinal injury.
   - "Triple flexion".
   - Flexion of the ankle joints.
   - Adduction.
   - Flexion of the toes.
4. Patterns of spasticity in stroke and brain injury.
   - Dynamic pattern.
   - Static pattern (equinovarus)
   - their combination with flexion of the toes.

Testing of the muscles of the lower limb is carried out in the supine position, on both limbs, consistently comparing flexion in the joints (to identify poor muscle extensibility not associated with spasticity) [18].

There are two main types of lower limb spasticity patterns in patients undergoing stroke: dynamic pattern (DP) and static pattern (SP), as well as their possible combinations with flexion of the toes and hip reduction. Patterns are proposed based on the principle of visual assessment of the limb position at rest and when walking [19].

In case DP manifestations of spasticity are determined only in the process of movement. In the resting position, the legs do not differ from healthy and its normal statics is kept (limb are visually full length, the joints are in the middle position, and toes are separated), the position of the fingers most often corresponds with the finger of these intact side. Walking is characterized by a peculiar pattern, in which in the phase of hip transfer and knee extension, before lowering the foot to the surface, there are oscillatory movements of the shin from side to side with possible flexion of the fingers. The cause of DP is increased tone and muscle-tendon contraction in the muscles of the back of the thigh (hamstrings), – mm. Semitendinosus (S/t), Semimembranosus (S/m), Biceps femoris (BF) and in *M. gracilis* (G).

Gait peculiarity in this type of spasticity is associated with the phylogenetic foundations of neurophysiology of movement in providing the act of walking and is realized through segmental connections, leading, in part, to its automatism [20–22]. As a result, the paretic limb, which tends to step of the same characteristics as the intact one, encounters hamstrings contraction, which leads to a push of the hip and knee backward and medially, stopping the inertia of the limb forward, shortening the step and, sometimes, bringing the hip and shin oscillatory movements [23–25].

SP is characterized primarily by equinecom and equinovarus that can be observed in standing and lying down. There may also be curvature of the pelvic position due to changes in limb length, and/or knee flexion. But more often there is flexion in the ankle joint with a possible compensatory tension of the anterior muscle group of the thigh. The gait in this case becomes circulatory with a slope contralateral to the paresis. This result toning any of the four muscles: m. Soleus (S), m. Gastrocnemius (G/c), m. Tibialis posterior (TP), m. Tibialis anterior (TA).

An additional phenomenon in SP and DP can be flexion of the toes, which is responsible for spasticity mm. Flexor digitorum longus (FDL), Flexor hallucis longus (FHL), Flexor digitorum brevis (FDB), and Flexor hallucis brevis (FHB).

1. Assessment of DP (**Figure 11**):

   A. For the differential diagnosis of posterior thigh muscle hypertonicity, the patient's straight leg is bent at the hip joint. At the limit of extensibility of spastic muscles, involuntary flexion of the leg in the knee joint is fixed. Fixing the leg at this level, use palpation and visually determine tense muscles of the back of the thigh. In difficult cases, for verification of spastic muscles, ultrasound diagnosis should be carried out.

   B. To test spasticity in the inner thigh muscles (adductors, G and m. Sartorius (Srt)), the leg is retracted to the tensile limit. After that spastic muscles are examined by palpation, visually, and optionally using ultrasonic equipment (**Figure 12**). To differentiate the tone increase in adductors and G, a gracilis test was also performed (**Figure 13**). To identify limitations in the diversion of the leg, it is made bending at the knee (the test must be performed on the edge of the couch). The ability to perform further hip abduction after flexion-indicates spasticity in G. The Lack of response to knee flexion indicates an increase in tone in the adductors.

2. Assessment of SP:

   A. To differentiate spasticity in m. Soleus (S) and in the heads of m. Gastrocnemius (G/c), a Silfverskiold test should be performed (**Figure 14**) [26].

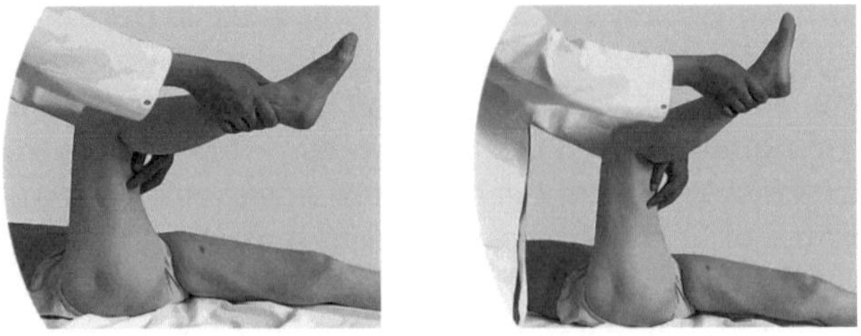

Figure 11.
Spasticity testing in posterior thigh muscles (mm. Semitendinosus, Semimembranosus, Biceps femoris, and Gracilis).

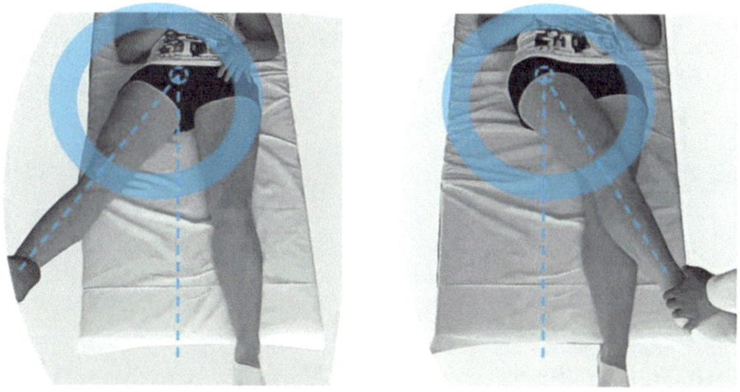

Figure 12.
Testing of spasticity in the hip adductor muscles.

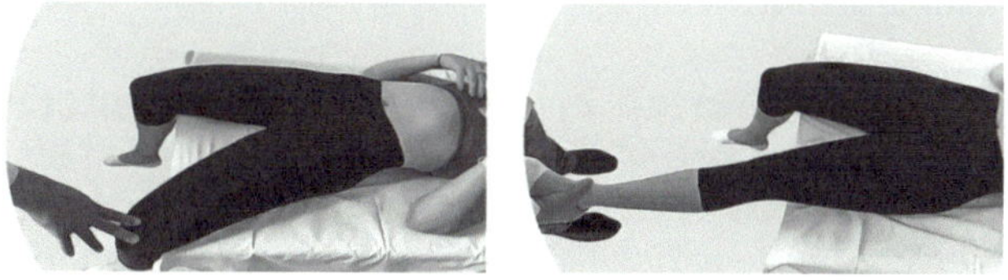

Figure 13.
Testing of spasticity in m. Gracilis (gracilis test).

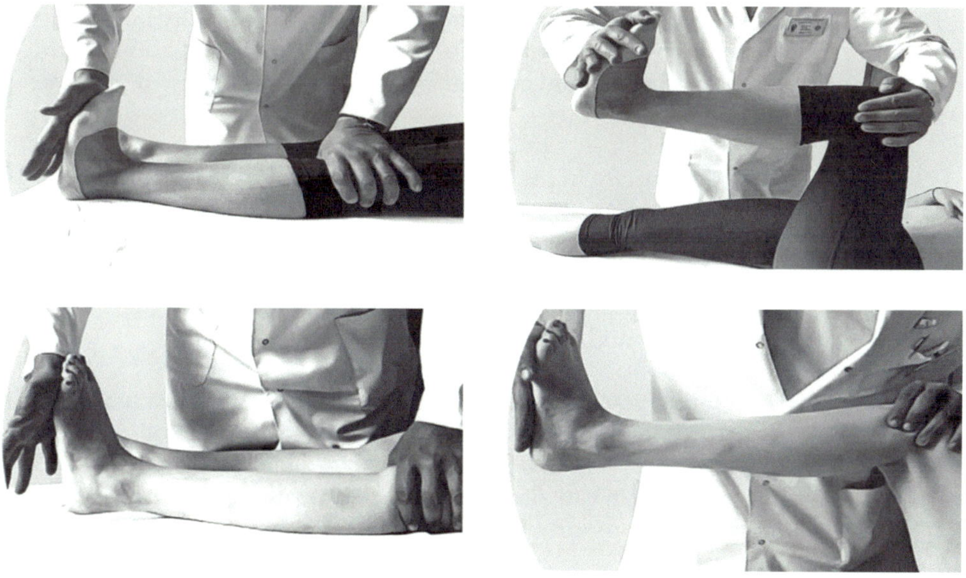

Figure 14.
Sequential test execution Silverskiold's to identify spasticity in m. Gastrocnemius and m. Soleus.

During the test, the angle of flexion of the foot is consistently determined with the leg straightened and bent at the knee. No change in the position of the ankle joint in response to flexion of the knee and the foot clonus testify the increase of tone in S. Marked decrease of the bending angle up to 80° or less while you straighten the legs indicates spasticity in G/c. Supination of the foot of any severity in the last phase of the rectification of the foot manifests the increased tone only in the medial head G/c. As an additional test when the leg is straightened, should be a passive extension of the foot

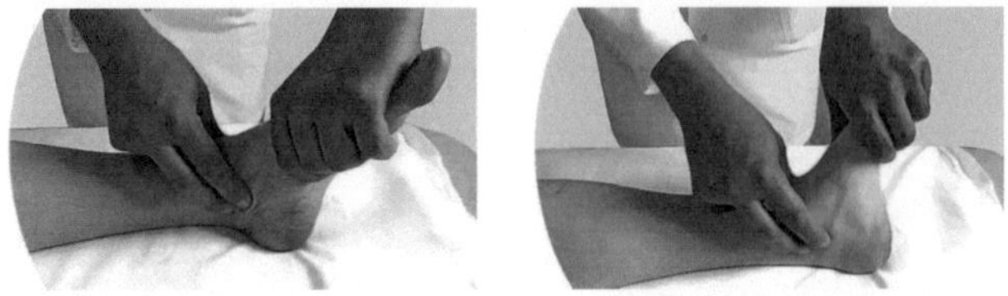

Figure 15.
Testing of spasticity in m. Tibialis posterior.

with simultaneous sharp proanation. Visually and by palpation fixed tension of medial head G/c confirms the increase of its tone. The presence of spasticity only in the medial head G/c leads to tension of the medial part of the Achilles tendon, which is manifested by pulling the heel bone back and up with a turn inward.

B. To determine the increase in tone *m. Tibialis* anterior (TA), it is necessary to make a rapid flexion of the foot followed by pronation. This maneuver provokes a stretch reflex in TA. The detected tension TA (visually and by palpation) and the contour of the tendon at the back of the foot is the evidence of increase of its tone.

C. To test spasticity in *m. Tibialis* posterior (TP), it is necessary to perform a rapid extension of the foot followed by pronation. This triggers the stretch reflex to TP. The muscle is not visually controllable, but its tendon runs along the lower edge of the medial ankle. Palpation recorded muscle tension and tendon contouring indicates an increase in its tone (**Figure 15**).

D. Diagnosis of spasticity in the flexors of the toes is made by performing sequential passive flexion and extension in the ankle joint:

- if there is simultaneous flexion of the toes during the extension of the foot, this indicates an increase in tone in m. Flexor digitorum longus (FDL) and/or m. Flexor hallucis longus (FHL);

- maintaining your posture of flexion, regardless of movements in the ankle joint demonstrates increased tone in m. Flexor digitorum brevis (FDB) and/or m. Flexor hallucis brevis (FHB). Tension in them can also be seen with palpation of the arch of the foot.

3. Scales for assessing spasticity and disorders of activity and participation

3.1 Rating scale for evaluating the condition of muscles

The main scales to assess the condition of the muscles are: the scale of muscle contraction force and volume of voluntary movements (MRCS), modified Ashworth scale (MAS) and the Tardieu scale (MTS) [27–30].

The scale of muscle contraction strength and volume of voluntary movements (Medical Research Council Scale (Oxford Scale), MRCS) allows to estimate the strength of muscle contraction and amplitude of active movements in the limb.

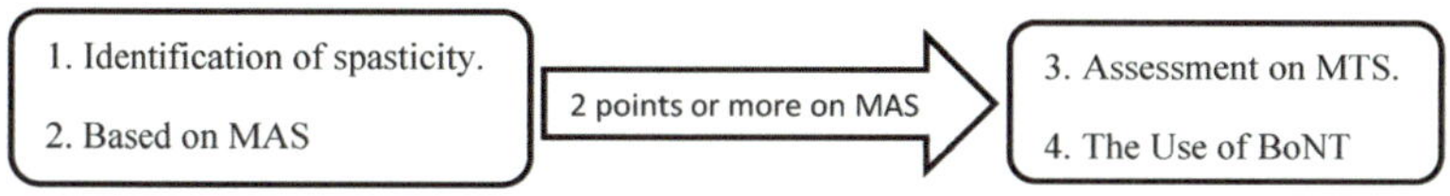

Figure 16.
Algorithm of diagnosis and treatment of spasticity.

The modified Ashworth Scale (MAS) serves to objectify muscle tone and is the most used to evaluate the effectiveness of treatment of spasticity of BoNT [31].

MAS allows, without resorting to special measuring tools and calculations, to assess the degree of mobility of the joints, associated with increased muscle tone when performing passive movement. At the same time, MAS does not reveal the nuances of spasticity, such as muscle reactivity, the dependence of its contraction on the rate of tendon stretching [13].

The modified Tardieu Scale (MTS) [29, 30, 32] allows the most complete assessment of all manifestations of spasticity: tone, stretch reflex (reaction to tendon stretching), and spastic co-contraction (inclusion of muscles antagonists to movement).

The capabilities inherent in the MTS assessment system allow not only to verify spasticity in more detail, but also to quantify muscle weakness, fatigue, and the state of deep sensitivity [33].

The following algorithm is used to diagnose and treat spasticity (**Figure 16**) [11]:

The measurement system incorporated in MTS is performed by a goniometer and must be performed at the same time of the day, and the tested limb must be placed in the same position during repeated testing (**Figure 17**) [11].

The peculiarity of MTS application is the assessment of changes in muscle tone and angles of movement in the joint in response to the provocation of spastic co-contraction (activation of muscles antagonists to movement) and stretch reflex (reaction to tendon stretching) obtained at different speeds of passive movement in the joint.

The speeds are selected according to the following characteristics:

- as slowly as possible (V1);
- speed equal to the speed of fall of a limb moving under the action of gravity (V2);
- as soon as possible (V3) (faster than the speed of natural fall of the limb segment under gravity).

In recent years, in the professional community, there is a refusal to assess the rate V2 [31, 33], which leaves two fundamental indicators (**Figure 17**):

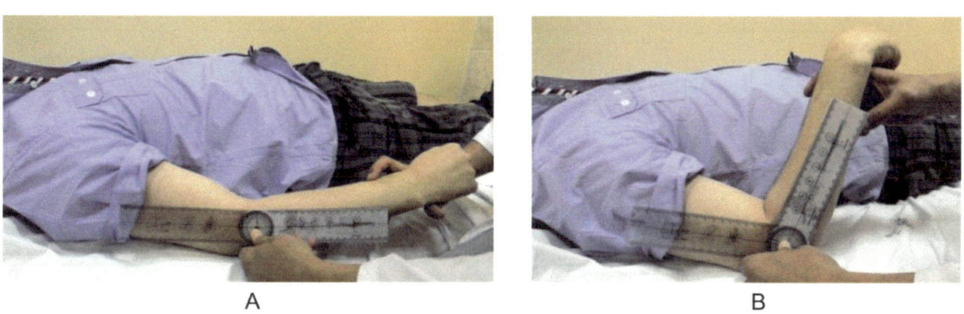

Figure 17.
(A) Slow passive extension, X_{V1} and (B) fast passive extension, X_{V3}.

X_{V1} – angle measured at speed V1.
X_{V3} – the angle measured at the speed V3.

The Tardieu scale offers a flexible evaluation system that allows you to use different approaches in the diagnosis of spasticity, opens the possibility of choosing evaluation parameters, provides options for both rapid evaluations based on one or two parameters, and a full-scale study of spasticity and paresis with the calculation of indices and coefficients, which makes it possible to register the minimum rehabilitation dynamics.

There are two main ways to use MTS. The first of them involves taking into account the score, which reflects the characteristics of the reaction of muscles and tendons in response to their stretching, the other option is based on taking into account the angle of the movement end, without a special assessment of the nuances of the muscle reaction. It is also possible to combine the use of both options or the use of separate elements from each of them.

In the 1st variant of MTS application, the assessment is based on two parameters: the degree of muscle reaction (Y) in points and the angle at which the muscle reaction (X) in degrees is achieved.

To score the degree of muscle reaction (Y), a table of scores and their interpretations is used (**Table 1**).

The estimated home value of 1st version of evaluation is **Index Tardieu** (IT)—the ratio Y (point) to X (degrees) achieved at different speeds of movement in the joint:

$$\text{IT (V1, V2, V3)} = \text{Y (score)/X (angle in degrees)}. \quad (1)$$

Thus, if the angle at which the reaction occurs and/or the score varies with the velocity, we get three results. For example, in the elbow joint:

1. $IT_{V1} = 1/180 = 0.005$.

2. $IT_{V2} = 2/90 = 0.022$.

3. $IT_{V3} = 3/90 = 0.033$.

IT_{V1} characterizes increased muscle tone outside the reaction to the stretch reflex and demonstrates the degree of shortening of the muscle. The results obtained at V2 and V3 rates characterize the degree of muscle reaction to the tendon stretching rate and are different degrees of stretch reflex provocation.

A significant difference between $IT_{V1–V3}$ (2.5 times or more) may indicate the degree of dynamism of the muscle-tendon contracture or its absence, which allows us to count on a good result when using BoNT. A slight difference in the values of it

Points	Interpretation
0	No resistance throughout passive movement
1	Slight resistance throughout with no clear catch at a precise angle
2	Clear catch at a precise angle, followed by release
3	Fatigable clonus (10 s) occurring at a precise angle
4	Unfatigable clonus (>10 s) occurring at a precise angle
5	Joint immobile

Table 1.
Quality of muscle reaction.

(1.5–2 times or less), with severe limitation of movement in the joint indicates a worse prognosis and the need for active exercises on muscle stretching or diagnosis of joint contracture [13].

The 2nd variant of application of MTS actually does not assume the use of the table of a point estimation and is based on variety of measurements of angles of movement in a joint and change of a scope of movements depending on manifestations of spasticity, register:

- X_{V1}—angle range of passive movement of a limb at a slow speed (angle arrest);
- X_{V3}—angle stop movement of the limbs at high speed (angle catch);
- X_A—angle muscle power (corner of the active movement in the joint by working the antagonist muscles spasticity (active motion));
- X_{A15}—angle fatigue of the muscle (measured after 15 s of working the antagonist muscles spasticity).

The main calculated value in the 2nd variant of MTS application is the spasticity angle (X_S):

$$X_S = X_{V1} - X_{V3}. \tag{2}$$

As part of the diagnosis and treatment, it is also necessary to know the X_N – angle of the normal volume of movement in a particular joint. This is necessary not only to understand the degree of spasticity but also to calculate the coefficients proposed in the scale and characterizing the state of the muscles. Such factors are: (1) velocity factor (C shorting) muscle C_{SH}, (2) ratio of spasticity (spasticity C) C_S; (3) the coefficient of weakness (weakness C) muscle C_W; and (4) coefficient of fatigue (fatigue C) C_F:

1. $C_{SH} = (X_N - X_{V1})/X_N$.
2. $C_S = (X_{V1} - X_{V3})/X_{V3}$.
3. $C_W = (X_{V1} - X_A)/X_{V1}$.
4. $C_F = (X_A - X_{A15})/X_A$.

Measuring X_A and X_{A15} and calculating C_F and C_W fill another important gap in neurology—the ability to fully quantify paresis, thereby significantly complementing the use of MRCS [33].

There is also a muscle reaction angle (x): measured as the difference between the forced position of the joint and the angle of the normal anatomical position of the limb and its segments (applies to all joints except the hip) [32, 34].

In a complete evaluation system for the Tardieu scale includes not only the motion estimation but also sensitivity. Verification of deep sensitivity disorders is achieved by measuring the proprioception angle (X_P). Normally, the brain fixes the angular displacement in the joints to 2–3°.

At neurological examination, as a rule, it is considered sufficient to reveal only the fact of violation of muscular-articular feeling. But, for the prognosis of spasticity, qualitative diagnosis of proprioception disorders and evaluation of rehabilitation dynamics is not enough. This provision has a pathophysiological justification. One version of the pathogenesis of spasticity is the activation of muscle contraction in response to afferentation insufficiency [7]. Obtaining information about the degree of proprioception impairment allows us to predict the subsequent development of spasticity, suggesting the effectiveness and assessing the dynamics of rehabilitation. That in turn makes it possible to talk about such a definition as "rehabilitation potential" and plan the volume, structure and timing of rehabilitation of the patient.

Full use of all the features of the Tardieu scale actually allows you to make a "passport" of a certain muscle. In cases where we cannot isolate the function of a single muscle, differentiating it from the synergists, we identify the effect of spasticity of movement in the joint as a whole. An example of this is the work of the muscles of the back of the thigh, where we cannot separate the function of m. Semitendinosus and m. Semimembranosusand assess the degree of their isolated effect on movement in the joint [35].

The "passport" of spastic muscles or restrictions of movements in the joint can be presented in the form of a table:

Muscle/joint	X_{V1}	X_{V3}	X_S	X_A	X_{A15}	X_P	C_{SH}	C_S	C_W	C_F

Especially important for the use of the Tardieu evaluation system is the understanding of the principles of measuring motion in the joint, in particular, the selection of the reference point of the angle of motion. In this case, the measurement system is different from that adopted in orthopedic practice. The reference point is the point is opposite to the studied movement or, in other words, the measurement is carried out from the extreme points of flexion/extension, reduction/withdrawal, pronation/supination, that is, the points to which the co-contraction tends [11]. The point is selected along the axis of the limb segment under study, regardless of whether the segment reaches this point or not. The main task is to make a movement from the point of greatest muscle relaxation to the point of maximum muscle stretching. A good example of this is the study of the movement during the extension of the ankle joint with spasticity in its flexors (**Figure 18**) [12].

Angles are measured from the point lying on the continuation of the axis line of the shin outside the limits of possible flexion in the ankle joint, that is, the count of extension in the joint a priori begins with 45°. The entire range of extension in the joint measured from the line of continuation of the Shin, that is, to the angle of 115°, is estimated. Thus, the movement is carried out in the direction of maximum stretching of the flexors of the joint. In the presented example (**Figure 18**), the

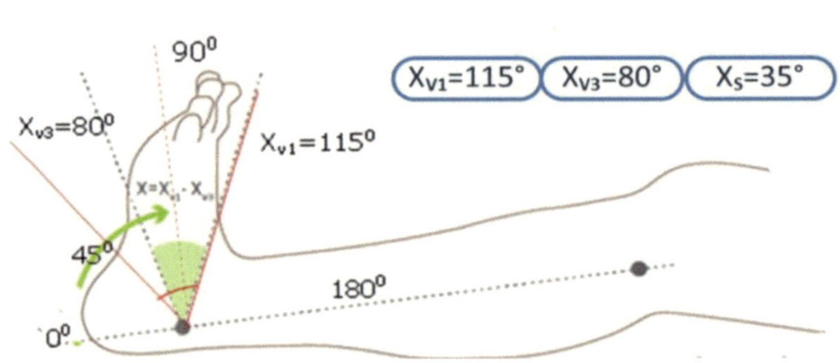

Figure 18.
Measurement of the volume movements of the MTS with increasing tonus of flexors of the ankle joint.

DOI: http://dx.doi.org/10.5772/intechopen.91046

slow-speed stop (V1) occurs at the extreme point of extension in the joint 115°, which indicates the absence of muscle contractures. Stopping at a fast speed (V3) occurs at 80°, which characterizes the stretch reflex and co-contraction of the ankle flexor muscles. The calculated spasticity angle in this case will be 35°.

In the case where it is necessary to evaluate the extensor muscles of the joint, the movement is carried out in the opposite direction-toward their maximum stretching and flexion of the joint. The starting point is the point lying on the shin axis, but since the maximum extension of the foot reaches 115°, the movement begins only from the position 65°. The entire range of flexion in the joint is estimated, that is, up to 135°.

Most often, spasticity limits the following movements: flexion and retraction in the shoulder joint, extension in the elbow, wrist and wrist joints, supination of the forearm, extension/flexion of the hip and knee joints, hip abduction, extension and pronation of the foot, and extension of the toes [19, 35]. Accordingly, the reference point for measuring the volume of these movements will be located at the point of maximum contraction of the muscles that prevent this movement (**Figures 19–25**) [11].

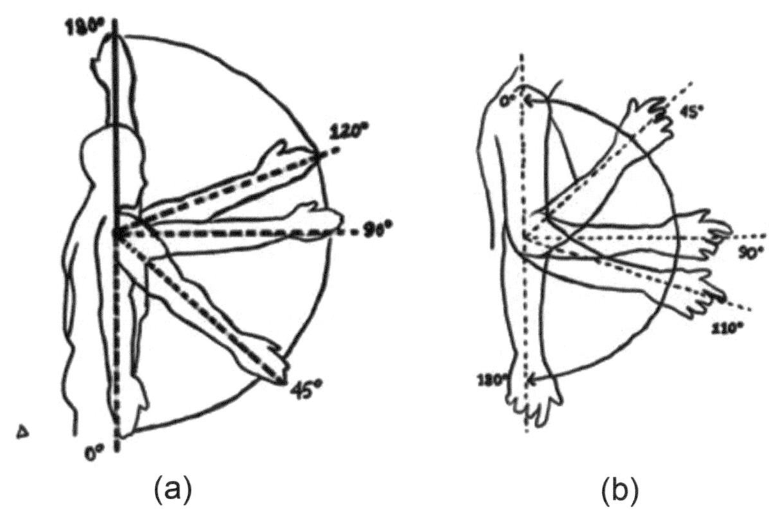

Figure 19.
Measurement of MTS range of motion in the shoulder (a) and elbow (b) joints in typical spasticity patterns.

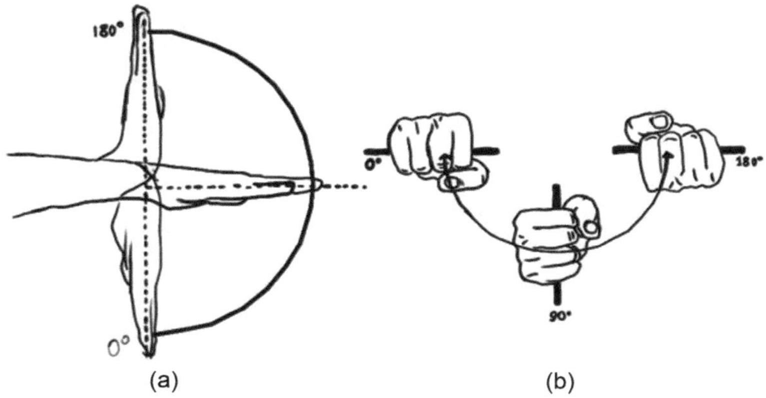

Figure 20.
Measurement of range of motion of MTS in the wrist joint in extension of wrist (a) and supination of the forearm (b) when the typical patterns of spasticity.

Considering the treatment of spasticity as part of the rehabilitation process and, given that the therapeutic effect on spasticity has the ultimate goal of normalizing the life and activities of the patient, Graces recommends the following step-by-step strategy for the use of the tardier scale [33].

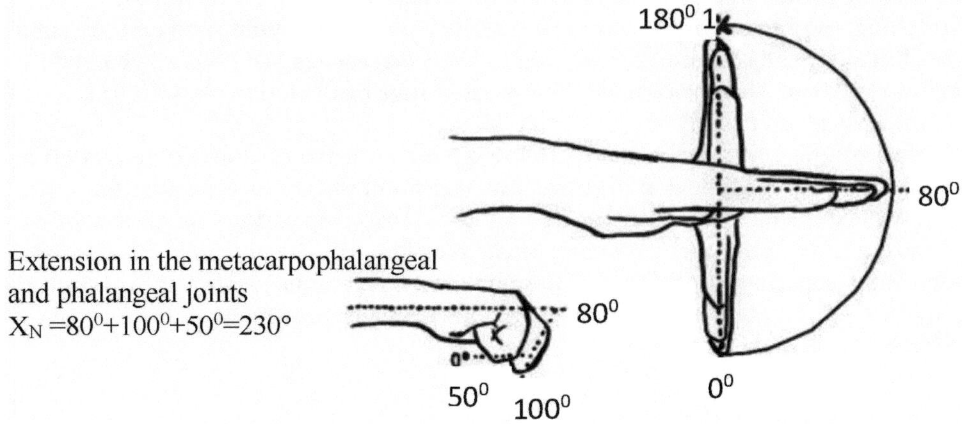

Figure 21.
Measuring the volume of movements by MTS in typical spasticity patterns in the joints of the hand.

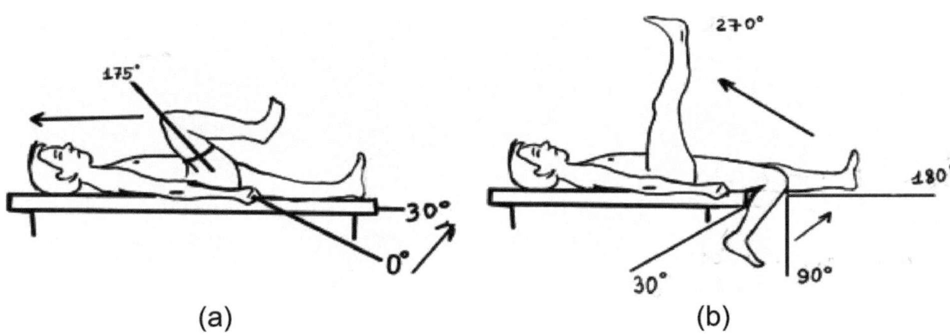

Figure 22.
Measurement of MTS range of motion in the hip and knee joints with gluteus maximus (a) and hamstrings (b) spasticity.

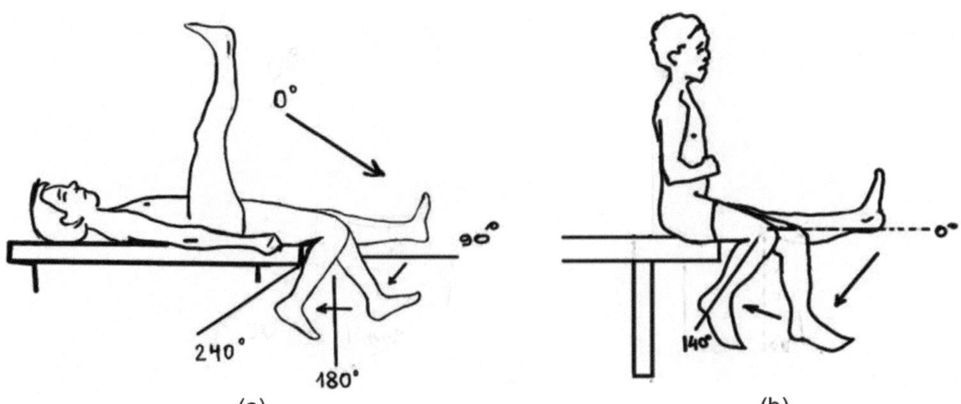

Figure 23.
Measurement of range of motion at the MTS when spasticity in the rectus (a) and lateral vastus, and medial, intermediomedialis et lateralis of m. Quadriceps femoris (b).

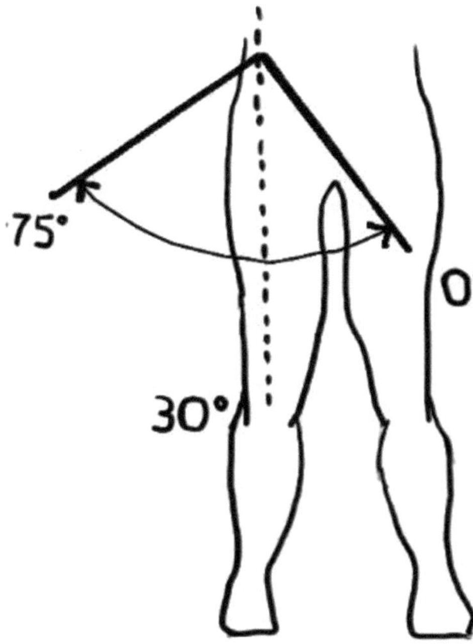

Figure 24.
Measuring the volume of movements by MTS in adductor spasticity.

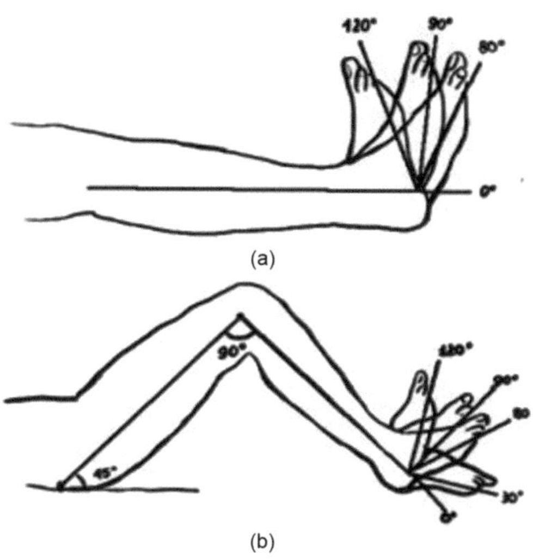

Figure 25.
Measurement of the volume of movements by MTS in the ankle joint with spasticity of Gastrocnemius (a) and Soleus (b).

Step 1: Maximum volume of passive movement (PROM-passive range of motion) in the joint at slow speed, assessment of the degree of muscle shortening (angle arest) = X_{V1}.
Step 2: Passive movement in the joint at fast speed, evaluation of spasticity (Y and/or angle catch) = X_{V3}.
Step 3: Active joint movement, strength score = X_A.
Step 4: Active and rapid movement in the joint for 15 s. With the subsequent angle measurement, assessment of fatigue = X_{A15}.
Step 5: Assessment of limb function and human activity (various activity and participation tests) (LASIS, Frenchay, 10 m walk test, etc.) = F (limb function).

The place and role of MTS in rehabilitation is demonstrated in the following algorithm of rehabilitation approach to patients with spastic paresis (**Figure 26**) [34]. It involves testing the patient, identifying the problem, selecting the rehabilitation goal, developing an intervention plan, and then analyzing the outcome with the selection of the new rehabilitation goal.

It is possible to use MTS in the most limited form. It is enough to measure V1 and V3 and calculate X_S. Registering these three parameters and their changes will

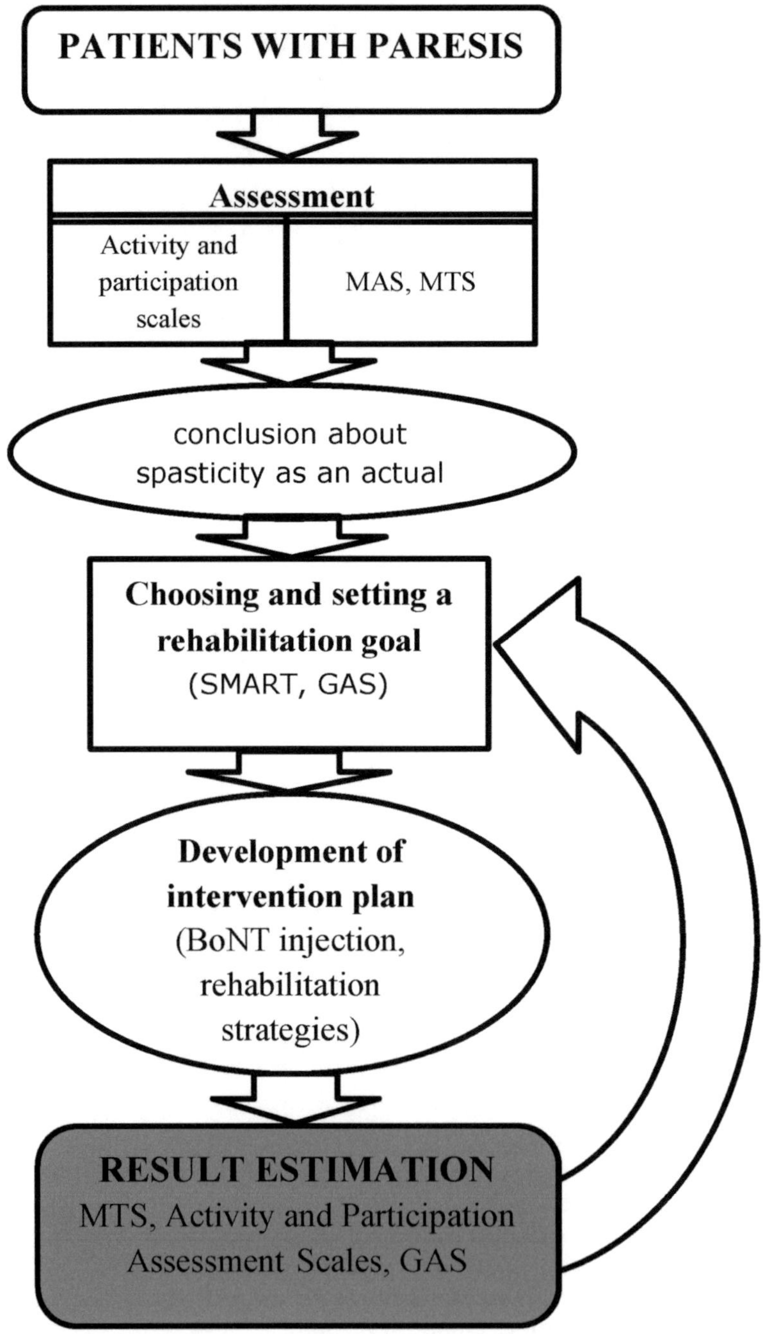

Figure 26.
Algorithm of diagnosis and treatment of a patient with spastic paresis.

allow to sufficiently assess the effectiveness of botulinum therapy and rehabilitation dynamics.

In the treatment of spasticity, the use of MTS allows us to conclude how the introduction of BoNT had an impact on the rehabilitation of the patient. The choice of a specialist drug BoNT for the treatment of spasticity is based on the experience and analysis of many factors, among which one of the most significant is pharmacoeconomics. On average, the duration of various drugs BoNT in patients with spasticity reaches 12–14 weeks [11].

Thus, the stages of application of MTS in the treatment of spasticity BoNT are:

1. testing before injection;

2. testing 3–4 weeks after injection, which demonstrates the effectiveness of BoNT;

3. testing 12–20 weeks after injection of BoNT. Evaluation at this time interval shows the effectiveness of rehabilitation, as well as being a baseline assessment for deciding on the next injection session.

Thus, the modified Tardieu scale (MTS) is convenient for full-scale diagnosis of the main elements of the clinical picture of the central nervous system damage, such as paresis, spasticity, proprioception disorders and allows to qualitatively and quantitatively assess the dynamics of treatment and rehabilitation.

3.2 Activity and participation scales

Spasticity has an extremely negative impact on daily and professional activities, severely restricts independent movement, self-service, reduces the role of the individual in the family and society. The therapeutic effect on spasticity has the ultimate goal of normalizing the life and activity of the patient and with a favorable outcome provides the return to the original standard of living [36].

The Hauser walking index (HAI) and the Rivermead mobility index (RMI) are used to verify self-mobility and self-service violations. Since these scales are not sensitive enough to small changes in mobility, they should be supplemented by a quantitative test to assess walking: distance, time, and independence [36–38].

The concept of self-service includes not only movement but also its assessment should be supplemented by the analysis of the degree of influence of spasticity in the hand on daily activities. The most convenient and informative tool for this analysis is the Leeds scale of influence of spasticity of the hand on the activity (LASIS) [34, 39, 40].

3.2.1 Movement assessment

The Hauser Ambulation Index (HAI) includes the ranking of patients by 10 gradations depending on the need for external assistance, the use of devices for movement, and the time of passing the test distance [34, 36].

Index of Rivermead mobility (Rivermead Mobility Index, RMI) [37, 38]. The value of the mobility index, developed at the Rivermead center, Cambridge University, is the sum of the points: 1 point for each positive response.

The range of values of the scale of the index can vary from 0 points (the inability to perform any of these actions on their own) to 15 points (the ability to run 10 m), which corresponds to normal human mobility. Of particular value for assessing the impact of spasticity on human activity, this test acquires due to the fact that it includes tasks similar to those performed by a person in everyday practice (that is, it has a high "environmental friendliness"). Also, this test can be used to assess the effectiveness of the use of BoNT in relation to the improvement of movement [41].

Walking assessment tests. A common feature of these tests is the lack of assessment of walking quality. Unfortunately, walking quality cannot be reliably assessed without the use of laboratory gait analysis techniques. But it must be borne in mind that it will always be more important for the patient to be able to reach the object he needs safely and quickly than to walk "beautifully." Therefore, the above scales and tests do not lose their relevance in clinical practice, despite the development of instrumental methods for diagnosing walking disorders.

3.2.2 Evaluation of hand productivity

For a quick (less than 10 min) evaluation of the possibility of manipulation (capture, lifting and transfer) objects of different sizes, you must use the "Test with nine pegs" (objects with a diameter of about 1 cm), the test "Box and blocks" (box and Block Test) (cube edge 2.5 cm), the test ARAT (Action Research Arm Test) (manipulation of objects with different sizes, shapes, and weights), Frenchay test (evaluation of functional movements: fixing the ruler, manipulation of objects of different sizes, pinch grip, as well as the ability to touch the top of the head), and Leeds Arm Spasticity Impact Scale (LASIS) [42–45].

This scale was developed at the University of Leeds to measure the effect of spasticity on the functionality and care procedures for paresis of the hand [44]. The daily activities of the patient or the caregiver during the preceding 7 days shall be taken into account.

In each case, the respondent, the patient and/or the caregiver are asked if the action is feasible or not. The difficulty is evaluated on the scale from 0 to 4.

Modified scale Frenchay (Modified Frenchay Test MFS) allows to estimate the functional state of hands. The concept of "functional state" indicates how the sick hand is adapted to everyday life and participates in it [46].

4. Treatment of spasticity

4.1 Methods of injection of BoNT in spasticity

The effectiveness of treatment of spasticity BoNT depends on the accuracy of the introduction into the target muscle and thus is directly related to the skill of a particular specialist and possession of his methods of navigation [47].

4.1.1 Ultrasonic navigation in the treatment of spasticity

Representations of the injection point and depth of the target muscle, based on the knowledge of anatomy, are often incorrect. The location of muscles and bones relatively to each other, their volume is individual, and the presence of vessels and nerves at the injection site is unpredictable. Only 15–20% of individual anatomical structure corresponds to that presented in the relevant atlases. Any pathology, associated with the distortion of movement, exacerbates the differences in the relative position and volume of muscles. Thus, the orientation to the generally accepted anatomical guidelines in the introduction of BoNT makes the treatment of spasticity extremely ineffective. Ultrasound scanning is the main navigation method for BoNT injections in the treatment of spasticity [17].

Ultrasound scanner. To navigate the muscles in botulinum therapy, it is enough to have a black and white ultrasound scanner. The use of the Doppler effect and

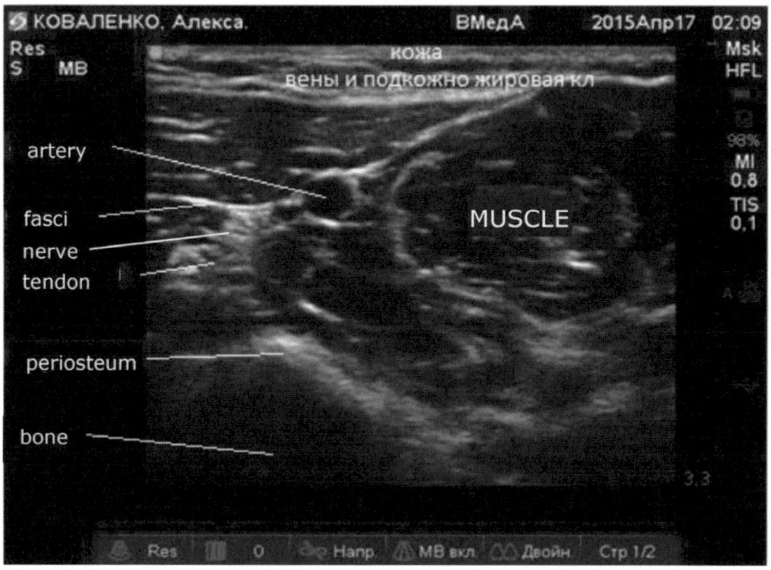

Figure 27.
Indicative ultrasound picture with symbols. Screen view of Edge (FujiFilm SonoSite Inc.'s handheld ultrasound machine).

color staining is effective, but practically not required for work on the limbs and in fact is only necessary for the ultrasound of tissues on the body and neck.

Ultrasonic sensor. Optimal, generally accepted and convenient for muscle visualization is a linear sensor with a width of about 38–50 mm and an operating frequency of 3–16 MHz. Sensors of smaller width narrow the ultrasound picture, thereby reducing the orientation space, some key points fall out of sight. This is especially noticeable when working on large muscle arrays, such as the thigh muscles.

Ultrasound picture of tissues (**Figure 27**).

1. Skin and bones represent the most superficial and deepest layers obtained by ultrasound navigation. Due to their acoustic properties, they tend to be hyperechogenic, that is, look light, bright. Tendons look almost the same.

2. Tendons are hyperechogenic. They have a characteristic fibrillar striated structure in the longitudinal and granular in the transverse section.

3. Arteries and veins. Anechoic (black) tubular structures. Arteries are pulsating and round, veins can be round or oval. A distinctive feature of veins is their easy compression when pressed by the sensor.

4. Muscle tissue is hypoechoic, compared to bones or tendons; its structure is flooded with bright spots. If these points are traced along the muscle, you can see how they come together and form tendons.

5. Nerves. With good resolution, you can see the structure of the nerve. Due to the presence of nerve fibers, its cut is similar to a honeycomb. The nerve, as a rule, is located next to the blood vessel and is considered as part of the neurovascular bundle.

Workplace organization. It is necessary to pay serious attention to the workplace, achieving its convenience, the correct location of the elements necessary for work.

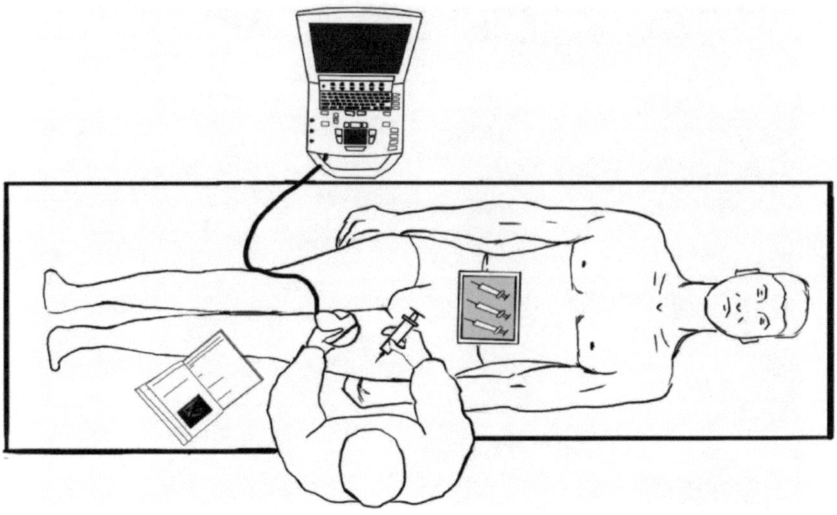

Figure 28.
Example of workplace organization for injection under ultrasound control.

The task of the doctor is not just to locate and verify the muscle, but also to make an injection. It should be borne in mind that the positioning of the limbs may be difficult due to spasticity and disturbance of the patient's consciousness. Picturing the muscles can be distorted by muscle contraction, etc. Therefore, it is preferable to use portable ultrasound scanner that allows you to easily move the machine around the patient. The most convenient location of the patient is between the doctor and the screen, the doctor does not have to turn around in order to study the ultrasound picture, and he can place all the necessary tools directly in front of him/her (**Figure 28**).

4.1.2 Operating procedure on the ultrasound machine

Pairing and orientation of ultrasound image and sensor. Coordination of needle and sensor movements, verification of the resulting image and orientation in the tissues of the body are developed over time. With the necessary experience, no problems in the orientation of the image will arise. For beginners, determining the coincidence of the sides of the sensor and the image on the monitor is an elementary but mandatory rule to get started. To do this, different simple methods are used: palpation of tissues, tapping on the edge of the working surface of the sensor, and positioning the label on the basis of the sensor.

Work with instrument settings. The skill of working with the parameters of the device also plays an important role. If for examining of some muscles (quadriceps femoris), special settings are not required, and then when scanning some other – the quality of the settings can affect the effectiveness of the injection. Additional image adjustment may require the location of the long extensors of the thumb and toes, the posterior tibial muscle, as well as the study of the muscles of the foot.

There are several basic settings for ultrasound imaging. Depending on the instrument, adjustments can be made manually or partially automatically.

The main adjustment parameters include:

1. Imaging modes:

- B-mode – the main imaging mode in which anatomical tissues and organs are displayed in real time.

- Musculoskeletal (Msk) mode, optimal for muscle examination.

2. Depth in most cases, the optimal depth is greater than the depth at which the target muscle is located. This is because when scanning, it is necessary to focus on the surrounding markers—vessel, bone, tendon, etc. for examination of the upper limbs in adults; the average depth are the following:

    - Muscles of the shoulder girdle-up to 4 cm.
    - Shoulder muscles-up to 4–6 cm.
    - Upper third of the forearm 3.3–4 cm.
    - The middle and lower third of the forearm-3.3 cm.
    - Muscles of the hand-up to 2 cm.

3. Frequency (frequency/THI) – the wave frequency is directly related to the ability to penetrate into tissue. It should be remembered that the higher the frequency, the faster the tissue absorption and shallower penetration of the signal, the lower the frequency, the greater the signal immersion. On average, the optimal frequency for the muscles of the shoulder girdle, shoulder, and forearm is 7–8 MHz, for the muscles of the hand from 10 MHz.

4. Focus (focus). Focus on a specific object from the overall scan pattern, allowing for higher contrast and resolution of the object.

5. Brightness (gain). This is the ability to amplify all signals from the entire image. It is perceived as the increased brightness of the picture. It should be noted that with excessive amplification, tissue boundaries may be fuzzy and interference may occur.

In addition to the basic adjustments, there are additional ones that can be used to change the power of the ultrasonic wave, improve the quality and overview of the image, change its profile, remove image interference, etc.

4.1.3 Types and methods of needle insertion under ultrasound control

1. Way to № 1. Transversely to the ultrasound beam.

    The needle is inserted at an angle to the plane of the sensor and, accordingly, transversely to the plane of the ultrasonic beam. The thickness of the ultrasound beam is 2–3 mm. Therefore, when moving the needle, the researcher sees only the displacement of tissues from it and only that part of it, or the slice that passed through the beam (**Figure 29**). This method, despite the limitations of needle visibility, is convenient, easy to learn and most often used in practice.

2. Way to № 2. In the plane of the ultrasonic beam (longitudinally). Introduction of the needle from the end of the working surface of the sensor at an angle. In this case, the entire needle is in the plane of the beam and is fully visible (**Figure 30**).

    This method has some limitations: even a slight change in the angle of the sensor relatively to the skin or its displacement leads to the loss of the needle from the plane of the beam and, accordingly, its image on the screen. In addition, it creates the need for the passage of the needle through the adjacent muscles and other formations.

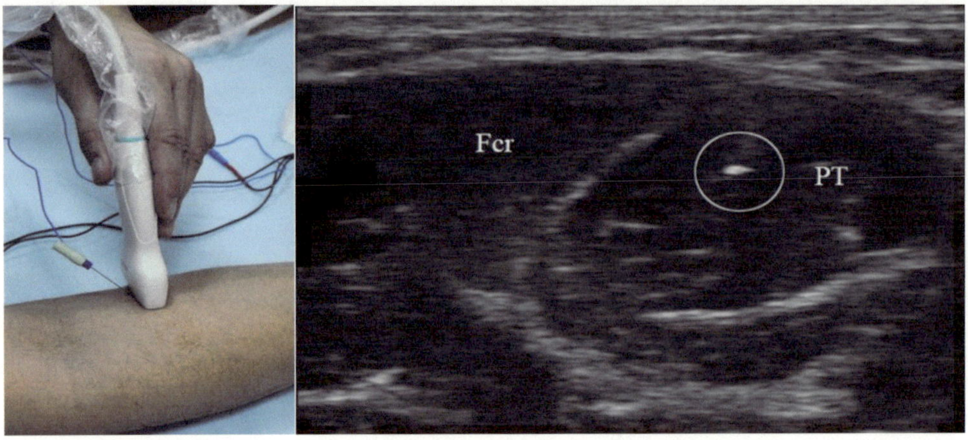

Figure 29.
Relative positions of the needle and the sensor introduction in a transverse slice of the needle as a point in the round pronator.

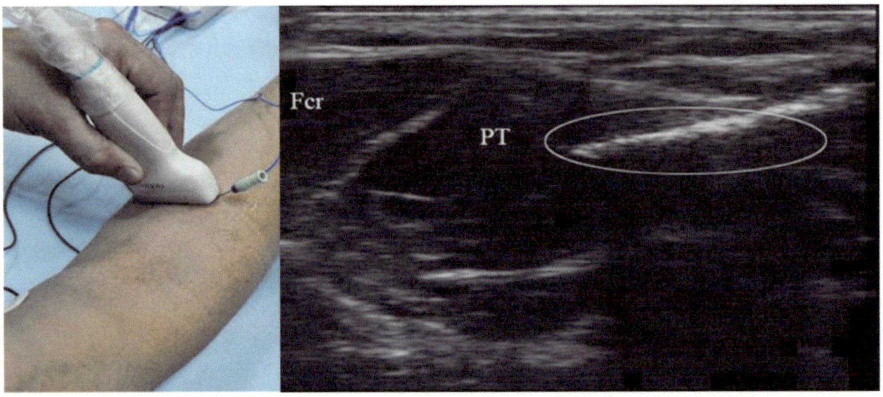

Figure 30.
The relative position of the needle and sensor in the longitudinal introduction and the needle along the ultrasound beam in a circular pronator.

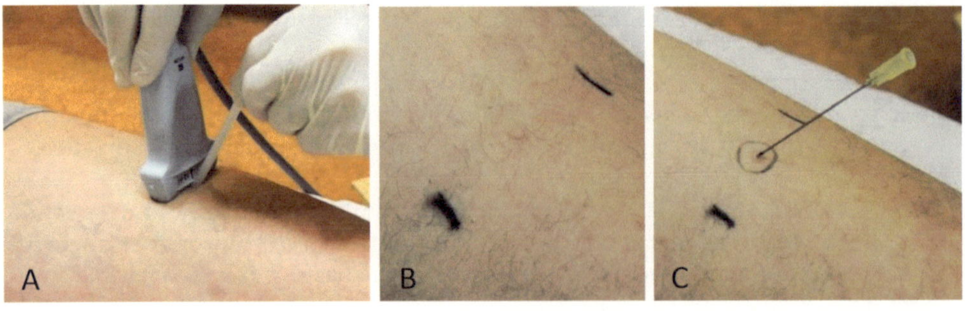

Figure 31.
(A) Tissue marking, (B) needle cap pressure mark on skin, and (C) inserting the needle into the center of the marking.

3. Way to № 3. Needle insertion after ultrasound control.

 In a situation where it is impossible to simultaneously hold the sensor and insert the needle into the tissue, you can use the following method:

 Determine the sensor object and depth of injection. Without removing the sensor, put a mark on the edge of the sensor. It is very convenient to use a sterile tip of the cap from the injection needle as a marker (**Figure 31A**). When you press the cap, a clear imprint in the form of a circle remains on the skin (**Figure 31B**). The needle is inserted into the circle on the skin to a measured depth (**Figure 31C**).

Tissue traction. Sometimes, for various reasons, it is impossible to get a full image of the needle on the screen of the ultrasound machine. In this case, you should focus on the tissue traction that occurs when the needle passes. This effect can be enhanced by light oscillating movements of the needle. This technique allows with a certain degree of error to understand at what depth and in what place on the screen the end of the needle is.

Aseptica. Introduction of drugs under ultrasound control requires compliance with the rules of asepsis. To do this, there are several different methods of treatment and protection: sterile gloves for the performer, sterile covers for the sensor, sterilizer for the sensor, sterile gel, aseptic solutions for the sensor, and the patient's skin.

For practical execution of the procedure, the scanner sensor can be protected by a sterile disposable cover, which has an adhesive base inside for fixing to the working part of the sensor. The adhesive base itself in this case also replaces the gel for ultrasound. Sterile cover can be replaced with a sterile glove, and instead of the adhesive base, you can use usual gel, which is applied to the working part of the sensor and the inner surface of the glove. Fixation of the glove on the handle of the sensor is performed using a patch (**Figure 32**).

Gel. Sterile ultrasonic gel is used for invasive manipulations under ultrasound control. Release form is sachets of 15 g, so when conducting the therapy even on one limb, you must have a few packages.

Treatment of the injection field. The patient's skin should be treated with a solution of 0.015% chlorhexidine.

Sensor processing. Treatment of the sensor with alcohol is undesirable. This causes damage to the rubber coating of the work surface and premature failure of the sensor. To sterilize the sensor, special solutions of the Sani-Cloth series are used and chlorhexidine can be used.

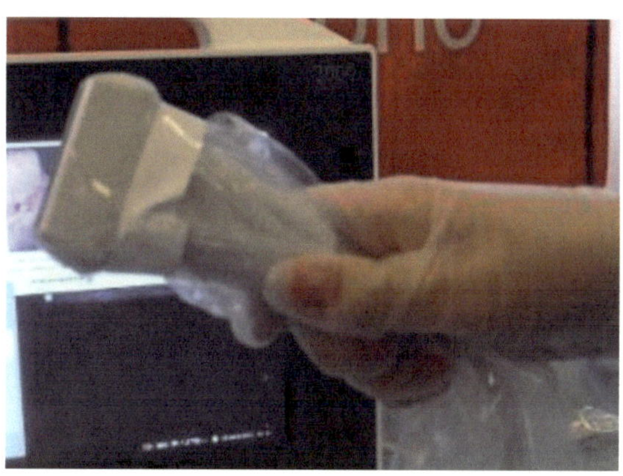

Figure 32.
Sensor in sterile case.

4.1.4 Methods of administration of BoNT in the intramuscular motor endpoint

Neuromuscular transmission is carried out by axon terminals in limited areas of intramuscular motor endpoint (IME). Accurate introduction to IME makes botulinum therapy more effective. The distribution of IME in the left and right limbs is identical; it does not depend on gender and age. The number of muscle motor points depends on the complexity of its functions and does not depend on its mass [47].

After finding a muscle using ultrasound navigation to orient the IME projection of the corresponding muscles on the human body, use the location map or find them using electroneuromyography (EMG). A cutaneous bipolar stimulating electrode is used to search for muscle IME. The study is carried out at a current strength of 5–10 mA and a frequency of 2 Hz [47–49]. The use of location maps in combination with ultrasound navigation significantly increases the effectiveness of treatment (**Figures 33–40**) [47].

4.1.4.1 Complex treatment of spasticity

Given the timing of the development of spasticity and the risk of complications, which in the future significantly reduces the effectiveness of rehabilitation and increases the cost of treatment, treatment of spasticity should be started when just its first signs appear. The period requiring special attention for early diagnosis and treatment is between 3 and 12 weeks after brain damage. In severe paresis, the period of occurrence of spasticity may coincide with the first signs of muscle strength and purposeful movement [50, 51].

Basically, all the drugs BoNT produced in the world are standardized to the 100-unit equivalent of Botox. The only drug that stands out from this series is Dysport. All drugs, except for Dysport, are similar in dosage of introduction to the relevant muscles and multiples of 100 Units. The drug Dysport is 500-unit drug and is

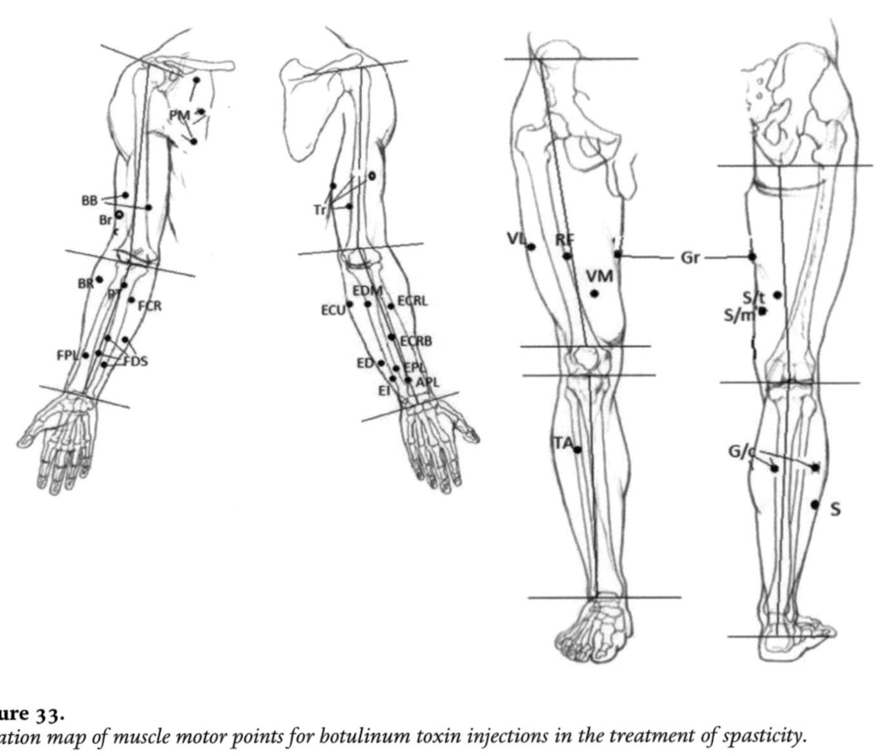

Figure 33.
Location map of muscle motor points for botulinum toxin injections in the treatment of spasticity.

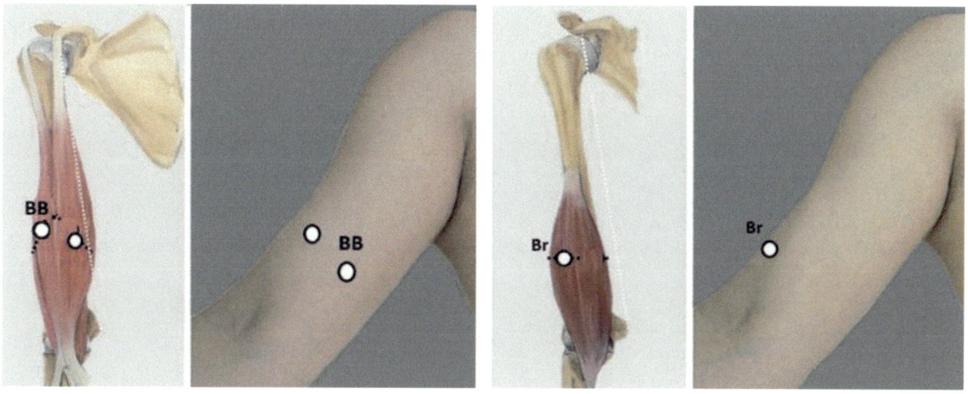

Figure 34.
Image of anatomy m. Biceps brachii (BB) and m. Brachialis (Br) and projections of their IME on the surface of the body.

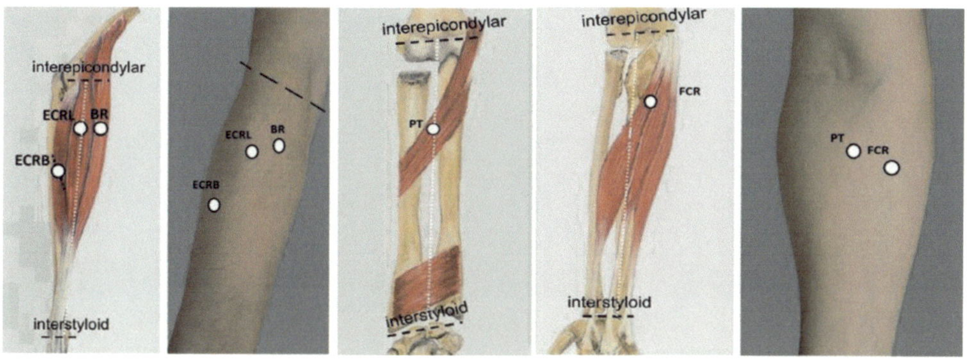

Figure 35.
Image of anatomy of m. Brachioradialis (BR), Extensor carpi radialis longus (ECRL), Extensor carpi radialis brevis (ECRB), Flexor carpi radialis (FCR), m. Pronator teres (PT), and projections of their IME on the surface of the body.

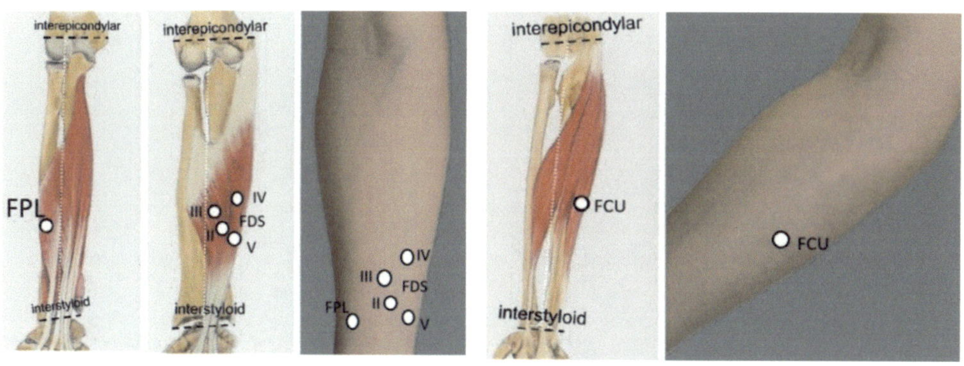

Figure 36.
Image of anatomy of m. Flexor pollicis longus (FPL), m. Flexor digitorum superficialis (FDS), m. Flexor carpi ulnaris (FCU), and projections of their IME on the surface of the body.

significantly different from the 100 individual drugs, dosage of the injection in the muscle (**Tables 2** and **3**) [7, 50–54].

To optimize the calculation of drug consumption and prognosis of needs, it is advisable to use models of patients based on the frequency of participation in the

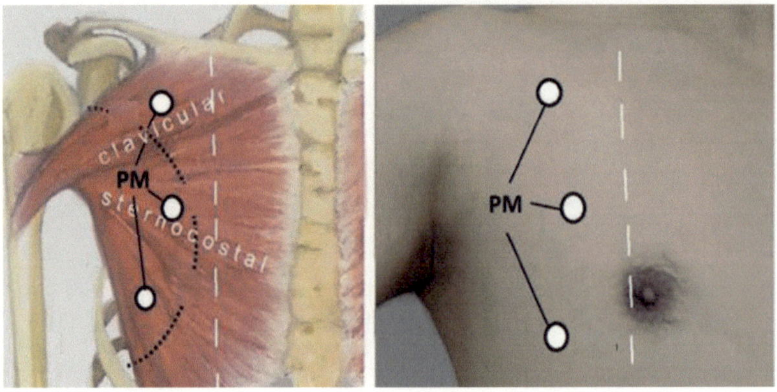

Figure 37.
Image of anatomy m. Pectoralis major (PM) and projections of their IME on the surface of the body.

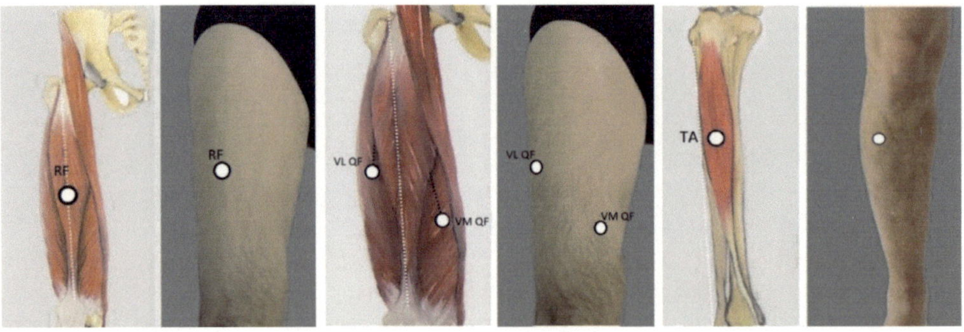

Figure 38.
Image of anatomy mm. Vastus lateralis (VL), Vastus medialis (VM), m. Rectus femoris (RF), m. Tibialis anterior (TA), and projections of their IME on the surface of the body.

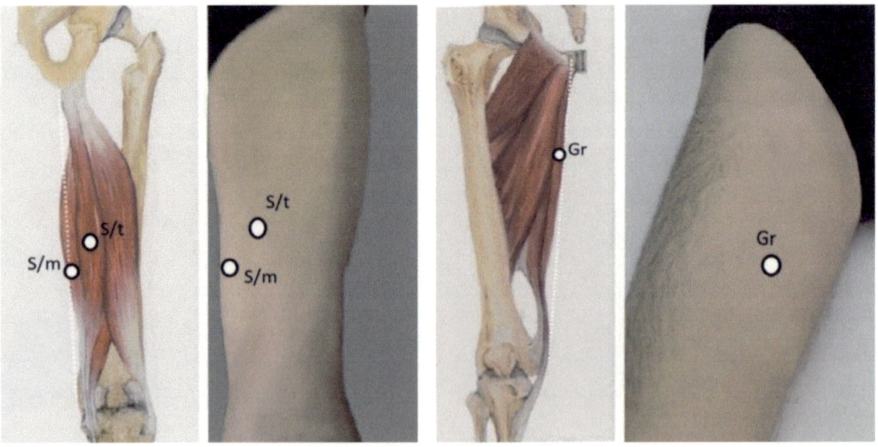

Figure 39.
Image of the anatomy of m. Semimembranosus (S/m), m. Semitendinosus (S/t) m. Gracilis (Gr), and projections of their IME on the surface of the body.

formation of a pattern of specific muscles (**Tables 2** and **3**). The use of these models allows you to accurately determine the required amount of the drug and the cost of treatment of spasticity.

DOI: http://dx.doi.org/10.5772/intechopen.91046

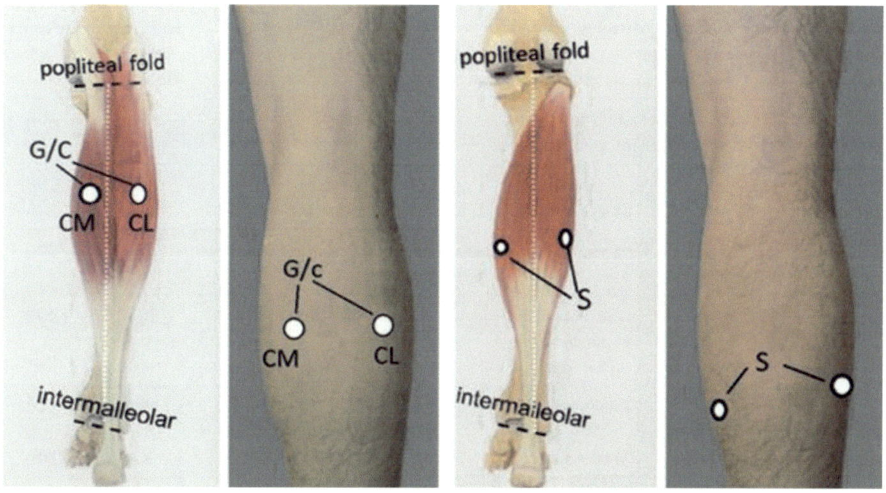

Figure 40.
Image of anatomy mm. Gastrocnemius (G/c), Soleus (S), and projections of their IME on the surface of the body.

Model	Pattern of spasticity	Muscles		100 Units of the BoNT, U	Dysport, U
1A	Flexion of the wrist, fingers and thumb	Flexor digitorum superfacialis		60	200
		Flexor digitorum profundus		60	200
		Flexor pollicis longus		20	60
				140	**460**
2A	Flexion of the wrist, fingers and thumb	Flexor digitorum superfacialis		60	200
		Flexor digitorum profundus		60	200
		Flexor pollicis longus		20	60
	Pronation of the forearm	Flexor carpi radialis	*Sometimes one of two*	60	200
		Pronator teres		30	80
				230	**740**
3A	Flexion of the wrist, fingers and thumb	Flexor digitorum superfacialis		60	200
		Flexor digitorum profundus		60	200
		Flexor pollicis longus		20	60
	Pronation of the forearm	Flexor carpi radialis	*Sometimes one of two*	60	200
		Pronator teres		30	80
	Elbow flexion	Brachialis	*More often one-two from three*	80	300
		Brachioradialis	*(BB less often than others)*	100	400
		Biceps brachii (BB)		100	400
		Very rarely are all muscles involved, so most often the average dosage		**410**	**1600**
4A	Flexion of the wrist, fingers and thumb	Flexor digitorum superfacialis		60	200
		Flexor digitorum profundus		60	200
		Flexor pollicis longus		20	60
	Pronation of the forearm	Flexor carpi radialis	*Sometimes one of two*	60	200
		Pronator teres		30	80
	Elbow flexion	Brachialis	*More often one-two from three*	80	300
		Brachioradialis	*(BB less often than others)*	100	400
		Biceps brachii (BB)		100	400
	Impossibility of shoulder retraction and arm extension	Pectoralis major		100	400
		Very rarely are all muscles involved, so most often the average dosage		**530**	**1600**

Table 2.
Models of patients with spasticity in the upper limb.

Model	Pattern of spasticity	Muscles		100 Units of the BoNT, U	Dysport, U
1L	Dynamic	Semitendinosus Semimembranosus	*Almost always*	80 100	300 400
		Gracilis Biceps femoris	*Often* *Very rarely*	80 140	200 500
		Very rarely are all muscles involved, so most often the average dosage		**250**	**800**
2L	Static	Gastrocnemius caput mediale (G/c c.m.)	*Almost always*	100	400
		Tibialis posterior Soleus Tibialis anterior	*Most often one of the muscles in combination with G/c c. m.*	100 80 80	400 300 300
		Very rarely are all muscles involved, so most often the average dosage		**200**	**700**
3L	Dynamic + Static	Semitendinosus Semimembranosus	*Almost always*	80 100	300 400
		Gracilis Biceps femoris	*Often* *Very rarely*	80 140	200 500
		Gastrocnemius caput mediale (G/c c.m.) Tibialis posterior Soleus Tibialis anterior	*Almost always* *Most often one of the muscles in combination with G/c c. m.*	100 100 80 80	400 400 300 300
		All muscles are never involved, so the average dosage is		**450**	**1500**
4L	Static + Flexion of fingers and big toe	Gastrocnemius caput mediale (G/c c.m.) Tibialis posterior Soleus Tibialis anterior	*Almost always* *Most often one of the muscles in combination with G/c c. m.*	100 100 80 80	400 400 300 300
		Flexor digitorum longus (FDL) Flexor halucis longus (FHL) Flexor digitorum brevis (FDB) Flexor halucis brevis (FHB)	*FDL and FHL are more common than FDB and FHL, and FDL is more common than FHL.* *A rare combination of long and short flexors of the fingers.*	40 40 100 30	140 140 400 100
		All muscles are never involved, so the average dosage is		**300**	**1000**
5L	Dinamic+ Static + Flexion of fingers and big toe	Semitendinosus Semimembranosus	*Almost always*	80 100	300 400
		Gracilis Biceps femoris	*Often* *Very rarely*	80 140	200 500
		Gastrocnemius caput mediale (G/c c.m.) Tibialis posterior Soleus Tibialis anterior	*Almost always* *Most often one of the muscles in combination with G/c c. m.*	100 100 80 80	400 400 300 300

DOI: http://dx.doi.org/10.5772/intechopen.91046

Model	Pattern of spasticity	Muscles		100 Units of the BoNT, U	Dysport, U
		Flexor digitorum longus (FDL) Flexor halucis longus (FHL) Flexor digitorum brevis Flexor halucis brevis	*FDL and FHL are more common than FDB and FHL, and FDL is more common than FHL.* *A rare combination of long and short flexors of the fingers.*	40 40 100 30	140 140 400 100
		All muscles are never involved, so the average dosage is		**500**	**1500**

Table 3.
Models of patients with spasticity in the low limb.

The treatment scheme of spasticity with the complex use of peripheral muscle relaxants (BoNT) and central muscle relaxants (baclofen) action may also be effective. Baclofen should be prescribed 25 ± 3 days after the introduction of BoNT. This treatment scheme provides a sufficient clinical effect for 110 ± 10 days after the injection session, which is 14–25 days longer than the action of BoNT in monotherapy. With an average spasticity treatment time of 2 years, this combination reduces the number of injection sessions from 7 to 5.

Author details

Alexander Kovalenko[1,2*], Viktor Misikov[3], Konstantin Sinelnikov[4], Valeriy Shamigulov[5], Dmitrii Iskra[1,6], Svetlana E. Khatkova[7] and Denis V. Kovlen[8]

1 Department and Clinic of Neurological Diseases, Medical Military Academy, Saint-Petersburg, Russia

2 Department of Adult Neuro-Rehabilitation, Adult Botulinum Toxin Center, Russia

3 Department and Clinic of Neurology, Moscow Regional Research and Clinical Institute n.a. M.F. Vladimirsky, Moscow, Russia

4 Pokrovskaya City Hospital, Saint-Petersburg, Russia

5 Medical Military Academy, Saint-Petersburg, Russia

6 Northwestern Association for the Study of Pain, Russia

7 Federal State Hospital for Treatment and Rehabilitation Ministry of Health Russia, Moscow, Russia

8 Medical-Military Academy n.a. S.M. Kirov, Saint-Petersburg, Russia

*Address all correspondence to: kvlnko73@gmail.com

References

[1] Lance J. The control of muscle tone, reflexes, and movement: Robert Wartenberg Lecture. Neurology. 1980; **30**(12):1303-1313

[2] Bhadra N. Neuroprostheses for spasticity control. In: Kilgore K, editor. Implantable Neuroprostheses for Restoring Function. Cambridge: Elsevier; 2015. 331 pp

[3] Ertzgaard P, Anhammer M, Forsmark A. Regional disparities in botulinum toxin A (BoNT-A) therapy for spasticity in Sweden: Budgetary consequences of closing the estimated treatment gap. Acta Neurologica Scandinavica. 2017;**135**(3):366-372. DOI: 10.1111/ane.12610

[4] Zorowitz R, Gillard P, Brainin M. Poststroke spasticity: Sequelae and burden on stroke survivors and caregivers. Neurology. 2013;**80**:45-52. DOI: 10.1212/WNL.0b013e3182764c86

[5] Maynard F, Karunas R, Waring W. Epidemiology of spasticity following traumatic spinal cord injury. Archives of Physical Medicine and Rehabilitation. 1990;**71**(8):566-569

[6] Rizzo M, Hadjimichael O, Preiningerova J, Vollmer T. Prevalence and treatment of spasticity reported by multiple sclerosis patients. Multiple Sclerosis. 2004;**10**(5):589-595. DOI: 10.1191/1352458504ms1085oa

[7] Iskra DA, Kovalenko AP, Koshkarev MA, Dyskin DE. Spasticity: From pathophysiology to treatment. Zhurnal Nevrologii i Psikhiatrii Imeni S.S. Korsakova. 2018;**118**(10):108-114. (in Russ.). DOI: 10.17116/jnevro201811 8101108

[8] Kovalenko AP. Pathophysiology of spastic paresis. The "incomplete movement" hypothesis. Vestnik Russian Voenno-medicinskoy Academy. 2019;**4**(68):235-239 (in Russ.). ISSN: 1682-73924

[9] Foust A, Popovic M, Zecevic D, McCormick DA. Action potentials initiate in the axon initial segment and propagate through axon collaterals reliably in cerebellar Purkinje neurons. Journal of Neuroscience. 2010;**30**(20): 6891-6902. DOI: 10.1523/ JNEUROSCI.0552-10.2010

[10] Khatkova SE, Orlova OR, Botsina AY, et al. The basic principles of managing the patients with impaired tone after focal brain damage. Consilium Medicum. 2016;**18**(2.1):25-33. Available from: https://con-med.ru/magazines/consilium_medicum/consilium_medicum-02.1-2016

[11] Kovalenko AP, Misikov VK, Iskra DA, Koshkarev MA, Sinelnikov KA. Tardue scales in the diagnostic of patients with spasticity. Zhurnal nevrologii i psikhiatrii imeni S.S. Korsakova. 2019;**119**(9):83-90 (in Russ.). DOI: 10.17116/jnevro20191 1909183

[12] Delgado MR et al. Abobotulinumtoxin A for equinus foot deformity in cerebral palsy: A randomized controlled trial. Pediatrics. 2016;**137**(2):e20152830

[13] Brashear A, Elovic E. Spasticity: Diagnosis and Management. 2nd ed. New York: Demos Medical Publishing; 2016. 139 pp. ISBN 978-1-62070-072-3; ISBN 978-1-61705-242-2 (e-book)

[14] Royal College of Physicians, British Society of Rehabilitation Medicine, Chartered Society of Physiotherapy, Association of Chartered Physiotherapists Interested in Neurology. Spasticity in adults: Management using botulinum toxin. In: National Guidelines. London: RCP; 2009

[15] Dietz V. Spastic movement disorder. Spinal Cord. 2000;**38**(7):389-393

[16] Aluru V, Lu Y, Leung A, Verghese J, Raghavan P. Effect of auditory constraints on motor learning depends on stage of recovery post stroke. Frontiers in Neurology. 2014;**23**(5):106. DOI: 10.3389/fneur.2014.00106

[17] Kovalenko AP, Misikov VK. Atlas of ultrasound imaging of muscles for botulinum toxin therapy. In: Spasticity. Diagnostic and treatment. Methodological Guidance. M: St-Spb.; 2020. 264 pp. ISBN: 978-5-9909968-0-9

[18] Hefter H, Jost WH, Reissig A, Zakine B, Bakheit AM, Wissel J. Classification of posture in poststroke upper limb spasticity: A potential decision tool for botulinum toxin A treatment. International Journal of Rehabil Research. 2012;**35**(3):227-233. DOI: 10.1097/MRR.0b013e328353e3d4

[19] Khat'kova SE, Akulov MA, Orlova OR, Usachev DY, Orlova AS, Krylova LV. Botulinum toxin treatment of lower extremity spasticity. Nervno-mishechnie Bolezni. 2017;7:27-35 (in Russ.). DOI: 10.17650/2222-8721-2017-7-3-21-35

[20] Bernstein NA. Essays on Physiology of Movements and Physiology of Activity. M.: Science; 1990. 496 pp. ISBN: 5020052345

[21] Granit R. The Basis of Motor Control. London: Academic Press; 1970 368 pp

[22] Sukhanov VB. General System of Symmetric Locomotion of Terrestrial Vertebrates and Peculiarities of Movement of Lower Tetrapods. L.: Science; 1968. 225 pp

[23] Janson HA. Biomechanics of the Lower Limb of Man. Riga: Zinatne; 1975 324 pp

[24] Zajac FE, Neptune RR, Kautz SA. Biomechanics and muscle coordination of human walking. Part I: Introduction to concepts, power transfer, dynamics and simulations. Gait Posture. 2002; **16**(3):215-232

[25] Zajac FE, Neptune RR, Kautz SA. Biomechanics and muscle coordination of human walking: Part II: Lessons from dynamical simulations and clinical implications. Gait Posture. 2003; **17**(1):1-17

[26] Simeonidis P. The silverskiold test. Foot Ankle International. 2014;**35**(8): 838. DOI: 10.1177/1071100714535202

[27] Van der Ploeg RJ, Oosterhuis HJ, Reuvecamp J. Measuring muscle sleight. Journal of Neurology. 1984;**231**:200-203

[28] Bohanon R, Smith V. Interrater reliability of a modified Ashworth scale if muscle spasticity. Physical Therapy. 1987;**67**:206-207

[29] Mehrholz J, Wagner K, Meissner D, Grundmann K, Zange C, Koch R, et al. Reliability of the Modified Tardieu Scale and the Modified Ashworth Scale in adult patients with severe brain injury: A comparison study. Clinical Rehabilitation. 2005;**19**:751-759. DOI: 10.1017/CBO9780511995590

[30] Tardieu G, Tardieu C, Colbeau-Justin P, Bret M. Effects of muscle length on an increased stretch reflex in children with cerebral palsy. Journal of Neurology, Neurosurgery and Psychiatry. 1982;**45**(4):348-352

[31] Mackey AH, Walt SE, Lobb G, Stott NS. Intraobserver reliability of the modified Tardieu scale in the upper limb of children with hemiplegia. Developmental Medicine and Child Neurology. 2004;**46**(4):267-272

[32] Gracies J-M, Marosszeky JE, Renton R, Sandanam J, Gandevia SC, Burke D. Short-term effects of dynamic lycra

splints on upper limb in hemiplegic patients. Archives of Physical Medicine and Rehabilitation. 2000;**81**(12):1547-1555. DOI: 10.1053/apmr.2000.16346

[33] Gracies J-M, Bayle N, Vinti M, Alkandari S, Vu P, Loche CM, et al. Five-step clinical assessment in spastic paresis. European Journal of Physical Rehabilitation. 2010;**46**(3):411-421

[34] Kovalenko AP, Kamaeva OV, Misikov VK, Poleshchuk YR, Koshkarev MA. Scales and tests in the rehabilitation and treatment of patients with spasticity of the lower limbs. Zhurnal Nevrologii i Psikhiatrii Imeni S.S. Korsakova. 2018; **118**(5):120-128 (in Russ.). DOI: 10.17116/jneuro201811851120

[35] Kovalenko AP, Misikov VK. Botulinum toxin treatment of patients with brain damage coused lower limb spasticity. Zhurnal Nevrologii i Psikhiatrii Imeni S.S. Korsakova. 2018; **118**(9):28-34. (in Russ.). DOI: 10.17116/jnevro201811809128

[36] Wade DT. Measurement in Neurological Rehabilitation. Oxford University Press; 1992. 200 pp

[37] Collin FM, Wade DT, Robb GF, Bradshaw CM. The Rivermead Mobility Index a further development of Rivermead Motor Assessment. International Disability Studies. 1991;**13**. DOI: 10.3109/03790799109166684

[38] Belova AN. Neurorehabilitation: A Guide for Doctors. M.: The Antidoron; 2000. 736 c

[39] Levin MF, Kleim JA, Wolf SL. What do motor "recovery" and "compensation" mean in patients following stroke? Neurorehabilitation and Neural Repair. 2009;**23**(4):313-319. DOI: 10.1177/1545968308328727

[40] Kwakkel G, Kollen B, Lindeman E. Understanding the pattern of functional recovery after stroke: facts and theories. Restorative Neurology and Neuroscience. 2004;**22**(3-5):281-299

[41] Page SJ, Gater DR, Bach YRP. Reconsidering the motor recovery plateau in stroke rehabilitation. Archives of Physical Medicine and Rehabilitation. 2004;**85**(8):1377-1381. DOI: 10.1016/j.apmr.2003.12.031

[42] Rehab Measures: Box and Block Test. Available from: www.rehabmeasures.org. Rehabilitation Institute of Chicago. Archived from the original on 2 May 2016. [Accessed: 16 June 2016]

[43] Action Research Arm Test. Internet Stroke Center. 2018. Available from: http://www.strokecenter.org/wp-content/uploads/2011/08/action_research_arm_test.pdf

[44] Royal College of Physicians, British Society of Rehabilitation Medicine, Chartered Society of Physiotherapy, Association of Chartered Physiotherapists Interested in Neurology. Spasticity in adults: Management using botulinum toxin. In: National Guidelines. London: RCP; 2009. p. 72

[45] Ashford S, Slade M, Nair A, Turner-Stokes L. Arm activity measure (ArmA) application for recording functional gain following focal spasticity treatment. International Journal of Therapy and Rehabilitation. 2015;**21**(1):10-17

[46] Baude M, Mardale V, Loche C-M, Hutin E, Gracies J-M, Bayle N. Intra- and interrater reliability of the Modified Frenchay Scale to measure active upper limb function in hemiparetic patients. Annals of Physical and Rehabilitation Medicine. 2016;**59s**:e59-e60

[47] Kovalenko AP, Misikov VK, Sinelnikov KA, Karimov AN. Mapping of motor-points in the flexor muscles of the arm for the optimization of botulinum toxin injections in treatment of spasticity. Zhurnal Nevrologii i

Psikhiatrii Imeni S.S. Korsakova. 2017; **117**(7):47-52. DOI: 10.17116/jnevro20171177147-52

[48] Sinelnikov RD. Atlas of Human Anatomy. Vol. 1. Moscow; 1978. 472 pp

[49] Shevkunenko VN. Short Course of Operative Surgery with Topographic Anatomy. Leningrad; 1947. 567 pp

[50] Borg J, Ward AB, Wissel J, et al. Rationale and design of a multicentre, double-blind, prospective, randomized, European and Canadian study: Evaluating patient outcomes and costs of managing adults with post-stroke focal spasticity. Journal of Rehabilitation Medicine. 2011;**43**(1):15-22. DOI: 110.2340/16501977-0663

[51] Dashtipour K, Chen JJ, Walker HW, Lee MY. Systematic literature review of Abobotulinumtoxin A in clinical trials for lower limb spasticity. Medicine (Baltimore). 2016;**95**(2):e2468. DOI: 110.1097/MD.0000000000002468

[52] Misikov VK. The preparations of Botulinum toxin type A in the treatment of lower limb post-stroke spasticity. Clinical Observation. 2014;**3**:49-51. DOI: 10.17650/2222-8721-2014-0-3-49-51

[53] Gracies J-M, Esquenazi A, Brashear A, Banach M, Kocer S, Jech R, et al. Efficacy and safety of abobotulinumtoxin A in spastic lower limb. 2017. DOI: 10.1212/WNL.0000000000004687

[54] Wissel J, Ward AB, Erztgaard P, Bensmail D, Hecht MJ, Lejeune TM, et al. European consensus table on the use of botulinum toxin type A in adult spasticity. Journal of Rehabilitation Medicine. 2009;**41**(1):13-25. DOI: 10.2340/16501977-0303

Chapter 5

Rehabilitation Medicine Management of Spasticity

Seyed Mansoor Rayegani, Marzieh Babaee and Seyed Ahmad Raeissadat

Abstract

Spasticity is a poorly recognized but common symptom, present in a wide range of neurological conditions. It can have a major impact on those affected, much of which is potentially preventable. This chapter provides an excellent paradigm to incorporate many of the key elements fundamental to the management of chronic conditions and it is of relevance to those who work in spasticity rehabilitation.

Keywords: spasticity, rehabilitation, orthoses, drug, physiotherapy, occupational therapy

1. Introduction

Spasticity is one of the common symptoms in a wide range of neurological conditions, and it needs multidisciplinary approach for best management. This chapter provides an excellent paradigm to incorporate many of the key elements fundamental to the management of chronic conditions and it is of relevance to those who work in spasticity rehabilitation. This chapter presents a comprehensive view about rehabilitation with these subtitles:

- Assessment of the individual with spasticity
- Provision of education and promoting self-management
- Physical management of spasticity(physiotherapy or occupational therapy)
- Orthoses
- Pharmacological intervention
- Setting up a service

2. Assessment of the individual with spasticity

Accurate assessment of spasticity is the starting point to make a proper and valuable plan for this route. In addition to assessing physical changes, resistance to movement, weakness, and contractures, the impact of spasticity on the activities of daily life should be considered as well. These assessments should also be carried out in the follow-up visits. In some references, it is recommended to perform the assessments by a professional in this area in a multidisciplinary visit with a team of specialists and clinicians instead of assessments by different specialists in several visits. The assessment consists of two parts: history and physical examination.

2.1 History

The ultimate goal of assessment of history is to provide a thorough history that encompasses the impact of the disease on the patient's communications and interactions with the environment and also covers all aspects of the disease. Therefore, the provision of a checklist is recommended (Appendix 1). In addition to the suggested questions, the answers to these two questions are very important in history taking and should be included in the treatment plan: Does the spasticity contribute to improving your performance? And is this spasticity a local problem or a generalized one?

2.2 Physical examination

The physical examination involves three steps, as follows.

2.2.1 Observation

For observation, it is recommended to evaluate the items of posture, alignment, presence of spontaneous spasms, seating if applicable, movement patterns when moving (e.g., walking, transferring or picking up objects), and pressure sores. However, observation alone is not enough and outcome measurements (Appendix 2) such as timed 10-meter walk test and goniometry are useful.

2.2.2 Assessment of active movement, including range of motion and muscle strength

The grading scale of the Medical Research Council (MRC) (**Table 1**) can be used to assess both weakness and spasticity. However, its application in severe to moderate spasticity is difficult.

2.2.3 Assessment of resistance to passive movement, including assessment of the full range of motion and contracture identification

Trunk and limb spasms are evaluated in this step. This assessment is usually performed using the Modified Ashworth scale. However, it may fail to distinguish

Grade	Definition
0	No contraction
1	Flicker of contraction only
2	Active movement with gravity eliminated
3	Active movement against gravity
4	Active movement against gravity and resistance
5	Normal power

Table 1.
Medical Research Council (MRC) grading of muscle strength.

Perform three passive movements only and record the score of the resistance felt on the third movement
The score is taken within the available range
Move the limbs in the best alignment possible, record position and use when repeating measures
Regulate the speed by counting 1001, 1002, 1003

Table 2.
Recommendations to standardize the measurement of the Ashworth scale.

between neuronal and non-neuronal causes of spasticity [1]; thus, the items addressed in **Table 2** should be noted to avoid misinterpretation [2]. It is effective to use the Tardiu scale [3] to differentiate between the neuronal component and the non-neuronal one because of the evaluation at different velocities [4]; however, it is more time-consuming than the Ashworth test. It should be noted that the suggested tests are specified for spasticity evaluation in limbs, and if one of the patient's chief complaints is trunk spasticity, the verbal or visual analog scales can be used as well as measuring the distance between two fixed points on the trunk in fast and slow trunk flexions by using a tape.

It is important to use outcome measures in clinical evaluation; however, it is always challenging to maintain a balance between test simplicity and speed with its reliability and validity [5], so different tests and methods have been suggested with respect to the disease diagnosis. In this book, we recommend the outcome measure of the National Hospital of Neurology and Neurosurgery (NHNN) in London with a few modifications [2], which is typically used for patients with moderate to severe spasticity (Appendix 2).

When the assessment is over and the treatment plan is being outlined, any physician should ask himself an important question: "why should I treat this spasticity?" and the more important question is "what are the patient's expectations of this treatment?" So the ultimate goal should be discussed with the patients and their caregivers to expect a realistic outcome. Since these goals are different for each patient, the following desires can be addressed: sitting comfortably in a wheelchair, adequate and comfortable night sleep, easier catheterization for bladder drainage, etc.

Different algorithms [6–8] have been developed for the evaluation of and therapeutic approach to spasticity; one of the most applied of them has been developed by Stevenson et al. [2] and is presented in **Figure 1**.

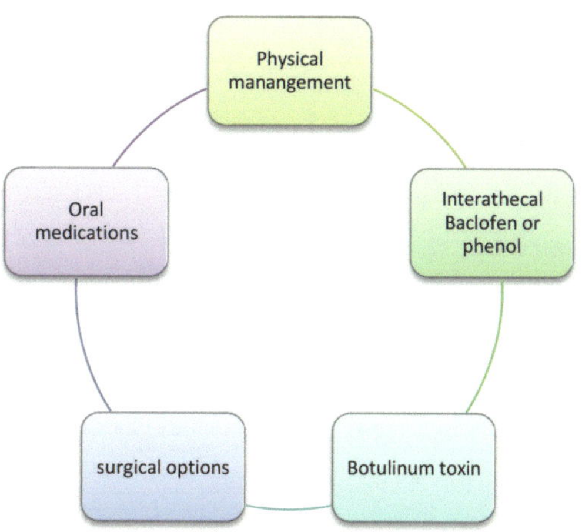

Figure 1.
Therapeutic approach to spasticity.

3. Provision of education and promoting self-management

Nowadays, it has been found that the patient's awareness of the disease and the situation he/she is dealing with promotes the therapeutic process and interventions. This view and its results have also led to the development of courses known as Expert Patient Programmes [9]. The patient and his/her caregivers' understandings of the medical conditions and therapeutic interventions are crucial and effective to the treatment and therapeutic protocol selection. This is especially because different therapeutic interventions for spasticity do not have a linear nature and several treatments are sometimes considered for the patient at the same time (**Figure 1**).

To improve the spasticity treatment efficacy, some instructions should be presented to the patient, either verbally or using a written material [10]. These instructions include the following:

A. Maintaining movement and adequate positioning and B) Recognizing and preventing factors that may aggravate or trigger spasticity and spasms.

B. Maintaining movement and adequate positioning:

A main factor in the spasticity treatment is to maintain the joints' range of motion, which should be performed by the patient or his/her caregiver. Moreover, maintaining muscle length is the second factor that is usually achieved by stretching or splinting [8]. Thus, sitting and standing positions are also critical.

C. Recognizing and preventing factors that may exacerbate spasticity and spasms:

Elimination of unwanted sensory triggers is an important factor in spasticity reduction. Naturally, cutaneous and visceral triggers (**Table 3**) regulate the interneuronal activity by signaling to the spinal cord. Elimination and dysfunction of some modulating pathways can inhibit polysynaptic reflexes (such as flexor withdrawal) and cause spasm [11].

Similarly, abnormal activities of spinal cord circuits induce discharges in motor neurons innervating several muscles, thereby causing a concurrent contraction of these muscles and aggravating spasticity [12, 13]. Sometimes, some patients are aware of such stimuli exacerbating their symptoms (e.g., bowel habit) while having no clue how to modulate or reduce them. The patients should consider the following:

1. Optimization of bladder and bowel management. Any defecation alteration including urinary retention, infection, constipation, or diarrhea can

Cutaneous stimuli	Visceral stimuli
Skin lesion (red or inflamed skin, broken skin, infected skin, pressure sores, ingrown toenails)	Bowel and bladder dysfunction: for example, constipation, overflow or diarrhea, infections, retention or incomplete emptying
Tight-fitting clothes or urinary leg bag straps	Any systemic or localized infection
Uncomfortable orthotics or seating systems	Deep-vein thrombosis

Table 3.
Sensory stimulations that may aggravate spasticity.

exacerbate the symptoms. Even the mild infection (e.g., Candida) can aggravate the symptoms.

2. Maintaining skin integrity. Avoiding any skin irritation, infection, and pressure sores is effective in spasticity reduction. So skin examinations, especially in the vulnerable areas including the areas under pressure or under orthosis, as well as preventing ingrown toenails and deep-vein thrombosis are needed.

Sometimes, there are individual factors that each patient gradually realizes (e.g., in some women, symptoms exacerbate during menstruation period). Knowledge of some of these risk factors is important in treatment choice. In some cases, elimination of some of these factors or waiting for a few days (e.g., in menstruation period) and or a temporary rise in the drug dosage is very effective in solving the patient's problem.

Another point of patient education is that the weakness and spasticity are concomitant [2]; so the patient should know that sometimes the weakness becomes more pronounced by medication use and subsequent spasticity reduction while patients consider this effect as a drug side effect or lack of response. So, in case the spasticity is an effective factor in preserving some of the patient's functions (e.g., standing up and going to the bathroom in the morning), the medication should be taken after the desired activity (going to the bathroom).

Patients should receive written information on the medication dosage, side effects, and follow-up tests for the response to treatment. There should be a telephone number in the form for convenient communication with the health care center or the physician.

4. Physical management of spasticity(physiotherapy or occupational therapy)

The key to a satisfying treatment for spasticity is to educate the patient properly and ensure that the patient follows the instructions correctly. Also, as spasticity changes during the treatment, treatment regimens should change with the patient's condition and be flexible. Proper patient management requires physiotherapy initiation immediately after the disease diagnosis and at regular intervals throughout the disease course, depending on the patient's condition and the diagnosis made by the treatment team. On the other hand, assessment and differentiation between the neuronal and non-neuronal (connective tissue, joint component, muscle, and tendon) causes of hypertonia are critical because the treatment of non-neuronal [14] (passive) causes involves physical therapies such as stretching and splinting; these problems do not respond to medical treatments.

4.1 Physical management strategies

The goal of physical management is to maintain and even improve the performance level and prevent the problems secondary to spasticity. In fact, spasticity reduction is not always a treatment goal, as in some cases maintaining the patient's function requires a little spasticity and increased tone. Therefore, physical management focuses on the performance, discomfort and pain relief, and prevention of secondary complications including contractures and pressure ulcers. The key goals of a physical management plan include the following [2]:

- Maintaining the viscoelastic characteristics of tissues including tendons, muscles, and joints to prevent contractures. This goal is achieved through active and passive movements as well as standing and stretching with splints.

- Controlling the spasticity and spasm so that they will not be self-perpetuating; for example, using techniques and methods in the situations and positions exacerbating the symptoms.

- Maintaining the individual's level of performance. It can be achieved by strengthening activities and keeping cardiovascular fitness.

- Evaluation of spasticity as a positive factor in the patient's function. But a balance should be maintained between the benefits and spasticity-induced complications.

- Generally, there is no single physical modality and the treatments are parallel and concomitant, depending on the patient's conditions. In the following, the treatment options will be discussed in detail.

4.2 Standing

Standing is considered as a therapeutic option since it activates the anti-gravity muscles, improves flexibility, reduces contractures, modulates the neuronal component of spasticity, reduces sensory inputs and lower limb spasms, and has positive psychological effects [15–18]. Regarding the duration and frequency of this physical therapy, studies have suggested a duration of between 30 minutes and 1.5 hours while most patients have performed this exercise for 40 minutes and with a frequency of three to four times a week [18–20]. Remember that the duration and frequency depend on the patient's condition; so, the decision should be made based on this factor. However, at least 30 minutes of standing seems to be reasonable. The best standing position is in an extended posture with neutral alignment of the trunk, pelvis, and lower limb joints, carried out actively by the patient himself/herself or by using standing aids including Oswestry standing frames, motorized or hydraulically assisted standing systems, standing wheelchairs, or at least a tilt table (according to the patient symptom severity respectively) [2]. In all these cases, hypotension is the most notable complication, which can be prevented by arrangements such as avoiding sudden position change or by using compression stockings.

4.3 Active exercise and promotion of optimal movement patterns

In most of the cases, patients with spasticity are advised for spasticity reduction and less attention is paid to muscle weakness, and sometimes strengthening exercises are not prescribed because of the concern for spasticity exacerbation [21]. It is recommended, to the extent possible, to perform active exercises in order to increase the strength, re-educate movement patterns, and improve cardiovascular fitness. The outcomes achieved by these exercises are not usually observed in passive exercises. Nowadays, it has been found that not only is antagonist muscle weakness effective in spasticity, but also an imbalance between agonist and antagonist muscles exacerbates the symptoms and causes atrophy [21]. The movement patterns should also change; in fact, proper movement patterns should be instructed. At the same time with limb exercises, the alignments of the trunk and pelvic girdle should be maintained. These exercises alter muscle functions and structures [22]. The strengthening recommendations should be realistic and close to the patient's daily life activities and include all the involved muscles [23, 24]. Although no specific protocol has been suggested for this kind of patients, most studies recommend the protocol adapted from the sport sources. These traditional training rates are a load of 60–80% of one repetition maximum (the maximum load that can be lifted once), three sets of 10 repetitions carried out three or four times a week.

Alongside these exercises, cardiovascular fitness exercises have been recommended in various papers [25, 26]. Because these exercises are being neglected in these patients due to their inactivity especially.

The task-focused active-use therapy techniques such as the constraint-induced movement therapy can sometimes be used for upper limbs. The techniques should be used in an intensive program over a short period (e.g., 4–8 weeks) [27].

4.4 Passive movement

When the patient cannot move his/her limb, passive movements can be carried out by another person. In passive movement, generally, all the body joints should be moved in their ranges of motion daily. According to the studies, it seems that using passive movements can be effective in changing spasticity pattern, alleviating secondary non-neuronal complications, and improving positioning [2]. It is recommended to perform the passive movements daily, and it can be carried out before the patient repositioning. These movements should be safe and comfortable for both the patient and caregiver. Spasmolytic medication taking in 20–30 minutes before the movements can be helpful [2]. Sometimes sudden stretching can exacerbate the spasm, so the movements should be performed at slow speed. Skin irritations can cause symptom exacerbation as well; thus, the best way is to desensitize the skin on a gradual basis or handling the limb on top of clothes. Grabbing and holding the ball of the foot should be avoided because it is usually a sensitive point for these triggers and better not to be touched [2]. Moreover, the movements should be carried out with the best alignments of the muscles and joints, overstretching should not occur, and stereotypical spasticity patterning (e.g., flexing the hip in the midline rather than in adduction and internal rotation) should be avoided.

The critical point is that after the movements are over, the patient should be positioned properly. The position should not be the same as the previous position caused by spasms to keep the benefits of the movements [2]. Usually, these movements are not performed by the physician or therapist because it is time-consuming and is not cost-effective. So in addition to providing written material on the right techniques for the patient and caregivers, assistance appliances such as continuous passive movement machines (CPMs) or lifters (hoist) can also be used [2].

4.5 Stretches

Typically, with a 2-day immobilization, muscle changes initiate, including muscle shortening and atrophy, muscle compliance reduction, and increasing the ratio of collagen to muscle fibers [21]. Following these changes, there will be an increase in the sensitivity of muscle spindles to stretching, which can exacerbate the neuronal component of spasticity and subsequently the non-neural component [28]. On the other hand, stretching induces actin and myosin synthesis; as a result, the number of sarcomeres as well as the muscle length increases [21, 29]. So far, there is no agreement on the duration and frequency of stretching exercises but the following protocol can be considered for the daily schedule [30, 31].

It is suggested to administer the stretching according to the patient's daily schedule and his/her posture [2]. The stretching can be carried out actively or passively (by someone else or with FES). We can use the positioning, for example standing, sitting, or lying down with using splints and orthosis, to achieve a prolonged stretching. Another important point is that while stretching a muscle, the antagonist muscle shortens, so there should be a balance in the stretching schedules for all the muscles [2, 32]. Regarding the duration of stretching, studies have suggested 20, 30, or even 60 minutes. So, there is no single protocol [30], but it seems that the efficacy increases with longer durations. Also, it seems that stretching before the exercises has a more favorable effect.

The patient should be given written instruction on stretching. Stretches should include the back muscles, quadriceps, hip flexors, hip adductors, hamstrings, calf muscles (gastrocnemius and soleus), wrists, and fingers, and should be performed actively or passively. The therapist should modify the stretching based on each patient's condition.

4.6 Positioning

As well as improving the effective stretching and subsequent maintaining of range of motion, correct positioning also helps in altering the spasticity pattern, modifying asymmetry, and decreasing the risk of pressure-induced skin injuries [33]. The golden key to good positioning is to change the position during the day. An ideal position is important in both lying and sitting; moreover, the presence of exacerbating factors and triggers (e.g., pressure sore, pain) is critical in position selection. Performing passive exercises before positioning is helpful; for example, when the patient tries to use a T roll for the leg flexion position, performing several knee and hip flexions and bending the hips and knees up toward the chest and abdomen facilitate this position [34].

In correct positioning, muscles should be stretched and longer than usual. For example, these are the suggestions to improve the positioning in a patient with continuous spasticity-induced hip adduction: The patient should monitor his/her sitting position and try to keep his/her knees apart while sitting so that he/she does not get accustomed to the wrong position. The impact of trunk and pelvis positions on the legs should be evaluated. In a flexed posture with a posteriorly tilted pelvis, the legs tend to be in internal rotation and adduction; so, having a firmer seat base, a contoured cushion, or extra trunk support may facilitate a more anteriorly tilted pelvis position, trunk extension, and better lower limbs alignment. In patients unable to reduce adduction, using aids including a pummel, rolled-up towel, cushion or T roll can help in reducing the adduction.

4.7 Wheelchair and seating

In patients suffering from spasticity, the sitting position should be modified to improve the performance, accommodate to contractures and deformities established, maintain comfort, and reduce fatigue [35, 36]. The main requirements for a good sitting position are a firm seat base and backrest with subtle changes by altering the seat base to promote an anterior tilt of the pelvis to help in achieving hip flexion, abduction, and external rotation as well as trunk extension.

Patients with weakness in the trunk and neck extensors can use the tilt-in-space systems [37, 38], where the patient seat has a reclining at the back and flexion at the hip. In this system, hip flexion decreases the extension tone and spasticity as well as providing support for the patient's back (by the backward movement of the backrest). Also, these seats improve kyphosis and breathing of the patients and reduce fatigue and pressure ulcers.

As the patient's spasticity status changes throughout the treatment, it is necessary to re-evaluate the patient's sitting position.

5. Orthosis

Orthoses or splints are tools for improving limb performance and preventing deformity. These appliances are usually custom-made [39]. Non-removable splinting devices made of plaster or casting tape are referred to as "casts." Casts are also a type of splint. Orthoses are used for the following treatment goals [27, 39]:

- Providing control over the joint's range of motion and thus improving its performance.
- Maintaining prolonged stretches on the muscle's tendon to alter or modify the changes occurred in tissues.
- Modifying deformities established (e.g., using heel raise in leg length discrepancy).
- Changing the neuronal component of spasticity through prolonged stretches and sensory input alteration.
- Increasing the patient's comfort.
- Correction of the posture.
- Correction of upper extremity performance.
- Improving walking efficiency.
- In children, preventing hip migration or slowing its progress.

In administering orthoses, in addition to discussing the treatment goals with patients, the method of use, duration, and times of use should be discussed as well. In each visit, the patient should be asked about pain, discomfort, and sleep disorder, while muscle wasting and the places under pressure by orthosis should be examined. Incorrect orthosis usage and feeling discomfort with orthosis use can exacerbate the symptoms and cause new deformities. There is no contraindication for administering orthoses; however, some problems addressed in **Table 4** can limit the use of splints, so these points should be noticed during the follow-up visits and proper solutions should be considered [2].

The most common splints based on the usage area are discussed here according to the evidence from different sources and guidelines. Evidence grading is according to **Tables 5** and **6** [40]. However, some of the splints are not mentioned here, we did not intend to deny their effects but only the splints with the best evidence are discussed.

Sensory impairment	**Uncontrolled epilepsy**
Unstable intracranial pressure	Heterotrophic ossification
Poor skin condition	Edema
Vascular disorder	Acute inflammation
Fracture or severe soft tissue injury	Medically unstable
Behavioral/cognitive disorders	Frequent spasms
Access to limb required for medical purposes	

Table 4.
Precautions for the use of splints or orthoses.

Quality of evidence	Grading	Characteristics
High	A	Based on consistent results from well-performed randomized controlled trials, or overwhelming evidence of an alternative source, for example, well-executed observational studies with strong effects
Moderate	B	Based on randomized controlled trials where there are serious flaws in conduct, inconsistency, indirectness, imprecise estimates, reporting bias, or some other combination of these limitations, or from other study designs with special strengths
Low	C	Based on observational evidence, or from controlled trials with several very serious limitations
Very low	D	Based on case studies or expert opinion

Table 5.
GRADE quality of evidence grading.

Strength	Grade	Benefits and risks
Strong	1. "It is recommended. .."	Benefits appear to outweigh the risks (or vice versa) for the majority of the target group
Conditional	2. "It is suggested. .."	Risks and benefits are more closely balanced, or there is uncertainty in likely service user values and preferences

Table 6.
Strength of grade.

5.1 Ankle

The following advice is suggested to correct contractures [40]:

- It is possible to use casts at the end of the range of motion for acute brain injury and stroke patients to improve the range of motion (2C). The cast should be replaced every 5–7 days. Use the cast for a 2- to 12-week period.

- In severely spastic patients, we can use casts with botulinum toxin injection (2B). The cast should be replaced every 5–7 days. Use the cast for a 2- to 12-week period.

- Using adjustable ankle splints at the end of the range of motion improves the joint's range of motion (2C). Splints are used 6–23 hours a day for

2–12 weeks and should be adjusted with improvements at the end of the range of motion.

- While using non-custom-made splints, necessary precautions should be taken to prevent pressure sores (2D).

Contracture prevention [40]:

- Using ankle casts at the end of dorsiflexion range can prevent contractures in ABI patients (2C). Primary casts should be replaced every 5–7 days depending on the change in the range of motion until the patient can maintain the plantar grade position. The last cast should be used as a bivalved plantar grade cast for 18 hours a day until the splint can maintain the range of motion.

- The ankle splint can prevent the limitation of the ankle's range of motion when the ankle is at a plantar grade position (2B). The recommended duration of use for ankle splint is 6–10 hours at night for 2–5 weeks.

- While using non-custom-made splints, necessary precautions should be taken to prevent pressure sores (2B).

Performance improvement [41]:

- The plantar spasticity ankle foot orthosis (AFO) can be used for better walking. In the case of mild spasticity, the single midline posterior stop AFO is used. The type of AFO with pins in the posterior channels can be used for more severe cases. Moreover, in patients with weak extensors of hip or knee, the solid type is recommended while the hinged type is suitable for patients with adequate control. In patients with crouched gait and passive range of motion in hip joints and pelvis, a ground reaction force AFO can be used.

5.2 Knee

Contracture improvement [40]:

- It is possible to use casts at the end of range of motion for acute brain injury and stroke patients to improve the knee's range of motion (2D). The cast should be replaced every 5–7 days. Use the cast for 2–12 weeks.

- Short-term application of the cast (1–4 days) entails fewer complications compared to the longer uses (5–7 days) (2C).

Contracture prevention [40]:

- Using casts at the end of range of motion in acute brain injury and stroke patients can prevent contractures (2C). The cast should be replaced every 5–7 days. Use the cast for a 2- to 5-week period.

- Use this cast with caution in the patients with acute lesions (acute brain injury and stroke) and decreased level of consciousness for preventing secondary complications such as pressure sores (2C).

- Knee splints can be used for standing control and walking improvement as well.

5.3 Wrist and hand

Contracture improvement [2, 40]:

- Using splints for deformity correction in hand and wrists is not routinely advised for every patient (e.g., in stroke and acute brain injury patients). However, they can be used in certain cases in an optional way (2B). These splints are custom-made or serial and adjustable (10 degrees wrist extension and finger extension with MCP flexion, wrist at neutral, or maximal available range of movement). Most of them are used for 20 minutes to 12 hours a day for a 1- to 8-week period.

Contracture prevention [2, 40]:

- Using splints for deformity prevention in hand and wrists is not routinely advised for every patient (e.g., in stroke and acute brain injury patients). However, they can be used in certain cases in an optional way (2B). In the studies, the splints have been used in different positions (10 degrees wrist extension and fingers fully extended, wrist at neutral, or close to maximal available range of movement) with duration of 6–12 hours a day for a 1- to 8-week period.

- Using splints in combination with botulinum toxin in selected cases can be effective in reducing the spasticity that has resulted in range of motion loss (2C). The splint is used at the end of the available range of movement but is not adjusted daily. On the other hand, strapping is used at the end of available range of movement, with daily adjustment to maximal stretch for 6 days.

- Using electrical stimulation in combination with splints is not recommended for contracture prevention (2A).

- Custom-made hand and wrist splints should not be used routinely for prevention from spasticity exacerbation in acute brain injury and stroke patients (2B).

- A wrist splint at neutral position can be effective in hand pain prevention caused by joint malalignment (2A). These splints should be used for minimum 6 hours a day for 13 weeks.

Performance improvement [2, 42]:

- Sometimes, a splint is also used to improve performance (**Figure 2**) or prevent tissue damage (e.g., sheepskin palm protector).

- Using volar splints in children with cerebral palsy can reduce the spasticity and improve the range of motion and performance in upper limb. However, theses splints are not effective on the upper limb movements in stroke patients.

- Using dorsal splints has no effect on spasticity, range of motion, and performance of upper limb in stroke patients.

- Dynamic splints can improve the upper limb performance and accelerate spasticity reduction.

DOI: http://dx.doi.org/10.5772/intechopen.93008

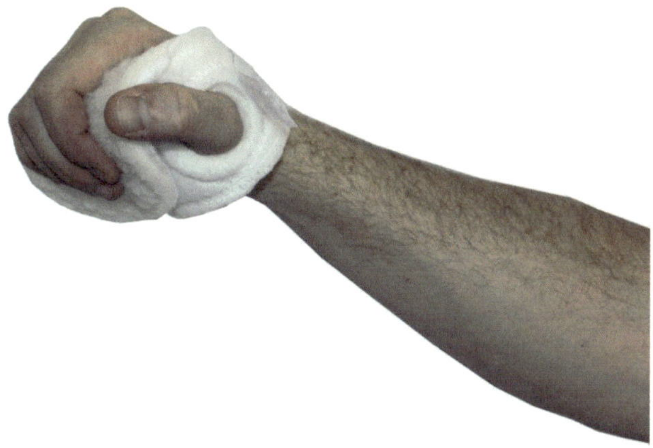

Figure 2.
sheepskin palm protector is used to prevent tissue damage.

- The use of C-Bar splint is an effective method to improve hand performance and range of motion while decreasing spasticity in upper limb of cerebral palsy children.

- Using anti-pronation splints can be an effective technique to improve the performance of upper limb, range of motion of forearm supination, and wrist extension, as well as reducing the severity of spasticity in forearms pronator muscles and wrist flexor muscles. These splints are also effective in improving the gripping and pinching ability in children suffering from spastic diplegia cerebral palsy.

- Extension splints are not helpful in the rehabilitation program of stroke patients.

- As a modern splint, SAEBO splints can be helpful in improving the upper limb of stroke patients.

- In general, volar, dorsal, anti-pronation, and C-Bar splints are effective in spasticity reduction and performance improvement of upper limb in children with cerebral palsy while SAEBO and dynamic splints are useful for performance improvement and spasticity reduction of upper limb.

5.4 Elbow

Contracture improvement [40, 42]:

- Using casts is recommended at the end of range of motion to modify the elbow's range of motion (2C). The cast should be replaced every 3–7 days. Use the cast for a 1- to 4-week period.

- Short-term application of the cast (1–4 days) entails fewer complications compared to the longer use (4–7 days) (2C).

- Enough studies for contracture correction by splint are not available.

Contracture prevention [40]:

- Enough studies for contracture correction by splints are not available.

Performance improvement [42]:

- Elbow gaiters are recommended to maintain extension and improve function.

5.5 Spinal braces

- Spinal braces are usually used in cases with muscle weakness. In the patients with spasticity being the predominant complaint, spinal braces are not frequently used. It is because they are difficult to fit on the patients, are not comfortable, and can induce breathing problems and sores [2]. In these cases, the use of customized seating with individualized truncal and pelvic support can be a more beneficial and comfortable option. The braces can be used in patients with kyphosis and scoliosis if it helps in sitting.

6. Pharmacological intervention

On the decision for the treatment of spasticity, considering goals is a critical point and pharmacological interventions should be considered with non-pharmacological treatment for optimizing the effectiveness of management [2]. Another important point in prescription of drugs is about the patient's situation and the dosage and timing should be considered according to it. For example, painful nocturnal spasms may best be managed with a long-acting agent taken at night-time that has sedative side effects. As a rule for all medication, "start low and go slow" [2]. Although it is time-consuming, this approach will limit any deleterious effects on function or unwanted side effects. For better discussion, pharmacological interventions are categorized according to spasticity pattern including, generalized, segmental, and focal.

6.1 Generalized spasticity

There are several oral treatments for management of generalized spasticity. However, there is more interest for some medications according to the country strategy (e.g., there is more discussion in American papers for Clonidine, but it is currently little used in the UK) [39]. Generally, these drugs are used more for spasticity management: baclofen, diazepam, tizanidine, dantrolene, gabapentin, and clonidine (**Table** 7). They may be used to provide systemic effect for modest spasticity severity. Choosing the drug is dependent on patient problems and goals [2, 39]. For example, if the neuropathic pain is a problematic as well as spasticity, gabapentin should be considered for this patient. Besides, some of the drugs are more recommended in papers for specific diagnosis; for example, gabapentin is also recommended as first- or second-line treatment for spasticity in the UK National Guidelines for Multiple Sclerosis [39].

There is no evidence-based consensus for combination drug regimes for oral treatment. However, they can be used according to associated features [2, 43]. There is no right or wrong way to titrate drugs in combination, and professionals suggest avoiding polypharmacy. If there is intolerance for maximum dose of first-line drug, continue the highest level the individual can tolerate comfortably and added the second-line drug and titrated upward. If the patient's problem has

Drug	Starting dose	Maximum dose	Side effects
Baclofen	5–10 mg daily	120 mg daily, usually in three divided doses	Drowsiness, weakness, paresthesia, nausea, vomiting
Diazepam	2 mg daily	40–60 mg daily, usually in three or four divided doses	Drowsiness, reduced attention, memory impairment Dependency and withdrawal syndromes
Tizanidine	2 mg daily	36 mg daily, usually in three or four divided doses	Drowsiness, weakness, dry mouth, postural hypotension Monitor liver function
Dantrolene	25 mg daily	400 mg daily, usually in four divided doses	Anorexia, nausea, vomiting, drowsiness, weakness, dizziness, paraesthesiae Monitor liver function
Gabapentin	300 mg daily (can start at 100 mg daily)	2400 mg daily, usually in three divided doses	Drowsiness, somnolence, dizziness

Table 7.
Drugs in spasticity treatment.

been decreased with this regime, the first drug can be cautiously withdrawn to see if monotherapy with the second-line drug alone is sufficient to achieve the goal of treatment. For optimizing the treatment, it is very important the patient has had written information about treatment goals and efficacy and side effects of drugs.

Evidence-based recommendations for choosing the drug are listed below:

Baclofen: It is more effective in patients with either multiple sclerosis (MS) [44] or spinal cord injury and few have concentrated on spasticity of cerebral origin, including stroke or traumatic brain injury [43].

Tizanidine: It reduces sign and symptoms in MS, spinal cord injury and stroke; no functional benefit has, however, been demonstrated in MS and spinal cord injury [45].

Dantrolene: It is the only available agent that works out of CNS with direct action on skeletal muscle. So, it can be prescribed for spasticity originating from both spinal and supraspinal lesions. It is effective in management of MS patient and has modest effect in spinal cord injury, stroke, and cerebral palsy [46–48]. It does not demonstrate any changes in function.

Diazepam: The efficacy of it in spinal cord injury, cerebral palsy, and MS has been proven. However, its side effects are more than those of other drugs in the studies [43].

Gabapentin: There is beneficial effect of gabapentin on measures of spasticity in MS and spinal cord injury [49, 50].

Clonidine: Its major use has been as an anti-hypertensive agent, but it is efficient in the spinal cord injury spasticity [43].

In children's spasticity, baclofen (for long treatment) and diazepam (for rapid onset) are recommended by NICE guideline [27].

6.2 For regional or segmental spasticity

This type of spasticity benefits from interathecal administration. This route of administration delivers the medication directly to where it is needed with less unwanted side effects like drowsiness and impaired cognition. Interathecal baclofen pump has been used since 30 years ago [39]. It is effective for lower limbs and trunk spasticity [51]. To manage changing needs, the dose and timing of drug delivery can be programmed over the 24-hour period. It has the beneficial effect in the autonomic storming in people with brain and spinal cord injury [39]. The risk of infection and the need to attend clinics every 3 months or so to have the pump refilled are its significant disadvantages.

The pump is recommended in children with severe motor function impairment (GMFCS level 3, 4, and 5) and bilateral spasticity affecting upper and lower limbs [27].

An intrathecal baclofen test to assess the therapeutic effect and adverse events is necessary before making the decision for intrathecal pump implantation. For evaluation of response, assessing the patient is necessary within 3–5 hours after sedation and recovery. Before pump implantation, written information is necessary including possible adverse effects, signs and symptoms suggesting the dose is too low or high, complications and follow-up appointments [27].

Implantation of the infusion pump can occur within 3 months of satisfactory response to intrathecal baclofen test [39].

Using intrathecal phenol injections is suggested in some studies too [52]. Compared with the intrathecal phenol, baclofen pump has complication of surgical procedure for implantation of pump, malfunction of pump, needing for dose adjustment and refilling the pump [52]. The advantages of intrathecal phenol include: less individual responsibility, low cost, no requirement of special equipment, and avoiding the regular clinical visits for refills. But the complications of this procedure are bladder and bowel incontinence, limb weakness, and paraesthesia, which are the reasons for intrathecal phenol not being considered for spasticity management routinely [52].

6.3 Focal spasticity

The most famous treatments that are used in this category are phenol neurolysis and botulinum toxin.

Phenol nerve block has been used for the treatment of spasticity since the 1960s and it has advantages in comparison with botulinum toxin including: faster onset of spasticity relief and greater degree of muscle relaxation for much longer and at much less expense [27, 39]. But it has disadvantages including, neurogenic pain or paraesthesia (if applied to a mixed motor/sensory nerve) and careful localization (needing for experienced hand), so some specialist prefer Botulinum toxin. However, it is appropriate for patients with troublesome spasticity and dystonia of hip adductors and calf muscles, especially for non-ambulant patients or "walkers" who are already dependent on an ankle-foot orthosis (AFO) [27, 39].

Botulinum toxin use has shown significant effects on improving the symptoms of patients with focal spasticity or dystonia [27, 39, 43]. The method of use and injection is discussed in detail in chapter x. Here is a brief explanation of its indications and contraindications.

There is more interest in botulinum toxin injection. This procedure for patients with focal spasticity in upper limb should be considered in the following cases [27]:

- Impeding fine motor function
- Compromising care and hygiene

- Causing pain
- Impeding tolerance of other treatments, such as orthoses
- Causing cosmetic concern to the child and young person

Botulinum toxin injection for patients with focal spasticity in lower limb should be considered in the following cases [27]:

- Impeding gross motor function
- Compromising care and hygiene
- Causing pain
- Disturbing sleep
- Impeding tolerance of other treatments, such as orthoses and use of equipment to support posture
- Causing cosmetic concern to the child and young person

Botulinum toxin is not recommended in the following cases [27]:

- Has severe muscle weakness
- Had previous adverse reaction or allergy to the botulinum toxin type A
- Is receiving aminoglycoside treatment

Administration of botulinum toxin should be done with caution in the following cases [27]:

The person has any of the following:

- Bleeding disorders for example due to anticoagulant therapy
- Generalized spasticity
- Fixed muscle contracture
- Marked bone deformity

There are concerns about people likelihood of engaging in post treatment adapted physical therapy treatment.

7. Setting up a service

Setting up a spasticity clinic or service depends on the local conditions and available resources. Setting up a clinic needs a team in which every member has certain tasks. Undoubtedly, the roles and duties will overlap, but it is important to understand the abilities and skills of each professional to evaluate what they can offer for the treatment process [2]. Thus, outlining the key skills and roles of each team member and providing a competency framework can help in making an efficient team.

In general, four professionals have roles in a spasticity clinic team including a physician (a pediatric or adult neurologist or a physical medicine and rehabilitation specialist), nurse, occupational therapist, and physiotherapist [2]. In the following, the tasks of each professional are briefly discussed.

Physician:

- Understanding the underlying condition, prognosis, natural history, associated features, and possible complications. Identifying the abnormal features or unexpected changes that may be caused by a secondary cause.
- Being experienced in neuromuscular history-taking and physical examination.
- Being able to perform necessary interventions including administering oral medications, botulinum toxin injection, intrathecal drug, and splint.

Nurse:

- Educating the patient and his/her caregivers to manage spasticity.
- Managing cutaneous and visceral triggers.
- Advising the patient on posture, moving, and handling.
- Managing psychosocial issues and considering the impact of spasticity on employment and social activities of the patient and managing it.
- Monitoring the patient's and caregiver's adaptations with the treatments and ensuring that they follow the protocols and guidelines properly.

Physiotherapist:

- Identifying the potential for movement patterns and functional ability to be improved.
- Identifying trigger factors of spasticity related to posture and movement.
- Identifying muscle weakness underlying the spasticity.

Occupational therapist:

- Assessing the patient for proper use of splints.
- Assessing the patient for posture and siting especially in a wheelchair.
- Assessing the impact of spasticity on the patient's performance.
- Evaluating the patient's access to work, home, and community environments.

Permanent presences of other specialists in the team are not necessarily needed, but they can be helpful in the treatment process. These specialists include orthopedics, neurosurgeons, speech therapists, orthotists, social workers, continence advisors, and psychologists.

One of the valuable points in setting up such services is their growth and development to provide better services. This goal is achieved through data collection, organization, and extraction so that effective and useful proposals will be presented. The development of these services based on this information results in optimizing the services as much as possible and targeted funding for treating these patients.

8. Conclusion

Spasticity is one of the common symptoms in a wide range of neurological conditions and it needs a multidisciplinary approach for best management. This chapter provided an excellent paradigm to incorporate many of the key elements that are fundamental, including: assessment of the individual with spasticity, provision of education and promoting self-management, physical management of spasticity (physiotherapy or occupational therapy), orthoses, pharmacological intervention, and setting up a service.

Conflict of interest

The authors certify that there is no conflict of interest with any financial organization regarding the material discussed in this chapter.

Appendix 1.

Demographic data and checklist for impact of the spasticity on the patient's communications and interactions with the environment.

Patient's name:	**Date of birth:**	**Date:**	**Diagnosis:**
Current medication	Please comment on dose, route, times, and any side effects experienced		
Other medication used in the past for spasticity: Why did they stop taking it (ineffective, not tolerated, other reason?)			
Primary difficulty: Is it attributed to spasticity: Yes/No		Severity rating out of 10	
Other difficulties related to spasticity:			
Spasticity	Please comment on site and severity of spasticity		
Not needing to be assessed			
Clonus	Please comment whether spontaneous		
Not needing to be assessed			
Spasms	Please comment on which muscles, extensors or flexors, severity, pain, frequency, and duration		
Not needing to be assessed			
Pain	Please comment on presence, severity, and management. Indicate if pain has been getting worse, better, or remains the same		
Not needing to be assessed			
Sleep patterns	Please comment on disturbances, positions, and quality		
Bed mobility	Please comment on how much, type of mattress used		
Not needing to be assessed			
Bladder	Please comment on current management		

Patient's name:	**Date of birth:** **Date:** **Diagnosis:**
Not needing to be assessed	
Bowel	Please comment on current management
Not needing to be assessed	
Skin	Please comment on the presence of pressure ulcers and the ability to relieve pressure, change position and sensation, and any aids used (Waterlow Tool)
Not needing to be assessed	
Mobility	Please comment on outdoor, indoor, aids, speed, and distance
Not needing to be assessed	
Toilet/bath/shower transfers	Please comment on ability and aids required. Indicate if this has been getting worse, better, or remains the same
Not needing to be assessed	
Transfers	Please comment on car, bed, chair, level of independence and assistance required
Not needing to be assessed	
Wheelchair	Please comment on posture, position, type, and make of chair and cushion
Not needing to be assessed	
Previous therapy and nursing input	Please comment on physiotherapy, OT, seating assessments, and nursing advice. Ensure details of time, date, and location of treatment obtained, including names, addresses, and contact details
Options discussed with patient	
Assessment by:	Signature:

Appendix 2. The outcome measures of spasticity

Name:	**Data**	
Goniometry to measure range of passive movement (Norkin and White 1985):	**Resting angle Right/left**	**Full range available Right/ left**
Hip flexion-extension		
Hip abduction-adduction		
Knee flexion-extension		
Ankle PF-DF		
Maximum distance between knees as measured during passive hip abduction (Hyman 2000):	Distance in mm:	
Modified Ashworth scale (Bohannon and Smith,1987):	Right	Left
Resistance to: hip and knee flexion in supine		
Resistance to: hip and knee extension in supine		
Resistance to: hip abduction in crook lying		
Resistance to: ankle dorsiflexion with knee extended		
Clonus and spasms score (self-report) (Smith 1994)*		

Name:	**Data**
Clonus	
Spasms	
Pain intensity by visual analogue scale(VAS)	
Seating posture score (please record 0 = yes, 1 = no)	
Are the feet well positioned on the footplates?	
Are the knees apart?	
Are the hips well aligned?	
Is the trunk posture symmetrical?	
Total	
Record the frequency of falls over the last month(0 = No falls, 1 = two to three falls per week, 2 = five to six falls per week, 3 = daily falls, 4 = more than one fall per day)	
10-metre timed walk (Wade 1987)	
No. of steps	
Time	
Aid used	
Identify the main problem that is amenable to treatment:	

0 = absent; 1 = Provoked by painful stimuli only; 2 = Provoked by touch, light pressure and/or occasionally spontaneous (5/day and/or < 2night); 3 = Provoked by passive movements (during physical therapy or nursing care) and/or frequently spontaneous (>5 day and/or 2/night).

Author details

Seyed Mansoor Rayegani, Marzieh Babaee* and Seyed Ahmad Raeissadat
Physical Medicine and Rehabilitation Research Center, Shahid Beheshti University of Medical Sciences, Tehran, Iran

*Address all correspondence to: rambabaee@yahoo.com

References

[1] Ashworth B. Preliminary trial of carisoprodol in multiple sclerosis. Practitioner. 1964;**192**:540-542

[2] Stevenson V, Jarrett L. Spasticity Management: A Practical Multidisciplinary Guide. Boca Raton: CRC Press; 2006

[3] Tardieu G. A la recherche d'une technique de mesure de la spasticite. Revista de Neurologia. 1954;**91**:143-144

[4] Barnes MP. Management of spasticity. Age and Ageing. 1998;**27**(2): 239-245

[5] Haas B, Bergström E, Jamous A, Bennie A. The inter rater reliability of the original and of the modified Ashworth scale for the assessment of spasticity in patients with spinal cord injury. Spinal Cord. 1996;**34**(9):560-564

[6] Barnes MP. An overview of the clinical management of spasticity. In: Johnson GR, Barnes MP, editor. Upper Motor Neurone Syndrome and Spasticity: Clinical Management and Neurophysiology. Cambridge: Cambridge University Press; 2008. pp. 1-8

[7] Ward A. A summary of spasticity management–a treatment algorithm. European Journal of Neurology. 2002;**9**: 48-52

[8] Thompson A, Jarrett L, Lockley L, Marsden J, Stevenson V. Clinical management of spasticity. Journal of Neurology, Neurosurgery and Psychiatry. 2005;**76**(4):459-463

[9] Tattersall R. The expert patient: A new approach to chronic disease management for the twenty-first century. Clinical Medicine. 2002; **2**(3):227

[10] Nicklin J. Improving the quality of written information for patients. Nursing Standard (through 2013). 2002; **16**(49):39

[11] Schmit BD, Benz EN, Rymer WZ. Reflex mechanisms for motor impairment in spinal cord injury. In: Sensorimotor Control of Movement and Posture. Boston, MA: Springer; 2002. pp. 315-323

[12] Norton JA, Wood DE, Marsden JF, Day BL. Spinally generated electromyographic oscillations and spasms in a low-thoracic complete paraplegic. Movement Disorders. 2003; **18**(1):101-106

[13] Sheean G. Neurophysiology of Spasticity. England: Cambridge University Press Cambridge; 2008, 2001

[14] Dietz V. Spastic movement disorder: What is the impact of research on clinical practice? Journal of Neurology, Neurosurgery and Psychiatry. 2003; **74**(6):820-821

[15] Edwards S, Charlton P. Splinting and the use of orthoses in the management of patients with neurological disorders. Neurological Physiotherapy. 2002;**2**:219-253

[16] Odeen I, Knutsson E. Evaluation of the effects of muscle stretch and weight load in patients with spastic paraplegia. Scandinavian Journal of Rehabilitation Medicine. 1981;**13**(4):117-121

[17] Tremblay F, Malouin F, Richards CL, Dumas F. Effects of prolonged muscle stretch on reflex and voluntary muscle activations in children with spastic cerebral palsy. Scandinavian Journal of Rehabilitation Medicine. 1990;**22**(4):171-180

[18] Eng JJ, Levins SM, Townson AF, Mah-Jones D, Bremner J, Huston G. Use of prolonged standing for individuals with spinal cord injuries. Physical Therapy. 2001;**81**(8):1392-1399

[19] Dunn RB, Walter JS, Lucero Y, Weaver F, Langbein E, Fehr L, et al. Follow-up assessment of standing mobility device users. Assistive Technology. 1998;**10**(2):84-93

[20] Walter SJ, Sola GP, Sacks J, Lucero Y, Langbein E, Weaver F. Indications for a home standing program for individuals with spinal cord injury. The Journal of Spinal Cord Medicine. 1999;**22**(3): 152-158

[21] Gracies J-M. Pathophysiology of impairment in patients with spasticity and use of stretch as a treatment of spastic hypertonia. Physical Medicine and Rehabilitation Clinics of North America. 2001;**12**(4):747-768

[22] Bruton A. Muscle plasticity: Response to training and detraining. Physiotherapy. 2002;**88**(7):398-408

[23] Dodd KJ, Taylor NF, Damiano DL. A systematic review of the effectiveness of strength-training programs for people with cerebral palsy. Archives of Physical Medicine and Rehabilitation. 2002;**83**(8):1157-1164

[24] White L, McCoy S, Castellano V, Gutierrez G, Stevens J, Walter G, et al. Resistance training improves strength and functional capacity in persons with multiple sclerosis. Multiple Sclerosis Journal. 2004;**10**(6): 668-674

[25] Hebert J. Impact of aerobic training on fitness and quality of life in multiple sclerosis. Journal of Neurologic Physical Therapy. 2000;**24**(4):161-162

[26] Rietberg MB, Brooks D, Uitdehaag BM, Kwakkel G. Exercise therapy for multiple sclerosis. Cochrane Database of Systematic Reviews. 2005;**1**:CD003980

[27] National Institute for Health and Care Excellence. Clinical Guidelines. In: Spasticity in under 19s: Management. London: National Institute for Health and Care Excellence (UK) Copyright (c) NICE 2018; 2016

[28] O'dwyer N, Ada L, Neilson P. Spasticity and muscle contracture following stroke. Brain. 1996;**119**(5): 1737-1749

[29] Goldspink G, Tabary C, Tabary J, Tardieu C, Tardieu G. Effect of denervation on the adaptation of sarcomere number and muscle extensibility to the functional length of the muscle. The Journal of Physiology. 1974;**236**(3):733-742

[30] Bovend'Eerdt TJ, Newman M, Barker K, Dawes H, Minelli C, Wade DT. The effects of stretching in spasticity: A systematic review. Archives of Physical Medicine and Rehabilitation. 2008;**89**(7):1395-1406

[31] Kalkman BM, Bar-On L, O'Brien TD, Maganaris CN. Stretching interventions in children with cerebral palsy: Why are they ineffective in improving muscle function and how can we better their outcome? Frontiers in Physiology. 2020;**11**:131

[32] Williams P. Use of intermittent stretch in the prevention of serial sarcomere loss in immobilised muscle. Annals of the Rheumatic Diseases. 1990; **49**(5):316-317

[33] Salazar AP, Pinto C, Ruschel Mossi JV, Figueiro B, Lukrafka JL, Pagnussat AS. Effectiveness of static stretching positioning on post-stroke upper-limb spasticity and mobility: Systematic review with meta-analysis. Annals of Physical and Rehabilitation Medicine. 2019;**62**(4):274-282

[34] Pope PM. Management of the physical condition in patients with chronic and severe neurological pathologies. Physiotherapy. 1992;**78**(12): 896-903

[35] Herman JH, Lange ML. Seating and positioning to manage spasticity after brain injury. NeuroRehabilitation. 1999; **12**(2):105-117

[36] Pope P. Posture management and special seating. In: Neurological Physiotherapy: A Problem-Solving Approach. 2nd ed. Edinburgh: Churchill Livingstone; 2002. pp. 189-217

[37] Chan A, Heck C. The effects of tilting the seat position of a wheelchair on respiration, posture, fatigue, voice volume, and exertion outcomes in individuals with advanced multiple sclerosis. Journal of Rehabilitation Outcomes Measurement. 1999;**3**(4):1-14

[38] Kheder A, Nair KPS. Spasticity: Pathophysiology, evaluation and management. Practical Neurology. 2012; **12**(5):289-298

[39] Physicians. RCO: Spasticity in adults: Management using botulinum toxin. Royal College of Physicia. 2018

[40] Therapists CoO, Neurology AoCPi. Splinting for the Prevention and Correction of Contractures in Adults with Neurological Dysfunction: Practice Guideline for Occupational Therapists and Physiotherapists. London: College of Occupational Therapists Limited; 2015

[41] Braddom RL. Physical Medicine and Rehabilitation e-Book. Philadelphia: Elsevier Health Sciences; 2010

[42] Pashmdarfard M, Amini M. Effect of different types of splinting on spasticity and function of upper exterimity of Cva and CP patients: A systematic review. The Scientific Journal of Rehabilitation Medicine. 2017;**6**(1):254-263

[43] Chang E, Ghosh N, Yanni D, Lee S, Alexandru D, Mozaffar T. A review of spasticity treatments: Pharmacological and interventional approaches. Critical Reviews in Physical and Rehabilitation Medicine. 2013;**25**(1–2):11-22

[44] Shakespeare D, Boggild M, Young CA. Anti-spasticity agents for multiple sclerosis. Cochrane Database of Systematic Reviews. 2003;**4**:CD001332

[45] Kamen L, Henney HR 3rd, Runyan JD. A practical overview of tizanidine use for spasticity secondary to multiple sclerosis, stroke, and spinal cord injury. Current Medical Research and Opinion. 2008;**24**(2):425-439

[46] Haslam RH, Walcher J, Lietman P, Kallman C, Mellits E. Dantrolene sodium in children with spasticity. Archives of Physical Medicine and Rehabilitation. 1974;**55**(8):384-388

[47] Ketel WB, Kolb ME. Long-term treatment with dantrolene sodium of stroke patients with spasticity limiting the return of function. Current Medical Research and Opinion. 1984;**9**(3): 161-169

[48] Katrak PH, Cole AM, Poulos CJ, McCauley JC. Objective assessment of spasticity, strength, and function with early exhibition of dantrolene sodium after cerebrovascular accident: A randomized double-blind study. Archives of Physical Medicine and Rehabilitation. 1992;**73**(1):4-9

[49] Mueller ME, Gruenthal M, Olson WL, Olson WH. Gabapentin for relief of upper motor neuron symptoms in multiple sclerosis. Archives of Physical Medicine and Rehabilitation. 1997;**78**(5):521-524

[50] Formica A, Verger K, Sol J, Morralla C. Gabapentin for spasticity: A randomized, double-blind, placebo-controlled trial. Medicina Clinica. 2005; **124**(3):81-85

[51] Furr-Stimming E, Boyle AM, Schiess MC. Spasticity and intrathecal baclofen. In: Seminars in Neurology.

Thieme Medical Publishers; 2014. pp. 591-596

[52] Anwar F, Antiga S, Mee H, Al Khayer A. Management of spasticity with intrathecal phenol injections: The past and the present. The Journal of the International Society of Physical and Rehabilitation Medicine. 2019;**2**(2):94

Chapter 6

Spasticity and Dystonia: A Brief Review

Vincenzo Cimino, Clara Grazia Chisari and Francesco Patti

Abstract

Spasticity and dystonia are two neurological conditions with a broad range of clinical manifestations that can emerge at any age. Although the spasticity and dystonia symptoms are caused by different pathophysiological mechanisms, both of them may cause functional impairment that contributes to a poor quality of life. Spasticity is characterised by a velocity-dependent increase in tonic stretch reflexes with exaggerated tendon jerks, resulting from hyperexcitability of the stretch reflex. It mostly occurs in disorders of the central nervous system (CNS) affecting the upper motor neurons, such as multiple sclerosis, amyotrophic lateral sclerosis, cerebrovascular diseases, cerebral palsy, traumatic brain injury, stroke, and spinal cord injury. Therapeutic options may combine, in various proportions, physical therapy, occupational therapy, self-rehabilitation, the use of orthoses and assistive devices, drug treatment, orthopaedic surgery, and neurosurgery. Dystonia is defined as a syndrome of involuntary movement that manifests as excessive muscle contractions that frequently cause twisting and repetitive movements or abnormal postures. It is often intensified or exacerbated by physical activity, and symptoms may progress into adjacent muscles. Dystonia has many different manifestations and causes, and many different treatment options are available. These options include physical and occupational therapy, oral medications, intramuscular injection of botulinum toxins, and neurosurgical interventions.

Keywords: spasticity, dystonia, treatments, oral drugs, rehabilitation

1. Introduction

According to Lance and colleagues, spasticity is a "...motor disorder characterised by a velocity dependent increase in the tonic stretch reflex with exaggerated tendon jerks, resulting from hyperexcitability of the stretch reflex, as one component of the upper motor neuron syndrome..." [1]. Over time, the interest of clinicians on spasticity has increased more and more, topics ranging from pathophysiology to clinical relevance and treatment options [2–8].

However, in everyday management of patients' spasticity symptoms, much more complex situation would be there, full of clinical problems. In fact, other positive and/or negative signs may be observed together with increased muscle tone and deep tendon reflexes. Abnormal cutaneous reflexes, spasms, co-contraction, Babinski reflex, and also dystonia, are described as positive phenomena, and weakness, fatigability, and reduced dexterity are considered negative ones. In clinical practice each problem that we have to treat may have different pathophysiological explanations [9]. A central nervous system lesion determines the upper motor neuron syndrome, induced by an interruption of descending pathways, which connect the highest centres to the spinal cord. Alternatively, reactivity of spinal cord circuits may be modified by a direct damage, through a different way to elaborate the input from peripheral afferents. It is important to differentiate immediate to delayed consequences of damage to the highest centres in the CNS. The delayed consequences lead to a rearrangement of reactivity in spinal cord circuits, in which it is considered a basis of spasticity. Moreover, spasticity may itself be modified by the consequences of paresis and immobilisation, i.e. development of contractures. Several pathophysiological mechanisms may explain the development of spasticity due to CNS lesions. These mainly include defective inhibition, such as postsynaptic inhibition of alpha motor neurons or presynaptic inhibition of 1a afferents. There is also a defective excitation of inhibitory interneurons underlying reciprocal inhibition, autogenetic inhibition, or recurrent inhibition [10].

Dystonia is defined as a neurological disorder characterised by sustained or intermittent muscle contractions, determining unusual movements and postures or both. Typically dystonic movements are patterned and twisting and may be tremulous. Often, dystonic movements may be started by voluntary action, worsening with typically an overflow muscle activation (Consensus 2013) [11]. Dystonia classification is based on clinical characteristics and aetiology. Indeed, except for hereditary forms, dystonic syndromes may be caused by birth-related or other physical trauma, infection, and poisoning or due to pharmacological treatments, particularly neuroleptics. The clinical characteristics include age at onset, temporal pattern, body distribution, and coexistence of other movement disorders. The etiologic characteristics are the presence or absence of nervous system pathology and the pattern of inheritance [11].

Focal dystonia is a neurologic movement disorder, due to an incorrect sensorimotor modulation, determining involuntary, excessive muscle contractions. Writer's cramp is a specific type of focal dystonia that affects the fingers, hand, or forearm. Writer's cramp is a task-specific dystonia, characterised by hands twisting into odd postures. A specific task induces this sign. Other skilled task-specific movements may induce focal hand dystonia, such as playing a musical instrument, typing, or sewing. Writer's cramp is known also as musician's cramp, focal hand dystonia, arm dystonia, finger dystonia, task-specific dystonia, and occupational cramp or dystonia.

Task-specific dystonia like writer's cramp may appear in anyone. It usually appears between 30 and 50 years of age. Task-specific dystonia, particularly musician's cramp, is more common in men.

Two types of writer's cramp could be described:

1. Simple writer's cramp, which appears only during writing. The abnormal postures spring up soon after you pick up a pen. So, it only affects the ability to write.

2. Dystonic writer's cramp appears not only during writing but also during other activities with your hands, like shaving, dressing, or applying makeup.

Probably, repetitive movements determine a remapping of the brain's sensorimotor areas. Bad posture of the hands while holding a pen or pencil associated with overuse seems to cause simple writer's cramp. Dystonic writer's cramp is less common than simple ones and may represent a symptom of generalised dystonia. In this case, the involuntary movements can appear also during other non-writing tasks, such as using a fork or handwashing. Rarely, writer's cramp could be the early onset of a generalised dystonia, which is associated with the DYT1 gene [12].

1.1 Pathophysiology of spasticity and dystonia syndromes

Typically, spasticity is considered as a specific "pyramidal" sign; nevertheless, selective lesions of the primary motor cortex or corticospinal tract often induce hypotonia, deficit, or weakness in distal movements, without inducing spasticity [4]. Only the involvement of non-primary motor areas (premotor and supplementary areas) and the corticoreticulospinal fibres together with cortical lesions may induce spasticity. Corticoreticulospinal fibres sends through the dorsolateral reticulospinal tract descending just anteriorly to the corticospinal tract, a massive bilateral inhibitory projection to spinal motor neurons, which are located in the lateral funiculus of the spinal cord. So the fact that a selective lesion of the anterior limb or the genu of the internal capsula predominantly induces spasticity without an evident motor deficit and vice versa can be explained by the different courses of corticoreticular and corticospinal fibres in the internal capsula. Hence, a lesion involving the corticoreticulospinal fibres will lead to a decreased inhibition (or to an increased facilitation) of the spinal cord and ultimately to spasticity [13, 14]. Three fundamental phenomena occur after a lesion to the central motor pathways assigned to motor command execution:

1. *Paresis:* the quantitative lack of command directed to agonist muscles when attempting to generate force or movement.

2. *Soft tissue contracture and contractile muscle property changes:* shortened position induced by immobilisation due to paresis, causing soft tissue and muscle alterations. [13].

3. *Muscle overactivity:* as a consequence of corticospinal pathway lesion, which causes loss of motor command, brainstem descending pathways are activated. Most of these brainstem descending pathways tend to be constantly active, as a consequence a constant muscle activity is maintained. Releasing of growth factors locally is induced in the spinal cord level by the lack of regular descending excitation to the lower motor neurons. So these phenomena induce local sprouting from neighbouring interneurons, creating perfect conditions in order to synthetise new abnormal synapse network, leading to the creation of new abnormal reflex pathways [8, 9].

1.2 Spasticity

Among these changes, which gradually develop, spasticity represents the principal sign detectable. A simple definition of spasticity is an *increase in velocity-dependent stretch reflexes* [9, 10] which can be evoked at rest by muscle stretch or tendon taps.

Principal key points:

- A tonic stretch reflex.

- Mediated by type 1a fibre nerve, predominantly in the muscle spindle. Passive muscle stretch induces exciting of muscle spindle, which sends sensory input back to the spinal cord through monosynaptic way principally but also oligo- and polysynaptic reflexes, which at the end induce an efferent impulse to the muscle, causing contraction.

- Velocity-dependent.
- Length-dependent.

1.3 Spastic dystonia

The term "spastic dystonia" was coined by Denny-Brown in 1966 to define tonic-chronic muscle activity that is present in a spasticity pattern, during rest [15]. Thus, spastic dystonia could be described as a spontaneous overactivity at rest, not induced by a primary triggering factor [14–16]. It is easy to recognise it in patients with spastic paresis, as spastic dystonia causes specific bad postures in joints and body. For example, in the upper limb, the shoulder can stay internally rotated and adducted with a flexed and pronated elbow and flexed wrist and fingers. Equinovarus deformity represents a specific spastic dystonia in the lower limb, and it is characterised by plantar flexors and/or toe flexors, which may be painful and disabling during walking.

1.4 Spastic co-contraction

Spastic co-contraction is defined as an "unwanted, excessive, level of antagonistic muscle activity during voluntary command on an agonist muscle, which is aggravated by tonic stretch in the co-contracting muscle" [13]. Spastic co-contraction in spasticity pattern is a descending phenomenon, most probably due to misdirection of the supraspinal drive. It may be caused by loss of reciprocal inhibition during voluntary command [9, 10]. So, voluntary command of an agonist muscle is the first step, which induces spastic co-contraction. In patients with good or fairly good motor control, spastic co-contraction is certainly the most disabling form of muscle overactivity, because it obstacles muscle physiological muscle voluntary recruitment.

1.5 Clinical evaluation

1.5.1 Passive range of motion

For each movement evaluated, the corresponding muscles and joints are stretched at a very slow speed, in order to keep below the threshold for eliciting a stretch reflex. The angle at which soft tissue offers a maximum resistance is defined as the passive range of motion for that joint [17].

1.5.2 Angle of catch or clonus and spasticity grade

For each movement evaluated, the clinician should stretch the corresponding muscles and joints as fast as possible for the examiner. The spasticity grade is determined by the joint angle at which catch or clonus appears, according to Tardieu scale [18].

1.5.3 Active range of motion

For each passive movement evaluated at first, the clinician asks the patient to carry out an active movement at maximal range, until the active movement produced by the agonist muscles is contrasted by the passive resistance together with the spastic co-contraction of antagonist ones. This angle measure is the effective active range of motion [18].

1.5.4 Outcome measure

Tardieu score is a scale realised to measure spasticity that evaluates resistance to passive movement at both slow and fast speed. Individuals are evaluated both in in sit and supine position. There are two types of measures:

1. Quality of muscle reaction.

2. Angle of muscle reaction.

The quality of muscle reaction is scored as follows (range 0–4):

0. No resistance throughout the course of the passive movement.

1. Slight resistance throughout the course of the passive movement, followed by release.

2. Clear catch at precise angle, interrupting the passive movement, followed by release.

3. Fatigable clonus (<10 seconds when maintaining pressure) occurring at precise angle.

4. Infatigable clonus (>10 seconds when maintaining pressure) occurring at precise angle.

In order to consider joint angle, speed movement has to be defined:

- V1 is slow as possible.
- V2 speed of limb falling under gravity.
- V3 moving as fast as possible.

Regarding the joint angle, modified Tardieu describes:

- R1 as the angle of muscle reaction.
- R2 as the full PROM.

The angle of full ROM (R2) is defined at a very slow speed (V1). The angle of muscle reaction (R1) is detected when a catch or clonus appears during a quick stretch (V3) [19].

Ashworth scale, original version (1964), is a test which quantifies resistance to passive movement, with respect to a joint and with varying degrees of velocity. Scores range from 0 to 4:

0. No increase in tone.

1. Slight increase in tone giving a catch when the limb was moved in flexion or extension.

2. More marked increase in tone but limb easily flexed.

3. Considerable increase in tone, passive movement difficult.

4. Limb rigid, sometimes fixed in flexion or extension.

The modified Ashworth scale (Bohannon & Smith, 1987) is similar to the original one, except for a 1+ scoring category to indicate resistance through less than half of the movement [20].

2. Treatment options of spasticity

2.1 Indications for treatment

It's demonstrated that burden of care is higher in neurological patients who developed spasticity than that of those without it, in particular regarding treatment costs, quality of life, caregiver burden, and the effects of comorbidities [21]. The treatment of muscle overactivity may be considered when the condition is disabling. Muscle overactivity usually impairs motor command, so this itself justifies the treatment. Moreover, independently from the aetiological context, it contributes to impair patient's function [22]. Nevertheless, not all patients with muscle overactivity need a specific treatment. Treatment in spasticity should be carried out only after rigorous clinical analysis, in order to determine the severity of functional impairment. A multidisciplinary approach is necessary in order to obtain this specific assessment, being different according to patient's clinical condition; it may include variably physician, physical therapist, occupational therapist, nurse, and/or caregiver [22]. In order to obtain an individual, task-oriented therapeutic strategy, it is necessary to analyse a list of personal measurable objectives, which may be different for each patient. The clinical follow-up is required in order to show the benefits as well as adverse events. Muscle spasticity, which usually is responsive to drug treatment, is not the only motor impairment in spastic paresis. It is necessary also that physiotherapy is associated to drug treatment, in order to obtain maximum gain in paresis. For example, stretch programmes can be used to treat soft tissue shortening. Therefore, before treatment, the following three questions must be answered:

- Is muscle overactivity handicap an activity of daily living? Only after a detailed analysis of the functional impairment induced by spasticity, it is possible to carry out an appropriate treatment, which could be really effective to improve patient's quality of life.

- Is disability caused by muscle spasticity, or is it only a comorbidity? In the latter case, which components are involved? It is important to specify the quality of motor control and weakness. If motor impairment is induced or worsened by muscle overactivity, its treatment is to be considered mandatory, in order to be helpful to the patient [23].

- Does muscle overactivity involve one specific muscle group, or does it spread to other? The correct therapeutic approach depends on the answer.

Pharmacological interventions for spasticity can be divided into two groups: those that act systemically and those that act locally [24] with the locally acting treatments tending to be more invasive, systemically acting drugs used as a first step [24]. If a systematic approach, which includes baclofen, tizanidine, or dantrolene, is not successful, local treatment is allowed [25], such as muscle botulinum toxin (BTX) injection or peripheral neurolytic blockade with alcohol or phenol [26]. Surgery is to be considered as the final treatment option; however, it is rarely used. If the principal aim is to inhibit neurotransmitter activity at one or more sites within the central nervous system, a systemic approach with specific drugs is to be evaluated. Targeted therapy could regard pre- or postsynaptic sites in spinal interneurons (at varying levels of the upper motor neuron pathway), alpha motor neurons, as well as primary sensory afferent neurons. So, the central nervous system is influenced by inhibitory effects of the neurotransmitters [27]. Oral administration needs high drug dose in order to cross the blood–brain barrier; therefore, side effects like dizziness could occur. In order to reduce the probability for these negative effects, it is possible to introduce some drugs directly into the cerebrospinal fluid, for example, by an intrathecal pump. For drugs used peripherally via injection directly to the nerve or muscle, systemic side effects are fewer.

2.2 Physical therapy

Physiotherapy is the basic treatment for all patients with spasticity [28, 29]. It may help limit muscle contractures and reduce overactivity for a short period. Physiotherapy together with drug treatment is fundamental to obtain the best functional gain, in order to help patients adapt to changes. In all cases, physiotherapy must be considered as complementary to drugs and surgery. In fact, stretching is considered an import goal in a physiotherapy session, as largely demonstrated [30]. Functional electrical stimulation allows spasticity reduction in antagonists of the stimulated muscles. An interesting use of electrical stimulation is the stimulation of hand and finger extensors during prehension training and mixing of overactive flexor inhibition with extensor activation [31]. Finally, it is important to educate patient in self-rehabilitation sessions comprehensive of stretching postures and active exercises, eventually assisted by caregivers and/or orthoses.

2.3 Oral drugs

Pharmacologic approaches emphasise oral drugs, neuromuscular blocks, and intrathecal agents. Usually, antispastic therapy is initiated with oral drugs, even though adverse side effects are frequently reported as a systematic effect [32]. Treatment decisions on specific pharmacologic approach are influenced by chronicity, severity, and localisation of spasticity. It was demonstrated that pharmacologic treatments are most effective if used early, in order to avoid muscle shortening and contracture development [33]. However, the time to treat is the first problem to resolve, in particular for drugs. Correctly, spasticity treatment is recommended when it induces a significant functional impairment, in particular regarding daily living activities, or clinical disability such as bad posture, motor capacity, or nursing. When spasticity is diffusely distributed above all in lower limbs, often observed as a consequence of spinal lesions, its treatment is firstly indicated, than in cerebral lesions.

The general goal of medical treatment is to decrease spinal reflex excitability by reducing the release of excitatory neurotransmitters or by potentiating the activity of inhibitory circuits. In clinical practice it is important to differentiate objectives in giving spasticity drugs. The technical objectives are focused to induce tone reduction, in order to increase range of motion or ameliorating joint position and promote rehabilitative procedures. Nevertheless, we also have functional therapeutic objectives regarding gait improvement, daily living activity, self-care, and spasm and pain reduction. When we evaluate the real effectiveness of different drug approaches, it is important to differentiate these therapeutic objectives. In order to achieve these therapeutic goals, most of the drugs currently used in spasticity influence the activity of the CNS neurotransmitters. Inhibitory neurotransmitters (GABA or glycine), as well as excitatory neurotransmitters (glutamate or the monoamines), are the main target. Diazepam, baclofen, tizanidine, and dantrolene represent the principal drugs more frequently used.

2.3.1 Diazepam

Diazepam, probably the first and oldest drug used in treating spasticity [34, 35], is a GABA-A receptor agonist. Its binding, to GABA-A receptors diffused in the brainstem and spinal cord, acts in increasing presynaptic inhibition. Consequently, reduction in the resistance to stretch is the principal clinical effect, showing an objectively increasing range of motion. Other clinical effects are also a reduction of deep tendon stretch reflexes and painful spasms [36]. Nevertheless, significant side effects are to be considered. The depressant effect of the drug on the CNS is the principal side effect, causing an influence on cognitive-level, consciousness status, leading to sedation, drowsiness, and attention or memory impairment. The same physiological mechanism explains weakness and motor discoordination caused by diazepam. Tolerance or dependency phenomena are often observed [37, 38]. Spasticity caused by spinal cord lesion, above all incomplete ones like in patients with multiple sclerosis (MS), is the principal indication to use diazepam, since the drug binding is mainly in the brainstem. Less literature are available for the use of diazepam in spasticity caused by cerebral accident, such as traumatic brain injuries, cerebral palsy, and stroke. In literature, a double-blind protocol is available showing the antispastic efficacy of diazepam, only in spinal cord lesions [39]. However, a possible strength and gait deterioration was also shown consistently in placebo-controlled studies.

2.3.2 Gabapentin

Gabapentin is approved as an antiepileptic drug. It is indicated also for postherpetic neuralgia treatment and as add-on therapy in partial seizures. GABA-B receptors are its target. Moreover, it is quietly safe. In a prospective, double-blind, placebo-controlled, crossover study, conducted on multiple sclerosis patients, a statistically significant reduction of spasticity was shown in gabapentin-treated patients compared to placebo [40]. The most efficient and safe dose range is still an open question. A dose range between 2700 and 3600 mg/day, as therapy for spasticity due to upper motor neuron syndrome, was found as efficient and safe. However, doses of 400 mg orally three times a day, in another double-blind, placebo-controlled crossover study, were shown to be effective in the treatment of spasticity and muscle painful cramps in patients with MS [41]. Nevertheless, considering the magnitude of the effect and the good tolerability of the drug, the evidence is on a weak recommendation for using gabapentin to reduce spasticity in MS [42].

2.3.3 Oral baclofen

Baclofen is another common drug diffusely used in spasticity. This drug is a GABA-B receptor agonist. Its physiological effect is a suppression of excitatory neurotransmitter release and, as a consequence, a potentiation of presynaptic inhibition. The main clinical effects are related mainly to the reduction in flexor-extensor spasms and mono- and polysynaptic reflexes. Obviously, related to its mechanism of action, this drug may induce dose-dependent side effects, quite similar to those seen with diazepam [43], although less frequent and less severe. However, sedation, confusion, dizziness, drowsiness, fatigue, and ataxia have been described as the common side effects observed in baclofen studies. Spasticity due to spinal cord lesions is the main indication to treat with baclofen. Unfortunately, in literature, there are very little studies focused on functional changes, so as a consequence, there is no evidence for effectiveness on functional activities such as gait, ambulation, or daily living activities. Moreover, also for oral baclofen, a weak recommendation for treatment of spasticity in MS has been shown [42]. It's notable that there is no evidence of significant differences between diazepam, tizanidine, and oral baclofen, regarding therapeutic effects on spasticity [43, 44].

2.3.4 Tizanidine

Tizanidine, an imidazole derivative approved for the treatment of patients with spasticity [45], acts as an alpha-2 agonist, both in the spinal and supraspinal level. Presynaptic activity reduction of the excitatory interneurons represents the main physiological effect of this treatment. The coeruleo-spinal pathway, because of its involvement in the control of spinal cord activities, was shown as the main target in order to induce clinical effect during tizanidine treatment [46]. Consequently, reduction in tonic and stretch polysynaptic reflexes can be observed. Because of co-contraction reduction, which is observed, a possible effect on reciprocal inhibition is questionable. Possible side effects include sedation, dizziness, and dry mouth. Nevertheless, with respect to diazepam or baclofen, weakness is not reported as a great problem [47]. From the literature, the indications for its use are mainly in spasticity due to spinal cord lesions [48]. It has been particularly used in multiple sclerosis patients [49]. In spasticity caused by cerebral lesions, its efficacy is less well documented in literature. However, there are a certain number of reports regarding its antispastic efficacy, also in controlled studies vs. placebo. In the treatment of spasticity due to cerebral lesions, there are some evidences of its greater efficacy than diazepam [47]. However, there is very little information about the possible functional changes resulting from this treatment, i.e. quality of life and self-care. In fact, although it has been shown to have an antispastic effect, we do not know whether this will translate into long-term functional benefit for the patients. In clinical practice, tizanidine is usually well-tolerated. Drowsiness and dry mouth are the most common although are rare side effects. A range of 24–36 mg is normally the therapeutic dose (20% mean reduction in muscle tone), usually divided in three daily doses [50]. Like oral baclofen and diazepam, there is a consensus for a weak recommendation for the use of tizanidine [42].

2.3.5 Dantrolene

Among the oral dugs, dantrolene is the only one which acts outside the central nervous system [51]. It acts on the inhibition of calcium release from the sarcoplasmic reticulum, so, as a final effect, it reduces in muscle the excitation-coupling reaction between actin and myosin fibres. The documented clinical effects are a reduction of muscle tone and phasic reflexes, reduction of spasm, and an increased range of passive motion. Unfortunately, a frequent occurrence of side effects is described with this drug, such as gastrointestinal symptoms, weakness, and sedation although this is less than that seen with other treatments. Over all, a serious side effect with the use of dantrolene is hepatotoxicity, which occurs frequently [51]. In patients with spasticity due to cerebral lesions, dantrolene is the only drug with evidence of efficacy, so from a pure clinical point of view, this is very disappointing. In fact, dantrolene in approved in patients with stroke, cerebral palsy, traumatic brain injuries, and spinal cord lesions. As shown for baclofen, also for dantrolene, there are many evidences of efficacy and safety of its antispastic effect proven vs. placebo, but no studies focused on functional changes in activities of daily living. It's notable that dantrolene is also used to prevent muscle stiffness and spasms caused by malignant hyperthermia (a rapid rise in body temperature and severe muscle contractions) that can occur during surgery with certain types of anaesthesia [52].

2.3.6 Cannabinoids

It is known, from many evidences, that the psychoactive ingredient in cannabis, delta-9-tetrahydrocannabinol (delta-9-THC), is able to treat muscle spasticity and pain. Two types of cannabinoid receptors can be described: CB1 and CB2. CB1s are located both in the central and peripheral neurons. CB1 and CB2 receptors are equally activated by delta-9-THC, a cannabinoid receptor agonist [53, 54]. On the contrary, cannabidiol, a natural cannabinoid, is inactive on the CB1 receptor. Some studies reported that cannabis extracts, containing approximately equal concentrations of delta-9-THC and cannabidiol administered through sublingual way, can significantly reduce spasticity. During the last years, several studies investigated and argued on the efficacy and safety of oral cannabinoid administration in MS patients as an add-on treatment for spasticity. A multicentre, double-blind, placebo-controlled trial showed that in MS spasticity treatment, cannabinoid may help to treat MS-related spasticity and pain [53]. However, according to the results from clinical trials, it is not allowed to use cannabinoids in MS as a general use. In a recent study, 630 MS patients affected by muscle spasticity were randomised to be treated with oral delta-9-THC, cannabis extract, or placebo for up to 12 months. The results showed a controversial effect; in fact, there was a small treatment effect on muscle spasticity and disability as functional independence measure, but patients' sensation was that these drugs were helpful in treating their disease [54]. Adverse side effects are generally mild, in particular dry mouth, somnolence, dizziness, nausea, and rarely intoxication. However, there is a need of longer-term studies to evaluate other, well-known, adverse side effects of cannabinoid such as risks of lung cancer and other respiratory dysfunctions. A recent multicentre observational study confirmed the efficacy and safety of delta-9-THC in clinical practice, as an effective and safe option for patients with MS with moderate to severe spasticity resistant to common antispastic drugs [55]. In a recent consensus, a significant recommendation for the use of cannabinoids in spasticity emerged, particularly for oromucosal spray nabiximols, as treatment of spasticity in MS; the strength of the recommendation is strong [42].

2.4 Botulinum toxin

BTX type A is considered as the first-line treatment of multifocal muscle overactivity, thanks to its better efficacy and safety profile with respect to systemic approach with drugs. Different from baclofen or tizanidine, the efficacy of BTX type A has been demonstrated in self-care improvement (in particular for washing and dressing) and in active movements for the leg, with gait improvement if possible. Except for using kinematic analysis, no improvement was possibly shown in active movement or function in the upper limb. Pain was also reduced by BTX treatment as demonstrated in literature. Four forms of BTX are currently available in Europe: three type As (BOTOX®, Allergan; Dysport®, Ipsen-Pharma; Xeomin®, Merz) and one type B (Neurobloc®, Elan-Pharma). It is absolutely recommended to keep in mind that the units of these four toxins are different, being specific for each one. Injection sites are better detected, using electrical stimulation, as anatomical markers alone may induce to an inaccurate target. The use of ultrasound guidance, particularly in children, in identifying muscle site injection, is an interesting study object; however, this technique has not been evaluated with respect to electrical stimulation guidance for its efficiency. Generally, there are no immediate postinjection complications (except for a little pain as a side effect related to injection itself). Above all, during the first 3 weeks after each injection treatment, there would be a low risk of adverse events (swallowing disorders and botulism-like syndrome), so patients and caregivers must be warned as well as encouraged to eventually consult if necessary. The effects of treatment could be assessed 1–6 weeks after the injection, based on personalised goals decided before treatment. The effect of the toxin is not permanent, so repeated injections are often needed; nevertheless, a long-lasting effect is also observed. No repeated treatment is recommended without a specific assessment. When and if needed according to functional evaluation, a minimum delay of 2–3 months between injections must be respected, in order to reduce the risk of an immunologic reaction that may induce a permanent inefficacy of subsequent treatments. Each subsequent treatment should be planned after an accurate functional evaluation according to the pre-therapeutic identified goals and task, as well as tolerance. So, a review of the dose and treated muscles could be scheduled. If therapeutic effects continue to be evident, repeated injections can be planned [33, 56–60]. Physical therapy has to be considered after BOTOX injections. Regarding maximum doses, according to European Consensus, it should be considered:

- Per session: 1500 MU Dysport® 600 U BOTOX®.
- Per site: 125 MU Dysport® 50 U BOTOX®.

It is notable that these dosages are identified relatively to acceptable side effects, in order to be safe. Moreover, each product could be effective with different doses for each patient, in terms of both efficacy and safety [61]. As well as the cannabinoid, there is a strong recommendation of the use of BTX to reduce muscle tone in spasticity do to multiple sclerosis [42].

2.5 Alcohol and phenol

Localised and loco-regional spasticity may effectively be treated by selective neurolysis. Coagulation and denaturing of proteins induced by phenol perineurally injected lead to cellular and axonal damage. Unfortunately, this chemical denervation is irreversible; moreover, the effects of phenol are not selective because also vascular and sensory structures can be destroyed [62]. In fact, the main recommendation choosing this approach is to identify preferably the nerves to be treated with a low sensory activity and a high motor predominance (i.e. obturator or musculocutaneous nerves, etc.). However, this focal treatment is usually not used as a first-line therapy, except in the case of particularly problematic overactivity affecting a big area under a single motor nerve control, for example, musculocutaneous nerve for biceps brachii muscle or obturator nerve for thigh adductor muscles. This may allow to use in the same patient BTX to treat other muscles, without the risk of an overdose. Electrical stimulation is used to identify a nerve, in order to perform injection on it. Firstly, a transient motor block may be a plan, in order to evaluate if chemical neurolysis might be significantly effective and safe. In fact, the efficacy and/or advantages eventually deriving from alcohol or phenol treatment could be evaluated before, in particular with respect to surgery (above all, tissue fibrosis induced by alcohol or phenol, which may hamper surgery approach). Advantages are the low cost and the long duration of effect. In clinical practice, 5–7% concentrations of phenol in aqueous solution are administered.

2.6 Intrathecal baclofen

Intrathecal baclofen (ITB) is a long-term treatment with continuous, intraspinal administration via an implanted pump that reduces spasticity, especially in spinal injury patients and in multiple sclerosis [63, 64]. For this reason, ITB has become the first choice in intractable generalised spasticity, especially when oral administration fails to be effective. ITB efficacy in reducing spasticity was demonstrated by several studies [65]. Through direct infusion into the cerebrospinal fluid, the baclofen can be concentrated regionally, avoiding liver metabolism, so it is totally available for its therapeutic effects. In fact, with respect to oral baclofen administration, the ITB, bypassing the blood–brain barrier entirely, needs much lower dose in order to obtain the same CSF concentrations; it has been determined that the ITB dose is 100–1000 times smaller than the oral daily dose. Depending on the pump model, it is possible to modify infusion rate, according to the patient's needs. In several studies ITB was shown as safe and effective in reducing spasticity. The complication rate was found to be low, and the efficacy was maintained over time [64]. A reduction in the Ashworth scale from 3 to 4 to 1 after ITB implantation was reported in several studies. Also spasm frequency significantly decreased. Some activities of daily living, in particular the ability to sit in a wheelchair and nursing care, improved after ITB implant. In some cases, authors showed that patients with less severe disability experienced an improvement in the ability to transfer, thanks to ITB effect [66]. Side effects, such as vertigo, nausea, nystagmus, dysmetria, mouth dryness, headache, amnesia, bladder, and sexual dysfunction, have been described in about 4% of patients and mainly are not life-threatening. As a red flag, it is notable that concerning gastrointestinal function, ITB could affect peristalsis, which could be severely slowed down to paralytic ileus. Nevertheless, constipation has previously been reported as an infrequent ITB-induced adverse effect, ranging from 3 to 10% of treated patients [67], rarely leading to death [68]. Therefore, recognition of constipation in patients treated with ITB is very important, not only because constipation is a possible side effect, being reported in some study, but also because it may be also a life-threatening complication. ITB has been used in patients with leg diffuse muscle overactivity. This type of treatment should be used above all in patients, in which muscle overactivity impaired posture, nursing, and personal independence or causes pain [63]. Several assessments are required before planning a definite pump implantation, performing drug test injection via lumbar puncture or via a temporary access device. Efficacy may be evaluated during the following 3–4 h. The first test dose is usually recommended up to 50 μg in adults, picking up gradually to a maximum dose of 150 μg, eventually reached after 3 days. A risk of overdose should be always evaluated, in particular regarding the effects on consciousness level and respiratory disorders. So, a specialised medical team is needed in order to monitor patient after and during the 4 h following the test. Only after the end of this test, if the treatment has been well-tolerated and effective, the team may make the decision to implant the pump. It is important to monitor the patient during the entire follow-up period, in order to prevent and/or detect collateral effects related to the procedure (displacement and/or obstruction of the catheter, infection, etc.), which may induce a serious withdrawal syndrome. ITB is often recommended for the treatment of spasticity, with a strong evidence of efficacy [42].

2.7 Surgery

Surgery may play an important role in the treatment of chronic muscle overactivity or for the after-effects induced by spasticity that become functional impairments (e.g. irreducible equinovarus foot), but it is not the first-line treatment. Because of its potential adverse events and its definite effects, surgical techniques should be reserved only in selected patients in order to reach different goals: hygiene, standing, transferring, walking, and the use of assistive devices. It involves neurosurgery and orthopaedic surgery. Surgical procedures may include one or more of the techniques described below. Peripheral neurotomy may include partial or segmental resection of a motor nerve, involving spastic muscles. In order to balance agonists and antagonists overlapping the muscle activity, a selective peripheral neurotomy is recommended to maintain a "functional" muscle tone. Collateral branches of the posterior tibial nerves and obturator nerves are commonly the main targets for the legs (e.g. ankle clonus, equinus, inversion of the foot). For the arms, neurotomy of the musculocutaneous, median, and ulnar nerves showed good results regarding efficacy and safety [69]. Other surgery techniques, such as rhizotomies, although used, have potential collateral effects and complications [70]. Musculoskeletal surgery, performed on the muscle or the tendon itself, aims to treat spasticity consequences, such as contracture and joint deformities. Tendon transfers (e.g. *tibialis* anterior) and lengthening are conservative treatments commonly proposed [69]. Tenotomy may be considered in the case of muscle contracture without active functional objectives [69]. Hip displacements and foot deformities induced by severe spasticity may be sometimes treated with osteotomies [69]. Arthrodesis may be the only solution to stabilise joints, notably ankle and foot joints in case of severe paresis associated with strong muscle overactivity and hypoesthesia [69].

3. Treatment options of dystonia

3.1 Indications of treatment

Treatment options of the management of dystonia include pharmacological therapies, injections, and surgical interventions. The main pharmacological therapies are anticholinergics (particularly trihexyphenidyl), baclofen, benzodiazepines (particularly clonazepam), and dopamine-related medications. However, medical therapy in dystonia is largely empiric and at times may seem anecdotal. Three main neurotransmitter systems are involved: cholinergic generally acting as antagonist at postsynaptic M1 receptor, GABAergic-like baclofen, and dopaminergic systems. Dopaminergic treatments can be divided into two: levodopa and dopamine reducing medications like presynaptic dopamine depleters such as tetrabenazine and postsynaptic dopamine-blocking agents, such as clozapine or neuroleptics. The therapeutic strategy, carried out by Fahn [71], is to "start low and go slow": medications should be started at a low dose and upped slowly to the lowest effective dose, in order to reduce symptoms without side effects. The rate of titration may depend on age: every 3–4 days in children, compared to every 1 week in adults. A combination approach is used when monotherapy achieves a "good" dose, but symptom control is incomplete. The question is which medications should be started first?

3.2 Cholinergic system agents

In 1952, beneficial effects of trihexyphenidyl in writer's cramp and "dystonia musculorum deformans" were first reported [72, 73]. The first open-label study of high-dose anticholinergics in dystonia using trihexyphenidyl and ethopropazine was conducted by Fahn [71]. Various forms of dystonia, both "primary and secondary," can be treated with anticholinergics, except for tardive dystonia and Meige syndrome. Studies showed a good effect in 61% of the children and 38% of the adults, with mean trihexyphenidyl doses of 41 and 24 mg, respectively. More benefit was demonstrated in children, possibly due to better tolerability, and in patients who received treatment earlier, within 5 years of disease onset [74]. Several studies have demonstrated that anticholinergic drugs may be useful to treat various forms of dystonia including focal [75], cranial [76], and secondary dystonia including dystonia in cerebral palsy [74], after ischemic stroke [77], and in tardive dystonia [78]. Side effects can be divided into central ones, which include sedation, cognitive slowing, confusion, memory impairment, psychosis and chorea, and autonomic side effects, which include blurred vision, due to mydriasis, dry mouth, urinary retention, and constipation.

3.3 GABAergic system agents

Baclofen was reported to be useful in tardive dystonia [79]. Just in 1988, Greene published a retrospective open-label study, showing that 20% of 108 patients had benefits from baclofen at a mean daily dose of 82 mg [80]. Later, Greene and Fahn also reported beneficial effects of baclofen in 7 of 16 patients with idiopathic childhood dystonia [81]. ITB was tried initially for spasticity and later in dystonia [82]. In 1991 Narayan and colleagues showed the efficacy of ITB in axial dystonia not responding to other drugs [83] and subsequently in dystonic cerebral palsy with lower extremity involvement [84]. Albright reported the use of intraventricular baclofen in two patients with dystonic cerebral palsy, one of whom previously failed ITB therapy and the other has a complex spinal anatomy precluding the intrathecal procedure [85]. Nevertheless, baclofen is generally considered as a second-line agent, due to its significant side effects like drowsiness, dizziness, fatigue, and nausea. Regarding benzodiazepines, diazepam therapy was described in "dystonia musculorum deformans progressiva" and spasmodic torticollis [86]. In 1988, the benefit of clonazepam was shown by Greene in 16% of 115 patients with dystonia, also including secondary dystonia [80]. Also in acquired hemidystonia, as shown in a report of 33 patients, clonazepam and diazepam were found to be the most effective drugs. Clonazepam and diazepam are the two most commonly used drugs, partly due to their relatively long half-lives. The side effects of benzodiazepines include sedation, depression, nocturnal drooling, and behavioural disinhibition. Benzodiazepines are considered a second- or third-line agent.

3.4 Dopaminergic system agents

In 1976 Segawa firstly used levodopa as a treatment in dystonia, showing a dramatic response to low-dose levodopa in two patients affected by "hereditary progressive dystonia with marked diurnal fluctuations" [87], later named Segawa syndrome. In dystonia therapy, levodopa is used (1) as an aetiology-specific treatment in dopa responder dystonia and (2) as a symptomatic therapy in other forms of dystonia where the dramatic response to levodopa is unfortunately not replicated. Levodopa may also be used to treat dystonia symptoms which may complicate a parkinsonian syndrome [88]. In clinical practice, levodopa or dopamine agonists are rarely used to treat dystonia symptomatically. The side effects of levodopa include nausea, orthostatic hypotension, and psychosis. In 1972, Swash reported only a slight benefit of tetrabenazine in spasmodic torticollis [89]. In 1982, a double-blind crossover trial by Jankovic demonstrated an improvement in 11 of 12 patients [90].

Tetrabenazine has been used in various forms of dystonia; however, benefits are greater in tardive dystonia than that of the other forms [91]. Tetrabenazine is rarely used as a first-line agent, except in tardive dystonia [92].

4. Conclusions

Spasticity and dystonia syndromes and their consequences negatively impact the quality of life of patients, so management of symptoms represents an important care issue. The best choice of antispastic treatments depends not only on the level of spasticity but also on the outcome achievable, according to a task-oriented rehabilitation programme. In this respect, it is important to underline the importance of the individualised rehabilitative project, which can be carried out only through a multidisciplinary approach, in which all available options must be targeted to the real needs of the patients, keeping into account that the final goal is the reduction of disability and improvement of the quality of life. With advances in diagnosis and treatment, therapeutic strategies for the management of spasticity and dystonia symptoms, including pharmacological treatments, have evolved. Progresses in other areas such as BTX, neuromodulation, and disease-specific treatment have changed the way patients are treated. Nevertheless, dystonia remains a challenging field in both diagnostic and therapeutic aspects. Further understanding of its pathophysiology may shed light on more specific therapies. In conclusion, the management of spasticity and dystonia may include a proper diagnosis and classification with an evaluation of the aetiology underlying the pathological features and a clinical assessment of the functional impairment. For both conditions, therapeutic approaches, usually limited to symptomatic therapy, must then be tailored to the individual needs of the patient.

Conflict of interest

Vincenzo Cimino has received grants for congress participation from Biogen Idec, Merck Serono, Novartis, Roche, Sanofi Genzyme, and TEVA.

Clara Grazia Chisari has received grants for congress participation from Almirall, Biogen Idec, Merck Serono, Novartis, Roche, Sanofi Genzyme, and TEVA.

Francesco Patti has received honoraria for speaking activities by Almirall, Bayer Schering, Biogen Idec, Merck Serono, Novartis, Roche, Sanofi Genzyme, and TEVA; he also served as an advisory board member of the following companies: Bayer Schering, Biogen Idec, Merck Serono, Novartis, Roche, Sanofi Genzyme, and TEVA; he was also funded by Pfizer and FISM for epidemiological studies; he received grants for congress participation from Almirall, Bayer Schering, Biogen Idec, Merck Serono, Novartis, Roche, Sanofi Genzyme, and TEVA.

Author details

Vincenzo Cimino[1], Clara Grazia Chisari[2] and Francesco Patti[2]*

1 Centro Neurolesi "Bonino Pulejo", IRCSS, Messina, Italy

2 Department "G.F. Ingrassia", Section of Neuroscience, University of Catania, Catania, Italy

*Address all correspondence to: fpatti@outlook.com

References

[1] Lance JW. Symposium synopsis. In: Feldman RG, Young RR, Koella WP, editors. Spasticity: Disordered Motor Control. Chicago: Year Book Medical; 1980. pp. 485-494

[2] Cramer SC. Editorial comment – Spasticity after stroke: What's the catch? Stroke. 2004;**35**:139-140

[3] Levin MF. On the nature and measurement of spasticity. Clinical Neurophysiology. 2005;**116**:1754-1755

[4] Sunnerhagen KS. Stop using the Ashworth scale for the assessment of spasticity. Journal of Neurology, Neurosurgery, and Psychiatry. 2010;**81**:2

[5] Lorentzen J, Grey MJ, Crone C, Mazevet D, Biering-Sorensen F, Nielsen JB. Distinguishing active from passive components of ankle plantar flexor stiffness in stroke, spinal cord injury and multiple sclerosis. Clinical Neurophysiology. 2010;**121**(11):1939-1951

[6] Gracies JM. Pathophysiology of spastic paresis. I: Paresis and soft tissue changes. Muscle & Nerve. 2005;**31**:535-551

[7] Pandyan AD, Gregoric M, Barnes MP, Wood D, van WF WF, Burridge J, et al. Spasticity: Clinical perceptions, neurological realities and meaningful measurement. Disability and Rehabilitation. 2005;**27**:2-6

[8] Sheean G, McGuire JR. Spastic hypertonia and movement disorders: Pathophysiology, clinical presentation, and quantification. The Journal of Injury, Function and Rehabilitation. 2009;**1**:827-833

[9] Sheean G. The pathophysiology of spasticity. European Journal of Neurology. 2002;**3-9**(Suppl 1):53-61

[10] Gracies JM, Fitzpatrick R, Wilson L, Burke D, Gandevia SC. Lycra garments designed for patients with upper limb spasticity: Mechanical effects in normal subjects. Archives of Physical Medicine and Rehabilitation. 1997;**78**(10):1066-1071

[11] Albanese A, Bhatia K, Bressman SB, et al. Phenomenology and classification of dystonia: A consensus update. Movement Disorders. 2013;**28**:863

[12] Goldman JG. Writer's cramp. Toxicon. 2015;**107**(Pt A):98-104

[13] Mayer NH. Clinicophysiologic concepts of spasticity and motor dysfunction in adults with an upper motoneuron lesion. Muscle & Nerve. Supplement. 1997;**6**:S1-S13

[14] Mayer NH, Esquenazi A. Muscle overactivity and movement dysfunction in the upper motoneuron syndrome. Physical Medicine and Rehabilitation Clinics of North America. 2003;**14**(4):855-883

[15] Lorentzen J, Pradines M, Gracies JM, Bo NJ. On Denny-Brown's 'spasticdystonia'-what is it and what causes it? Clinical Neurophysiology. 2018;**129**(1):89-94

[16] Marinelli L, Currà A, Trompetto C, Capello E, Serrati C, Fattapposta F, et al. Spasticity and spastic dystonia: The two faces of velocity-dependent hypertonia. Journal of Electromyography and Kinesiology. 2017;**37**:84-89

[17] Bethoux F. Spasticity management after stroke. Physical Medicine and Rehabilitation Clinics of North America. 2015;**26**(4):625-639

[18] Morris SL, Williams G. A historical review of the evolution of the Tardieu scale. Brain Injury. 2018;**32**(5):665-669

[19] Ansari NN, Naghdi S, Hasson S, Azarsa MH, Azarnia S. The modified Tardieu scale for the measurement of elbow flexor spasticity in adult patients with hemiplegia. Brain Injury. 2008;**22**(13-14):1007-1012

[20] Bohannon RW, Smith MB. Interrater reliability of a modified Ashworth scale of muscle spasticity. Physical Therapy. 1987;**67**(2):206-207

[21] Esquenazi A. The human and economic burden of poststroke spasticity and muscle overactivity. Journal of Clinical Outcomes Management. 2011;**18**(1):34-44

[22] Barnes MP. Management of spasticity. Age and Ageing. 1998;**27**(2):239-245

[23] Sheean G. Botulinum toxin treatment of adult spasticity: A benefit-risk assessment. Drug Safety. 2006;**29**(1):31-48

[24] Gormley ME, O'Brien CF, Yablon SA. A clinical overview of treatment decisions in the management of spasticity. Muscle and Nerve. Supplement. 1997;**20**(S6):S14-S20

[25] Bogey RA, Geis CC, Bryant PR, Moroz A, O'Neill BJ. Stroke and neurodegenerative disorders. 3. Stroke: Rehabilitation management. Archives of Physical Medicine and Rehabilitation. 2004;**85**(3):S15-S20. S34-S40

[26] Kocabas H, Salli A, Demir AH, Ozerbil OM. Comparison of phenol and alcohol neurolysis of tibial nerve motor branches to the gastrocnemius muscle for treatment of spastic foot after stroke: A randomized controlled pilot study. European Journal of Physical and Rehabilitation Medicine. 2010;**46**(1):5-10

[27] Gracies JM, Nance P, Elovic E, McGuire J, Simpson DM. Traditional pharmacological treatments for spasticity. Part II: General and regional treatments. Muscle & Nerve. 1997;**20**(S6):S92-S120

[28] Yelnik AP, Simon O, Parratte B, Gracies JM. How to clinically assess and treat muscle overactivity in spastic paresis. Journal of Rehabilitation Medicine. 2010;**42**:801-807

[29] Watanabe T. The role of therapy in spasticity management. American Journal of Physical Medicine & Rehabilitation. 2004;**83**:s45-s49

[30] Veerbeek JM, van Wegen E, van Peppen R, van der Wees PJ, Hendriks E, Rietberg M, et al. What is the evidence for physical therapy poststroke? A systematic review and meta-analysis. PLoS One. 2014;**9**:e87987

[31] He YL, Gao Y, Fan BY. Effectiveness of neuromuscular electrical stimulation combined with rehabilitation training for treatment of post-stroke limb spasticity. Medicine (Baltimore). 2019;**98**(39):e17261

[32] Pappalardo A, Castiglione A, Restivo DA, Calabrese A, Cimino V, Patti F. Pharmacologic management of spasticity in multiple sclerosis. Neurological Sciences. 2006;**27**:S310-S315

[33] Ks S, Olver J, Francisco GE. Assessing and treating functional impairment in poststroke spasticity. Neurology. 2013;**80**:s35-s44

[34] DeJak JJ, Lowry R. Use of diazepam (valium) for spasticity in spinal cord injury. Proceedings of Annual Clinical Spinal Cord Injury Conference. 1964;**13**:78-81

[35] Simpson CA. Use of diazepam for the relief of spasticity in multiple sclerosis. Annals of Physical Medicine. 1964;(Suppl):39-40

[36] Verrier M, Ashby P, MacLeod S. Diazepam effect on reflex activity in patients with complete spinal lesions and in those with other causes of spasticity. Archives of Physical Medicine and Rehabilitation. 1977;**58**(4):148-153

[37] Waldman HJ. Centrally acting skeletal muscle relaxants and associated drugs. Journal of Pain and Symptom Management. 1994;**9**(7):434-441

[38] Broderick CP, Radnitz CL, Bauman WA. Diazepam usage in veterans with spinal cord injury. The Journal of Spinal Cord Medicine. 1997;**20**(4):406-409

[39] Corbett M, Frankel HL, Michaelis L. A double blind, cross-over trial of valium in the treatment of spasticity. Paraplegia. 1972;**10**(1):19-22

[40] Cutter NC, Scott DD, Johnson JC, Whiteneck G. Gabapentin effect on spasticity in multiple sclerosis: A placebo-controlled, randomized trial. Archives of Physical Medicine and Rehabilitation. 2000;**81**:164-169

[41] Formica A, Verger K, Sol JM, Morralla C. Gabapentin for spasticity: A randomized, double-blind, placebo-controlled trial. Medicina Clínica (Barcelona). 2005;**124**:81-85

[42] Comi G, Solari A, Leocani L, Centonze D, Otero-Romero S. Italian consensus group on treatment of spasticity in multiple sclerosis. Italian consensus on treatment of spasticity in multiple sclerosis. European Journal of Neurology. 2019;**25**:445-453

[43] Cartlidge NE, Hudgson P, Weightman D. A comparison of baclofen and diazepam in the treatment of spasticity. Journal of the Neurological Sciences. 1974;**23**(1):17-24

[44] From A, Heltberg A. A double-blind trial with baclofen (Lioresal) and diazepam in spasticity due to multiple sclerosis. Acta Neurologica Scandinavica. 1975;**51**:158-166

[45] Bes A, Eyssette M, Pierrot-Deseilligny E, Rohmer F, Warter JM. A multi-Centre, double-blind trial of tizanidine, a new antispastic agent, in spasticity associated with hemiplegia. Current Medical Research and Opinion. 1988;**10**(10):709-718

[46] Coward DM. Tizanidine: neuropharmacology and mechanism of action. Neurology. 1994;**44**(11 Suppl 9): S6-S10

[47] Groves L, Shellenberger MK, Davis CS. Tizanidine treatment of spasticity: A meta-analysis of controlled, double-blind, comparative studies with baclofen and diazepam. Advances in Therapy. 1998;**15**(4):241-251

[48] Nance PW, Bugaresti J, Shellenberger K, Sheremata W, Martinez-Arizala A. Efficacy and safety of tizanidine in the treatment of spasticity in patients with spinal cord injury. North American Tizanidine Study Group. Neurology. 1994;**44** (11 Suppl 9):S44-S51. Discussion S51-S52

[49] Nance PW, Sheremata WA, Lynch SG, Vollmer T, Hudson S, Francis GS, et al. Relationship of the antispasticity effect of tizanidine to plasma concentration in patients with multiple sclerosis. Archives of Neurology. 1997;**54**(6):731-736

[50] Shakespeare DT, Boggild M, Young C. Anti-spasticity agents for multiple sclerosis. Cochrane Database of Systematic Reviews. 2003;**4**:CD001332

[51] Pinder RM, Brogden RN, Speight TM, Avery GS. Dantrolene sodium: A review of its pharmacological properties and therapeutic efficacy in spasticity. Drugs. 1977;**13**(1):3-23

[52] Krause T, Gerbershagen MU, Fiege M, Weisshorn R, Wappler F. Dantrolene—A review of its pharmacology, therapeutic use and new developments. Anaesthesia. 2004;**59**(4):364-373

[53] Vaney C, Heinzel-Gutenbrunner M, Jobin P, et al. Efficacy, safety and tolerability of an orally administered cannabis extract in the treatment of spasticity in patients with multiple sclerosis: A randomized, double-blind, placebo-controlled, crossover study. Multiple Sclerosis. 2004;**10**:339-340

[54] Zajicek JP, Sanders HP, Wright DE, et al. Cannabinoids in multiple sclerosis (CAMS) study: Safety and efficacy data for 12 months follow up. Journal of Neurology, Neurosurgery, and Psychiatry. 2005;**76**:1664-1669

[55] Patti F, Messina S, Solaro C, Amato MP, Bergamaschi R, Bonavita S, et al. Efficacy and safety of cannabinoid oromucosal spray for multiple sclerosis spasticity. Journal of Neurology, Neurosurgery, and Psychiatry. 2016;**87**(9):944-951

[56] Turner-Stokes L, Ward A. Botulinum toxin in the management of spasticity in adults. Clinical Medicine. 2002;**2**:128-130

[57] Suputtitada A, Suwanwela NC. the lowest effective dose of botulinum a toxin in adult patients with upper limb spasticity. Disability and Rehabilitation. 2005;**27**:176-184

[58] Gracies JM, Brashear A, Jech R, Mcallister P, Banach M, Valkovic P, et al. Safety and efficacy of abobotulinumtoxinA for hemiparesis in adults with upper limb spasticity after stroke or traumatic brain injury: A double-blind randomised controlled trial. Lancet Neurology. 2015;**14**:992-1001

[59] Turner-Stokes L, Fhedoroff K, Jacinto J, Maisonobe P. Results from the upper limb international spasticity study-II (ULIS-II): A large, international, prospective cohort study investigating practice and goal attainment following treatment with botulinum toxin A in real-life clinical management. BMJ Open. 2013;**3**:e002771

[60] Esquenazi A, Moon D, Wikoff A, Sale P. Hemiparetic gait and changes in functional performance due to OnabotulinumtoxinA injection to lower limb muscles. Toxicon. 2015;**107**:109-113

[61] Wissel J, Ward AB, Erztgaard P, Bensmail D, Hecht MJ, Lejeune TM, et al. European consensus table on the use of botulinum toxin type a in adult spasticity. Journal of Rehabilitation Medicine. 2009;**41**(1):13-25

[62] Carda S, Molteni F. Selective neuromuscular blocks and chemoneurolysis in the localized treatment of spasticity. European Journal of Medical Physics. 2004;**40**:123-130

[63] Penn RD, Savoy SM, Corcos D, et al. Intrathecal baclofen for severe spinal spasticity. The New England Journal of Medicine. 1989;**320**:1517-1521

[64] Middel B, Kuipers-Upmeijer H, Bouma J, et al. Effect of intrathecal baclofen delivered by an implanted programmable pump on health related quality of life in patients with severe spasticity. Journal of Neurology, Neurosurgery, and Psychiatry. 1997;**63**:204-209

[65] Coffey RJ, Cahill D, Steers W, et al. Intrathecal baclofen for intractable spasticity of spinal origin: Results of a long-term multicentre study. Journal of Neurosurgery. 1993;**78**:226-232

[66] Ben Smail D, Peskine A, Roche N, et al. Intrathecal baclofen for treatment of spasticity of multiple

sclerosis patients. Multiple Sclerosis. 2006;**12**:101-103

[67] Kofler M, Matzak H, Saltuari L. The impact of intrathecal baclofen on gastrointestinal function. Brain Injury. 2002;**16**:825-836

[68] Patti F, Pappalardo A, Lo Fermo S, Cimino V, Castiglione A, Zappia M. Life-threatening constipation induced by intrathecal baclofen therapy. European Neurology. 2008;**60**(2):95-96

[69] Chambers HG. The surgical treatment of spasticity. Muscle and Nerve. Supplement. 1997;**6**:S121-S128

[70] Farmer JP, Sabbagh AJ. Selective dorsal rhizotomies in the treatment of spasticity related to cerebral palsy. Child's Nervous System. 2007;**23**:991-1002

[71] Fahn S. High dosage anticholinergic therapy in dystonia. Neurology. 1983;**33**:1255-1261

[72] Ravina A. A case of writer's cramp cured by trihexyphenidyl. Bulletins et Mémoires de la Société Médicale des Hôpitaux de Paris. 1952;**68**:581-582

[73] Corner BD. Dystonia musculorum deformans in siblings; treated with artane (trihexyphenidyl). Proceedings of the Royal Society of Medicine. 1952;**45**:451-452

[74] Burke RE, Fahn S, Marsden CD. Torsion dystonia: A double-blind, prospective trial of high-dosage trihexyphenidyl. Neurology. 1986;**36**:160-164

[75] Lang AE, Sheehy MP, Marsden CD. Anticholinergics in adult-onset focal dystonia. The Canadian Journal of Neurological Sciences. 1982;**9**:313-319

[76] Nutt JG, Hammerstad JP, de Garmo P, Carter J. Cranial dystonia: Double-blind crossover study of anticholinergics. Neurology. 1984;**34**:215-217

[77] Vogels OJ, Maassen B, Rotteveel JJ, Merx JL. Focal dystonia and speech impairment responding to anticholinergic therapy. Pediatric Neurology. 1994;**11**:346-348

[78] Kang UJ, Burke RE, Fahn S. Natural history and treatment of tardive dystonia. Movement Disorders. 1986;**1**:193-208

[79] Rosse RB, Allen A, Lux WE. Baclofen treatment in a patient with tardive dystonia. The Journal of Clinical Psychiatry. 1986;**47**:474-475

[80] Greene P, Shale H, Fahn S. Analysis of open-label trials in torsion dystonia using high dosages of anticholinergics and other drugs. Movement Disorders. 1988;**3**:46-60

[81] Greene PE, Fahn S. Baclofen in the treatment of idiopathic dystonia in children. Movement Disorders. 1992;7:48-52

[82] Bonouvrie L, Becher J, Soudant D, Buizer A, van Ouwerkerk W, Vles G, et al. The effect of intrathecal baclofen treatment on activities of daily life in children and young adults with cerebral palsy and progressive neurological disorders. European Journal of Paediatric Neurology. 2016;**20**:538-544

[83] Narayan RK, Loubser PG, Jankovic J, Donovan WH, Bontke CF. Intrathecal baclofen for intractable axial dystonia. Neurology. 1991;**41**:1141-1142

[84] Butler C, Campbell S. Evidence of the effects of intrathecal baclofen for spastic and dystonic cerebral palsy. AACPDM treatment outcomes committee review panel. Developmental Medicine and Child Neurology. 2000;**42**:634-645

[85] Albright AL. Intraventricular baclofen infusion for dystonia. Report of two cases. Journal of Neurosurgery. 2006;**105**:71-74

[86] Bianchine JR, Bianchine JW. Treatment of spasmodic torticollis with diazepam. Southern Medical Journal. 1971;**64**:893-894

[87] Segawa M, Hosaka A, Miyagawa F, Nomura Y, Imai H. Hereditary progressive dystonia with marked diurnal fluctuation. Advances in Neurology. 1976;**14**:215-233

[88] Termsarasab P, Yang AC, Frucht SJ. Intermediate phenotypes of ATP1A3 mutations: Phenotype-genotype correlations. Tremor and Other Hyperkinetic Movements. 2015;**5**:336

[89] Swash M, Roberts AH, Zakko H, Heathfield KW. Treatment of involuntary movement disorders with tetrabenazine. Journal of Neurology, Neurosurgery, and Psychiatry. 1972;**35**:186-191

[90] Jankovic J. Treatment of hyperkinetic movement disorders with tetrabenazine: A double-blind crossover study. Annals of Neurology. 1982;**11**:41-47

[91] Jankovic J, Orman J. Tetrabenazine therapy of dystonia, chorea, tics, and other dyskinesias. Neurology. 1988;**38**:391-394

[92] Chen JJ, Ondo WG, Dashtipour K, Swope DM. Tetrabenazine for the treatment of hyperkinetic movement disorders: A review of the literature. Clinical Therapeutics. 2012;**34**:1487-1504

Section 3

Neuromodulation for Neurodegenerative Disease

Chapter 7

Intranasal Insulin as Promising Therapy for Preserving Pragmatic Competence in MCI and AD

Sara Schatz

Abstract

Our chapter contends that extended intranasal insulin administration can preserve pragmatic functioning even when there are temporal lobe and frontal lobe brain volume losses consistent with AD disease progression. CT scans of a patient receiving extended intranasal insulin 6 years after AD diagnosis are compared with his CT scans at the original MCI diagnosis. The results demonstrate that areas of the brain associated with pragmatic functioning were not as affected as expected in late-stage AD patients. This, along with linguistic evidence of preserved pragmatic competence, indicates the likely effectiveness of intranasal insulin treatment in enhancing neuronal activity in certain areas of the brain associated with pragmatic competence.

Keywords: MCI, intranasal insulin, brain atrophy, pragmatics

1. Introduction

This chapter explores, on a brain circuitry level, why patients receiving extended intranasal insulin therapy continue to be able to ambulate independently, pay attention, speak, and participate in jokes even throughout late-stage AD [1–3]. We find that extended intranasal insulin administration can preserve pragmatic functioning even when there are temporal lobe and frontal lobe volume losses consistent with Alzheimer's brain (AD) volume loss. A series of CT scans of a patient receiving extended intranasal insulin from mild cognitive impairment (MCI) diagnosis and those from the same patient 5.5 years after AD diagnoses are examined. At baseline, this patient's original MCI CT scans indicated no significant intracranial pathology and normal aging brain morphology. Over time, we show how this patient demonstrates slower atrophy rates in occipital and thalamic structures as compared with the structural imaging of patients with disease progression from MCI to AD not receiving intranasal insulin therapy. Enhancing neuronal activity in the areas of the brain associated with pragmatic competence reduces the likelihood of anomia typical of late-stage AD.

This chapter is structured as follows: Section 1 examines studies of the perfusion of intranasal insulin in older adults concerning neuropsychiatric tests of cognitive decline in MCI and AD. Section 2 discusses CT scans and the medical and social history of the patient case study used in this chapter. Section 3 examines CT scans at three distinctive points in the patient's MCI to AD progression (at MCI diagnosis and 3.5 and 5.5 years receiving intranasal insulin therapy). Section 4 suggests that results demonstrating extended intranasal insulin treatment may slow disease progression by reducing some areas of neuronal atrophy in the (thalamus) cortico-pulvinar projection system associated with the anomia typical of late-stage AD.

2. The perfusion of intranasal insulin in context

In MCI and AD, the intranasal delivery of insulin has been found to enhance brain insulin activity either through improved glucose metabolism or reducing hypothalamic inflammation [4]. The route of intranasal insulin to the central nervous system (CNS) is via the olfactory and trigeminal neural pathways which innervate the nasal cavity and provide a direct connection to the CNS [5]. Given the short time frame (15–30 minutes) by which intranasal insulin reaches the brain, it is assumed that extracellular delivery from the nasal mucosa, instead of axonal transport, is the main transport mechanism. Glucose metabolism abnormality is thought to play a critical role in pathophysiological alterations by inducing multiple pathogenic factors such as oxidative stress, mitochondrial dysfunction, glycolysis, and Krebs citric acid cycle [6]. By pharmacologically restoring disrupted brain insulin signaling that ensues from glucose insufficiency [7], intranasal insulin is thought to promote neurol survival.[1]

Recent studies of the perfusion of intranasal insulin into the regional areas of the brain cortex demonstrate two main regional cortical areas of penetration. Akintola et al. [10] found that, in older adults, intranasal administration of insulin significantly increased perfusion through the occipital gray matter by 6.5% ($P = 0.001$) when compared to the administration of placebo as well as perfusion into the thalamus ($P = 0.003$). Perfusion through the parietal gray matter was also increased by 4.3% after administration ($P = 0.034$) in older adults.

According to the authors, increased perfusion strongly suggests that intranasal insulin therapy might restore energy demand and neuronal activity in these regions. They note:

We observed that intranasal insulin application increased perfusion of the thalamus. The thalamus receives information from almost all sensory systems and relays the information to associated cortical areas. From literature, increased cerebral blood flow has been linked to vasodilatation around the active area due to increased energy demand [11]. Also, insulin has been shown to be a vasoactive modulator that regulates peripheral and cerebral blood flow possibly via a direct vasodilatory effect [12]. Taken together, our finding of increased perfusion in some brain areas would support the hypothesis that intranasal insulin application might restore energy demand and neuronal activity in these regions [4, 10].

2.1 The thalamus and occipital structures in language, attention, and visuospatial tasks in Alzheimer's disease

The thalamus is a central mechanism in understanding and formulating language [13]. It passes information from one cortical area involved in language generation to another, including semantic feature binding and the generation of

[1] Delivery of IGF-I to the CNS is thought to be beneficial in the treatment of Alzheimer's disease or stroke because of IGF-I's ability to potently promote neuronal survival [8]. In adult rat CNS, regions of the circumventricular organs (choroid plexus and median eminence), olfactory system (olfactory bulb, anterior olfactory nucleus, and primary olfactory cortex), frontal cortex, hippocampus, amygdala, cerebellum, and spinal gray matter exhibit the highest concentration of IGF-I binding sites [9]. In a recent study, Sami et al. show that intranasal insulin treatment moderately increases glucose uptake in the WT mouse hippocampus via activating the Akt2 signaling pathway.

lexical items [14]. Pragmatics, in particular, relies on both the left and the right hemispheres, and the thalamus mediates from the superior temporal cortex and posterior parietal cortex, or the "language eloquent cortex" in humans [15, 16].

The thalamus is also relevant to "cognition," which includes the capacity to pay attention and to process multiple channels of information at once, i.e., to engage in "intentionally guided attention" or "engagement in action" [17]. An explicit mechanistic model has even been developed for thalamic stimulation effects on language and cognition that incorporate modern activation and connectivity data called the "specific alerting response" (SAR). The SAR effect involves secondary switching in the striatum caused by the activation of thalamostriatal projections, whereas the "anomia effect" implicates the disruption of the cortical synchronization action of the pulvinar via the cortico-pulvinar-cortical projection system [18].[2] In this SAR model, the retained ability to speak (an "anti-anomic" effect) depends upon the preservation of nuclei within the thalamus to regulate the transmission of information to the cortex and between cortical areas [21]. As such, the thalamus acts as a "selective engagement mechanism" which suppresses right frontal cortical activity, preventing it from interfering with language [17]. As Crosson [22] notes:

> *"in other words, once an intention to act is formed, the frontal lobes engage the cortical nets relevant to the intended activity. For example, if one intends to engage in a conversation, frontal cortex associated with language, via the nucleus reticularis and the pulvinar, engages cortices related to understanding and formulating language. At the same time, areas not involved in the intended activity would be held in a state of relative disengagement so as to minimize attention to stimuli irrelevant to the intended task."*

In Alzheimer's disease, it is well recognized that the thalamus is essential for generating attention [23], and its anterior and medial nuclei are involved in declarative memory functioning [24]. Anatomic evidence from AD patients shows that thalamic volume reduction in Alzheimer's disease has been related not only to anomia but also to global cognitive decline in all of these areas: motor behavior, emotional, motivational, associative, and cognitive abilities [25]. Nevertheless, until de Jong et al. [26], the direct correlation between measurements of decreasing thalamic volume and cognitive functioning in Alzheimer's disease had never been reported in the literature.

Intranasal administration of insulin also significantly increased perfusion through the occipital and parietal gray matter in older adults [10]. The occipital lobe is the visual processing center of the mammalian brain containing most of the anatomical region of the primary visual cortex. It also contains the ventral stream of vision that enables ability to focus on motor actions in response to outside stimuli. The parietal lobe is a source of speech and reading. Next to the occipital lobe, the parietal lobe integrates sensory information among various modalities, including proprioception, mechanoreception, and visuospatial processing. The posterior parietal cortex, also referred to as the dorsal stream of vision, receives somatosensory and/or visual input that can be transmitted to motor signals [27].

In MCI and AD, impairments in the dorsal stream of visual perception and processing have been found to be a predictor of AD [28]. Increasing impairment in visuospatial skills, visual object processing, and visual recognition of human

[2] The functional and anatomic evidence supports the assertion that the connectivity of the pulvinar is the likely nucleus to mediate communication of information [18]. The pulvinar is heavily connected to the cortex and forms cortico-thalamo-cortical pathways. As a general principle, directly connected cortical areas will be indirectly connected via the pulvinar [19, 20].

emotion processing are common on test scores of AD patients as part of annual cognitive deterioration [29–31]. Previous studies of MCI and AD patients receiving extended intranasal insulin have demonstrated unusual patterns of relatively limited annual cognitive declines as measured by several years of neuropsychiatric batteries. This was the case in tests covering visuospatial skills and executive function and inference tests which required simultaneous attention and the processing of multiple sources of information in parallel such as the VOSP Number Location, Pentagons, Modified Rey, CATS-Fact, and Affect Matching tests [2]. Furthermore, the short-term administration of intranasal insulin (21 days) has been found to significantly improve response inhibition on discordant items of an executive function-attention test (the Stroop test) [32, 33]. In addition, visuospatial function was significantly improved in performance on the Benton Visual Retention Test (BVRT) after 40 IU of insulin detemir, regardless of apoe4 status [32, 34].

Observational data on one patient receiving extended intranasal insulin therapy showed that even 5.5 years after AD diagnosis, he was still able to walk independently, pay attention to his physical surroundings, process visual information, and make verbal inferences [2]. Another patient who began intranasal insulin at MCI/mild dementia diagnosis after having lost the ability to manage his finances, shop, or independently go to doctor's visits returned to being able to do all of these tasks and even to going skiing after 3 years on treatment.

3. CT scans and progression from MCI to AD

Computed tomography (CT) is a structural medical imaging method that employs computer-based tomographic reconstruction to delineate bodily structures based on their ability to block X-ray beams. CT images are used to identify structural abnormalities, such as space-occupying lesions or intracranial neoplasms, although CT images are less fine in detail than newer structural imaging technologies [35].

The key CT structural markers of disease development in the progression from MCI to AD include atrophy rate measurements in the hippocampus and medial temporal lobe (the inner part of the temporal lobe, near the divide between the left and right hemispheres) [36]. In addition, ventricular enlargement of portions of the lateral ventricles adjacent to the medial temporal lobe (MTL) is also a sensitive marker of the transition from MCI to AD [37–39]. Thus, in the disease progression from MCI to AD, hypometabolism in glucose uptake leads to increased atrophy rates of lateral ventricles adjacent to the MTL and to a reduction of hippocampal volume and then to the temporal neocortex. Finally, the disease progresses into adjoining association and primary sensory areas [40, 41].

The medial temporal lobe in particular is thought to be involved in declarative and episodic memory. Deep inside the medial temporal lobe is the region of the brain which includes the hippocampus, the amygdala, the cingulate gyrus, the thalamus, the hypothalamus, the epithalamus, the mammillary body, and other organs, many of which are of particular relevance to the processing of memory. Studies of single-dose intranasal insulin demonstrate that intranasal does reach the hypothalamus but these results did not reach statistically significant levels ([10]:793). Other single-dose studies of intranasal insulin to diabetics showed acutely increased resting-state functional connectivity between the hippocampal regions and multiple regions within the DMN, i.e., the medial frontal cortex; the medial, lateral, and inferior parietal cortex (IPC); and anterior (ACC) and posterior cingulate cortex (PCC). These are brain regions directly linked to interactive higher cognitive functions [42][3] including language. The uncus,[4] an anterior extremity of the parahippocampal gyrus, a deep structure within the limbic system of the MTL, is of central importance in protecting/rescuing hippocampal neurons from amyloid-induced neurotoxicity [43, 45, 46].

Conversely, patients on extended intranasal insulin should demonstrate slower rates of atrophy as the insulin restores energy demand and neuronal activity in occipital and parietal gray matter regions and the thalamus [10]. CT scans over the AD disease course of a patient receiving extended intranasal insulin can be hypothesized to illustrate patterns closer to "normal aging" of MCI even 5–6 years after AD diagnosis (see also Additional materials). Thus, it can be hypothesized that AD patients receiving extended intranasal insulin therapy may demonstrate slower atrophy rates in occipital and thalamic structures than MCI to AD patients not receiving this therapy.

3.1 Case study: social and medical history

A series of three CT scans were conducted on patient "AR" between May 2012 and April 2018. AR was between the ages of 82 and 88 during this time and was being treated by a Kaiser Permanente Neurologist who diagnosed him with Alzheimer's disease in December 2012 after a May 2012 diagnosis of mild cognitive impairment. The patient was moved out of state in September 2017 when his 82-year-old girlfriend developed Parkinson's disease. He subsequently lived near his daughter in an Alzheimer facility and was seen by a qualified university neurologist until his death in December 2018.

The patient initially became involved in the compassionate use of twice-daily intranasal insulin for the purposes of reducing cognitive decline in June 2013. This treatment was administered by nurses who also gave him his daily medications and reminded the patient to conduct daily or weekly hygiene (bathing, tooth brushing, correct dressing). The patient ate independently or with minor assistance throughout the course until the final months of his life when he needed assistance with cutting up his food (8/18–12/18). During the years of 2012–2017, AR was still able to live in his home with his 80-year-old girlfriend who cooked, shopped, and drove him to their social activities, and his financial and medical management was done

---

[3] Zhang et al. [42] found that intranasal insulin-treated diabetic subjects performed better on the visuospatial memory task (BVMT-R) and on verbal fluency naming tasks. The former tended to correlate with stronger connectivity between the left hippocampal region and PCC. Better performance on the verbal fluency naming task was associated with stronger coefficient of connectivity between the right hippocampal region and ACC and lesser connectivity between the left hippocampal regions and the MFC for a more difficult category switching task. As Zhang et al. [42] summarize: "Differences in relationships between cognition and connectivity between the right and left hippocampal regions were found which reflect a complexity of the large-scale verbal fluency network that comprises of verbal fluency and orthographic discrimination subnetworks...Set switching is a complex operation involving a number of different brain structures that usually include various parts of the dorsolateral and dorsomedial prefrontal cortex, as well as temporal regions where hippocampus is located."

[4] The uncus is a rudimentary, small area where the frontal lobe meets the temporal lobe and the area of cortex on the uncus of the parahippocampal gyrus (both belonging to the olfactory cortex). It is phylogenetically older (the so-called paleocortex) and is part of the limbic system. The uncus is connected to the olfactory tract through nerve fibers which bend abruptly toward it and is separated from the apex of the temporal lobe by a slight fissure called the incisura temporalis. Given its centrality in early MCI [43], it is necessary to ascertain potential structural and/or diffusional and cellular barriers to intranasal insulin penetration into the surrounding CNS tissue and significant clearance of CSF into the venous and lymphatic circulation [44].

by his daughter [2]. While residing in his Alzheimer residence facility (11/17–12/18), AR was still ambulatory, fed himself, ate with the early AD patients at the dining room, and was highly conversational even at this stage of disease progression [3].

AR's medical history at MCI diagnosis was (5/12) OSA, diverticulosis, tinnitus, lumbar stenosis, and BPH. His medications were memantine, donepezil, tamsulosin, multivitamin, and intranasal insulin (at 6/13). At 10/16, the same medications, all blood work normal.[5] At 4/18, the same medications, all blood work normal. At 4/18, 5.5 years after his original AD diagnosis and at age 88, his doctor stated to AR's daughter that the patient was still "very functional with good language skills" and, to the doctor's surprise, still possessed "the body of a 70-year-old" [3].

4. Results

4.1 At MCI diagnosis: before beginning intranasal insulin therapy

AR was diagnosed with MCI in May 2012 based on a Slums test score (24/30) and a mild cognitive impairment AD8 score = 0/8. His neurologists stated: "The patient came in because he had begun to not remember essential tasks, lost his keys and had begun to become disoriented at times. For example, he could not remember the proper freeway exit for the airport or where he was on the freeway despite having driven to that airport on that same route for over 40 years. Patient himself feels memory not so good. He was also beginning to forget the names of plants at the botanical gardens which he once knew he could. His girlfriend thinks his memory issue may be out of the ordinary in forgetting day to day conversations [47]."

CT scans were ordered due to this "altered level of consciousness." The initial CT findings of AR's neurologist at this time stated there was "no significant intracranial pathology" with "normal aging brain morphology." All other CT findings were also "normal," i.e., "intact (calvarium, central skull base, temporal mastoids: adequate; cellular, non-sclerotic, paranasal sinuses: well aerated; brain showed no acute intracranial bleed, large vessel territory infarct, or mass effect) (CT Results 5/12)."[6] B-12 and TSH levels were also in normal limits (5/12). Indeed, the overall assessment of AR's 5/12 CT scan was summarized succinctly as "changes of aging brain."

In terms of his memory loss, however, the neurologist's findings were more uncertain. He noted: "Robust looking man. Gait brisk, very cordial and engaging and gives detailed history but when asked his profession, he seemed to have to think awhile before he recalled he was a science teacher." Clearly AR's neurologist detected something was amiss when he stated: "While patient score is in the mild cognitive impairment range, and while he is very intellectually active: plays bridge, studies German, goes folk dancing still I think he should be scoring higher than he does. While I cannot make a diagnosis of Alzheimer's now, I think we need to follow up in 6 months and see how it goes [47]."

Nevertheless, CT at 5/12 *did* show markers of disease progression toward AD. AR's CT scan includes the following analysis: "Ventricles are 'prominent' as there are subarachnoid spaces within cerebrospinal fluid." Ventricular enlargement represents a feasible short-term marker of disease progression in subjects with MCI

[5] Full blood work results available upon request. (10/16): BP 121/58 mmHg | Pulse 84 | Temp(Src) 98.7°F (37.1°C) | Resp 18 | Wt 189 lb. 6 oz. (85.9 kg) | SpO2 98%. Ext: WWP; no leg swelling/asymmetry/edema; 2+ bilateral symmetric radial pulses; no calf swelling/TTP/cord [47].

[6] CT HEAD. Technique: Contiguous noncontrast transaxial images from the vertex to the skull base were obtained. Estimated phantom dose: CTDIvol (mGy): 29 DLP (mGy-cm): 501. Consider follow-up limited brain FDG-PET evaluation (PET scan) to work up dementia, if clinically indicated.

and subjects with AD because portions of the lateral ventricles are adjacent to the medial temporal lobe (MTL), structures that atrophy notably in the preclinical stages of dementia [38, 48]. Nestor et al. [49] even hypothesize that ventricular dilatation after 6 months would differentiate normal aging, MCI, and MCI to AD progressors and be a more sensitive measure of disease progression than cognitive scores. For example, they found subjects with AD had a 60% greater ventricular enlargement than subjects with MCI and a fourfold enlargement compared with normal aging as measured over a 6-month interval. Jack et al. [50] argue that hemispheric atrophy rates, measured by ventricular enlargement, correlate more strongly with changes on cognitive tests than medial temporal lobe (MTL) atrophy rates and capture significant variation between subjects with MCI and AD [37, 39]. The rate of ventricular volume change is also highly correlated with an increase in senile plaques and neurofibrillary tangles [51].

In AR's case such ventricle enlargement was, in fact, a sensitive measure of disease progression. Six months later in his follow-up visit (12/18), AR's Slums score had dropped by 4 points to 20/30, and his AD8 score increased by 1 point to 1/8. Even more disease progression was evident in cognitive measures of his short-term memory: AR scored 4/8 in story recall and had a 0/5 recall of objects 5 minutes later [47]. At this point in time, December 2012, AR's neurologist diagnosed him with early AD. He noted: "Impression and plan: It is now clear that this is early Alzheimer's. Will begin Aricept. Gave information on Alzheimer's disease and referral number of our incredibly skilled and compassionate memory clinical social worker. Follow up on 3–4 months [47]."

4.2 3 ½ years after diagnosis: 3 years on intranasal insulin: still looks more like MCI

AR, in conjunction with his family, made the decision to begin intranasal insulin therapy in June 2013, 6 months after his 12/12 AD diagnosis. At this point, his MMSE score was 24 (3/13), and his word recall after 10 minutes was 0/9 (3/13) [2]. The patient's functional abilities had also markedly deteriorated from a year previous at his 5/12 MCI diagnosis. AR could no longer manage his finances or his medical treatments and could no longer drive. His family also noticed the development of significant social and linguistic withdrawal, irritability, and flattened affect ([1]:331–333). For example, AR expressed very little positive emotion upon seeing his daughter and granddaughter at the airport after a 6-month separation. Furthermore, he was unable to participate in conversations or even access anything about himself such as how he was feeling, often remaining silent for extended periods of time, and withdrawing from social engagement ([1]:331–333).

The patient's family began compassionate use of intranasal therapy (6/13) at twice daily for AR (20 IU per dose). Over the subsequent 6–8 months of treatment, they noticed a marked return of pragmatic functioning, an increase in social and linguistic participation (even returning to telling and understanding jokes), self-awareness, and decreased irritability ([1]:333–35). AR himself reported just 2 days after beginning therapy that his head hurt less, spontaneously holding his head with his hand and stating to his daughter: "Oh, it is like I have had a terrible headache for a long time."

A return of meaningful linguistic interaction after intranasal insulin therapy and a stabilization of the further deterioration were also noted by other patient's family members after several months. This stabilization was reflected in his 2014 and 2015 neuropsychological battery of tests. These cognitive tests revealed a marked slowing of annual percent decline in executive function and visuospatial scores compared with average annual declines [2, 31]. AR also was able to use and respond affectively to humor in conversations, related areas of the brain typically associated with significant deterioration in AD progression [52].

A CT scan was taken on AR in October 2016, just over 3 years after the patient began receiving intranasal therapy (**Figure 1a** and **b**). Again, the overall neurologist's impression was "age-related volume loss." The record reads:

Comparison: "Comparison is made with 05/17/2012. There is no evidence of intracranial hemorrhage, mass, mass effect, large infarct or midline shift. Prominence of the ventricles and sulci are noted, likely age-related volume loss. Scattered periventricular white matter hypodensities are noted, most commonly seen with small vessel ischemic changes. Vascular calcifications are noted. Partial opacification of the ethmoid and sphenoid sinuses noted. Bones are unremarkable. Impression: No evidence of acute intracranial process. *Age-related volume loss*. Likely small vessel ischemic changes [47]."

This diagnosis of "age-related volume loss" after 3 years receiving intranasal insulin suggests some positive effects of extended therapy. AR's neurologist noted in his 10/16 comments that the patient was: "alert and oriented" with "5/5 strength in all 4 extensions with full distal sensation; no saddle anesthesia; 2+ symmetric reflexes throughout and ambulates without difficulty [47]."

Figure 1a and **b** shows evidence of AD disease stage progress. For example, in his 10/16 notes, AR's neurologist comments on the "prominence of the ventricles and sulci" which are more enlarged (the ventricles) and deeper (the sulci in the frontal lobe) (**Figure 1a**) than AR's 5/12 MCI diagnosis CT scan (**Figure 2**). Furthermore, AR's memory was very uneven; he stated that he quit smoking when he was 30 years old but did not remember his daughter who lived out of state.

Further clarification of the positive effects of intranasal insulin therapy at 3 ½ years after his AD diagnosis can be observed comparatively. **Figure 3** shows a structural MRI of the typical progressive atrophy (of medial temporal lobes and hippocampus) in an older cognitively normal (CN) subject, an amnestic mild cognitive impairment (aMCI) subject, and an Alzheimer's disease (AD) subject. In this disease progression from MCI to mild AD, the hippocampus of the subject in **Figure 3** shows marked atrophy as indicated by the white arrows. Hippocampal atrophy, especially left volumes, and its contribution to memory decline in the process of Alzheimer's disease have been often described and are widely accepted [53, 54].

In contrast, AR's CT scan (**Figure 1a**) shows a hippocampus size that is still relatively robust. As indicated by the white arrow in **Figure 1a**, AR's left hippocampus is similar to that of the patient in **Figure 3** at MCI disease stage. **Figure 1a** and **b** also shows significantly less overall frontal cortex atrophy, medial temporal lobe atrophy, and occipital lobe atrophy as compared with disease progression of the MCI to

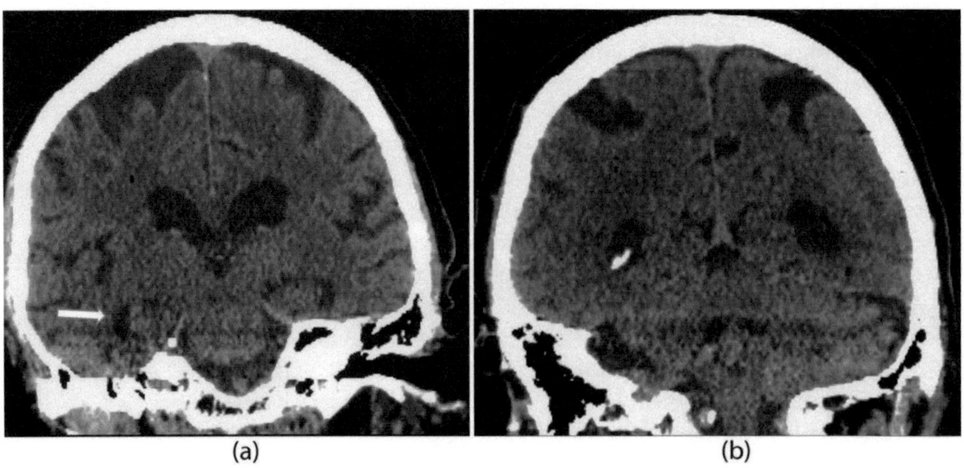

Figure 1.
(a) and (b): CT scans of patient AR, 10/16.

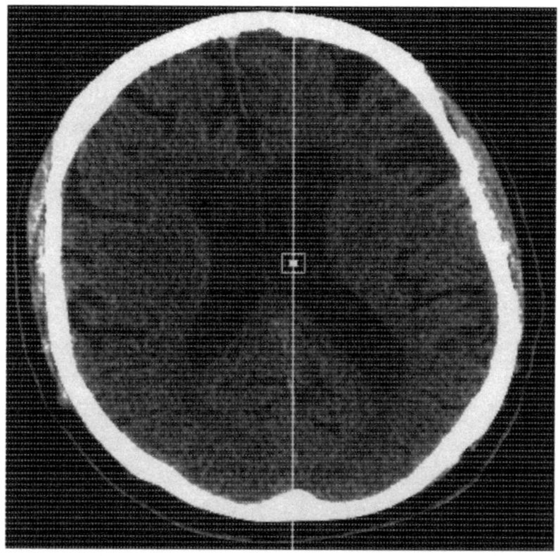

Figure 2.
CT scan of patient AR, 5/12.

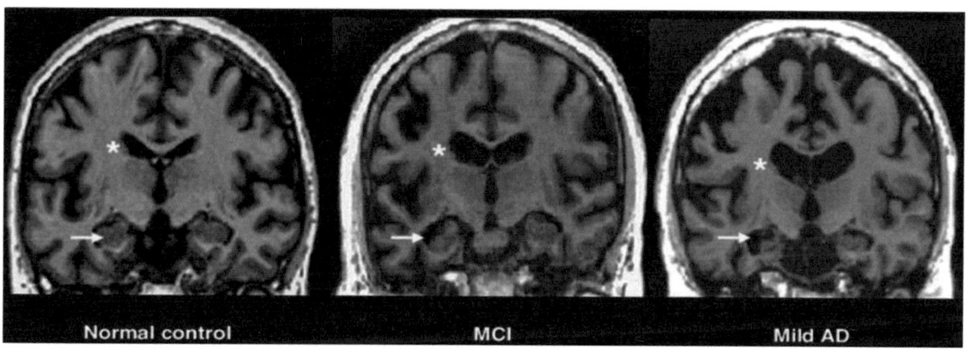

Figure 3.
Structural MRI of the typical progressive atrophy (of medial temporal lobes and hippocampus) in an older cognitively normal (CN) subject, an amnestic mild cognitive impairment (aMCI) subject, and an Alzheimer's disease (AD) subject.

AD patient (**Figure 3**). These are significant positive effects of extended intranasal insulin as illustrated in AR's 10/16 CT scan.

A return of meaningful linguistic interaction after intranasal insulin therapy and a stabilization of AR's executive functioning test scores also reflect his neurologist's overall interpretation of "age-related" (vs AD disease progression related) volume loss in his 10/16 CT scan. AR's executive functioning capacities at year 4 after AD diagnosis include still being able to actively watch a TV series in several 45-minute episodes. In addition, on one occasion, when a scratched DVD disk caused the episode to pause, AR was able to immediately alert his daughter of the need to fix the problem. This demonstrates that AR was actively paying attention [2]. Prolonged attention span was found across patients with Phelan-McDermid syndrome after 1 year receiving intranasal insulin [55].

Another patient diagnosed with mild AD improved his executive functioning area scores (immediate recall, delayed free recall, and animal recall scores) after 8 months receiving intranasal insulin [2]. As Sperling et al. [56] note, AD causes considerable damage to the neurobiological substrate of episodic memory, the hippocampal-entorhinal complex (located in the medial temporal lobes) early in the course of the disease. After several years receiving intranasal insulin therapy, the patient continued to demonstrate capabilities in visual processing skills (occipital and parietal lobe functioning) as well as improvements in executive functioning under targeted therapy. At 3 years, he had returned to being able to ski (2019) after having lost the ability to manage his finances, shop, or independently go to doctor's visits [2].

4.3 5 ½ years after AD diagnosis and 5 years on insulin therapy: less atrophy of occipital and thalamic structures

At year 5 ½ after AD diagnosis and at 5 years receiving intranasal insulin therapy (12/17–12/18), AR was still able to inferentially reason. He was also fully ambulatory, eating with the mild AD patients at his nursing home, and looked at books and TV while paying attention to both. His visual skills were also still intact. For example, one day AR was walking independently back to his room with his daughter and headed toward a large automatic opening and closing door to the Alzheimer wing which was being held open by a staff member. AR immediately turned to his daughter and asked: "Can we go through?" His daughter responded: "Yes." Then AR was able to remember, proceeded to analyze contextual information and to simultaneously warn her of possible impending danger, telling her: "Hurry up. It closes fast" [3].

Figure 4 is AR's CT scan at 5 years receiving intranasal insulin therapy (5 ½ years after AD diagnosis) (4/18). **Figure 5a** and **b** presents subcortical segmentation of MRI scans after boundary correction of a subject classified as MCI (4a) and of a subject diagnosed with probable Alzheimer's disease (4b) [26].

Consistent with our hypothesis that extended therapeutic usage should slow AD disease progression, AR's 4/18 CT scans demonstrate that his occipital lobe does not show a significant shrinkage of gray matter volume (indicated by black arrow, **Figure 4**). Similarly, AR's thalamus, indicated by the yellow arrow (**Figure 4**), is also not as atrophied in terms of volume loss as the AD patient (**Figure 5b**) despite his significant frontal volume loss and lateral ventricle enlargement consistent with late-stage AD [50].

AR's retained volume in the occipital and thalamic subcortical structures supports previous findings that intranasal insulin directly reaches the occipital cortical brain regions and the thalamus in older adults [10]. These results suggest such enhanced insulin action in these brain areas can, in fact, slow AD disease progression.

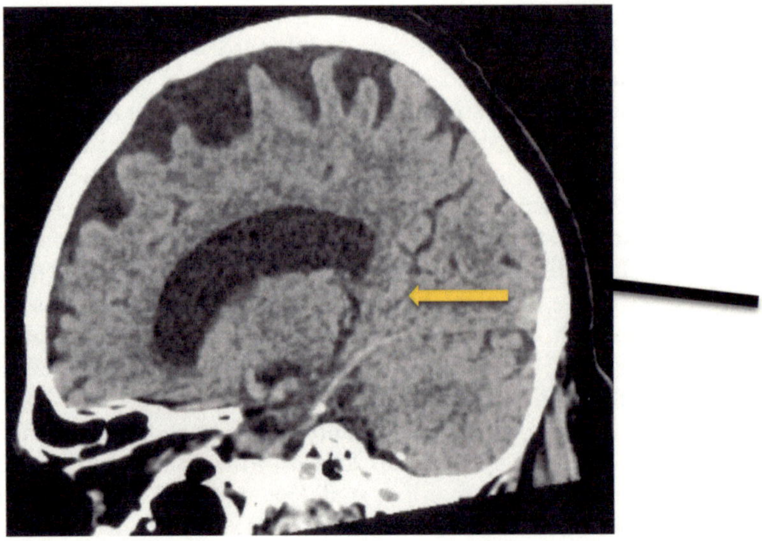

Figure 4.
CT scan of patient AR, 4/18.

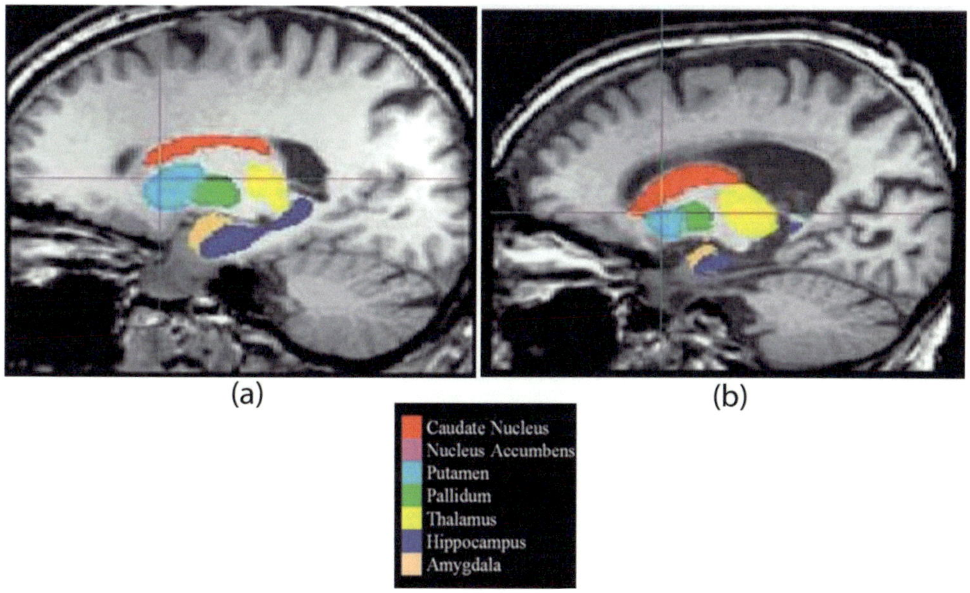

Figure 5.
(a) and (b): subcortical segmentation of MRI scans, after boundary correction, of a subject classified as MCI (a) and of a subject diagnosed with probable Alzheimer's disease (b) (sagittal view) [26].

Figure 6a and **b** demonstrates how AR clearly shows signs of advanced AD by 4/18. AR's neurologist noted of his 4/18 CT scan:

> *"Lateral ventricles are enlarged with disproportionate enlargement of the frontal horns. Temporal horns are both markedly enlarged, more so on the right. Third ventricle is moderately enlarged. Basel cisterns are enlarged, as are the sylvian fissures. Overall, findings are compatible with generalized volume loss, with disproportional frontal and temporal lobe volume loss. This includes medial temporal lobe volume loss with likely considerable hippocampal volume loss especially on the right. Sulci are not symmetrical on both sides [47]."*

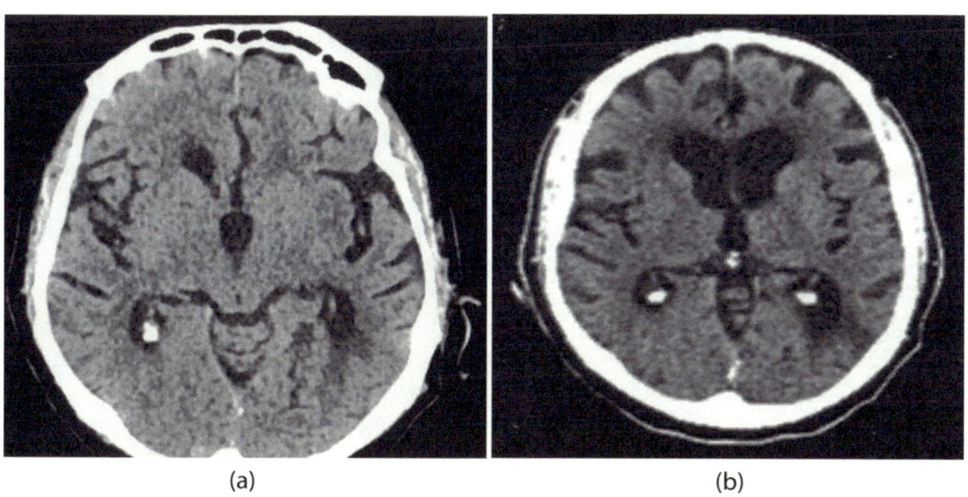

Figure 6.
(a) and (b): CT scans of patient AR, 4/18.

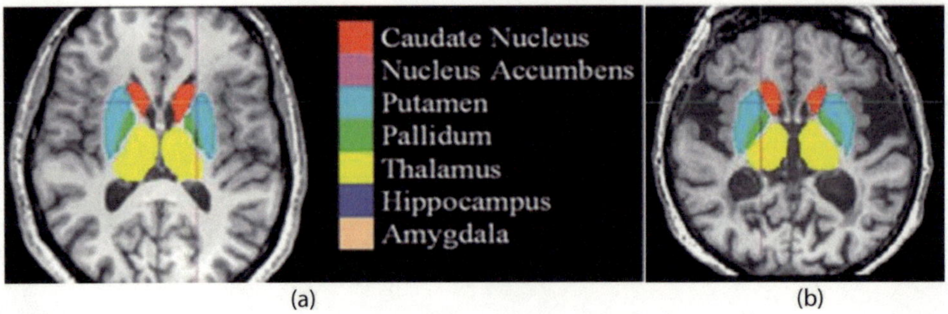

Figure 7.
(a) and (b): subcortical segmentation of MRI scans, after boundary correction, of a subject classified as MCI (a) and of a subject diagnosed with probable Alzheimer's disease (b) (axial view) [26].

Yet, as (again) compared with probable AD (**Figure 7b**), AR demonstrates less overall volume loss even with respect to the medial temporal lobe. Furthermore, in AR's case, left hippocampus atrophy is less pronounced than right (**Figure 6a** and **b**). This is also a significant finding because, as de Jong et al. [26] found in their Alzheimer's disease group, volume reduction of the *left* hippocampus, putamen, and thalamus formed the strongest predictors for declining cognitive performance in Alzheimer's disease progression.

5. Discussion

The potential of intranasal insulin to curb the development and progression of AD [57] is by avoiding decreases in cerebral glucose metabolic rate within a complex neuronal network which comprises the hypothalamus, hippocampus, thalamus, and cortical brain structures. A series of CT scan results of a patient receiving extended administered intranasal insulin usage shows delayed atrophy of key areas of the brain associated with cognitive, visual, executive, and pragmatic functioning as compared to disease progression in MCI to AD patients not receiving therapy. These findings, particularly those that demonstrate slowed atrophy of the thalamus and occipital lobe, strongly suggest that extended intranasal insulin treatment might slow disease progression by reducing some areas of neuronal atrophy in the (thalamus) cortico-pulvinar projection system [18] associated with the anomia typical of late-stage AD [58, 59]. They also highlight the importance of thalamic stimulation on language and cognition and the ability of the preservation of nuclei within the thalamus to regulate the transmission of information to the cortex and between cortical areas [21]. The reduced atrophy of the occipital lobes in this patient on extended intranasal insulin therapy is also significant because lesion studies have shown that the pulvinar is critically involved in visual perception, attention, and visually guided behavior [21], which can include directing visual attention to a cued location.

The slowing of atrophy of the thalamus is also consistent with the hypothesized medial pathway of insulin [2, 3, 60] in which the thalamus is reached via the olfactory tubercle. Future research is required to refine precisely how intranasal insulin promotes glucose utilization in these neuronal networks, i.e., through changes in hippocampal synaptic plasticity and/or by increasing synapse density and dendritic plasticity in structures that process visual input ([61]:216).

Future follow-up studies are needed to explore how intranasal insulin's potential effectivity for reducing transition rates from amnestic MCI to AD is related to preserving those neurological structures associated with pragmatic tasking.

Specifically, additional studies are required consisting of mapping out the bulk flow of intranasal insulin along the olfactory and trigeminal pathways between the nasal passages and the CNS into deeper structures within the medial temporal lobe (MTL) ([45, 62]:491). The region of the MTL showing the greatest atrophy in mild cognitive impairment is the entorhinal cortex, which is precisely part of the parahippocampal gyrus and is the same region that has been postulated by Braak and Braak [40] to be the site where AD pathology is first expressed.

Additional practical studies are necessary to understand the relationship between the olfactory system and the delivery route of intranasal insulin on such hippocampal structures within the MTL to further elucidate the potential of intranasal insulin therapy. AR's continuing pragmatic abilities including sarcastic utterances, utilizing empathic tone and pragmatic discourse markers [3] 6 years after AD diagnosis and 5 ½ years on intranasal insulin, point toward the partial effect of intranasal insulin on deeper hippocampal brain structures. The right parahippocampal gyrus, for example, has functions beyond the contextualizing of visual background stimuli and identifying social context such as the inclusion of paralinguistic elements of verbal communication resulting in the ability to employ sarcasm [63]. As Smith [43] notes:

Many years (up to 50) before the symptoms (of AD) occur, neurofibrillary tangles start to form in neurons in the parahippocampal gyrus. At some stage, this process is exacerbated, and many projection neurons in the MTL then start to die, leading to atrophy of the lobe and to early signs of memory deficits. Once denuded of their input from the MTL, neurons in the target areas of neocortex show reduced activity, leading to slower metabolism and a fall in local blood flow. They will no longer function properly in the neural networks underlying higher cognition [64].

The findings in this chapter also illustrate, on a brain circuitry level, AR's other continued pragmatic capacities even with late-stage AD [2, 3]. Several weeks before his death from a post-hip surgery-related heart attack, AR was still able to employ a bodily related metaphor: "I am tired. It seems like that is all I say. What a pain in the ass that is." This statement involves the capacity to abstract and inhibit literal interpretation, both of which are associated with executive functioning tasks. Other linguistic evidence of AR's preserved pragmatic competence even 5.5 years after his AD diagnosis include telling jokes and using humor to assert autonomy [1–3]. The capacity to detect, understand, and respond to humor deteriorates significantly in the progression of AD [65]. Scholarship on the neural basis of humor processing precisely suggests that humor engages a core network of cortical and subcortical structures, including temporo-occipito-parietal areas involved in detecting and resolving incongruity [66]. The temporo-parietal junction incorporates information from the thalamus, among other systems.

Treatment-induced improvements in neuronal activity in the thalamus and occipital and parietal lobes can bring moderate to significant improvements in communication exchanges with caregivers, thereby reducing the AD patient's social and communicative isolation, lessen caregiver stress, and improve executive functioning. Furthermore, AR's annual, standard blood tests did not reveal abnormalities or indicators of chronic intranasal insulin therapy leading to (further) desensitization of his brain insulin signaling [67] a concern expressed in the literature [57].[7]

The results contained in this paper are the first published CT scans of a patient receiving extended intranasal insulin use. Begun at early MCI diagnosis, the extended use of intranasal insulin could substantially impact sites along the

[7] Future studies can measure this potential through recent exosome biomarker tests derived from blood, plasma, and serum for the detection of brain insulin signaling resistance [68, 69].

olfactory pathway (hypothesized to be affected early on in AD).[8] This could potentially arrest the further spread of the disease process in the involvement of the hippocampus, areas of the neocortex in the parietotemporal and frontal lobes, as well as hypothalamic inflammation linked to age and disease-related declines in insulin sensitivity [4, 46]. One patient after 8 months of intranasal insulin was administered a series of pre- and post-therapy neuropsychological tests, including visuospatial skills, visual spatial ability, visual working memory, and executive functioning after beginning intranasal insulin [2]. Eight months later, his neurologist concluded that: "There was about a two-year reversal of cognitive impairment while receiving intranasal insulin, going from mild dementia to mild cognitive impairment [3]." A return to MCI from early AD is a significant therapeutic achievement that deserves further application and investigation.

Additional materials

Several previous studies on 153 MCI and AD patients involved in the short- (4 months) and medium-term (12 months) administration of intranasal insulin using the ViaNase device to deliver the drug confirm the findings of the preservation of *caregiver-rated functional ability* in MCI and AD patients. The first randomized, placebo-controlled pilot study of ViaNase delivered intranasal insulin consisted of 104 adults with amnestic mild cognitive impairment (n = 64) or mild to moderate AD (n = 40), all of whom were treated with 20 and 40 IU daily dosages of intranasal insulin for 4 months (9). The mean patient age was 71 years old, and the mean 3MSE score was 83.7–84.3 [20 IU/40 IU]. 50–57% were positive for the high-risk apolipoprotein E epsilon-4 allele. The following results were reported: "Treatment with 20 IU of insulin *improved delayed memory* ($P < .05$), and both doses of insulin (20 and 40 IU) *preserved caregiver-rated functional ability* ($P < .01$). Both insulin doses also preserved general cognition as assessed by the ADAS-cog score for younger participants and functional abilities as assessed by the ADCS-ADL scale for adults with AD ($P < .05$). Cerebrospinal fluid biomarkers did not change for insulin-treated participants as a group, but, in exploratory analyses, changes in memory and function were associated with changes in the Aβ42 level and in the tau protein-to-Aβ42 ratio in cerebrospinal fluid. Placebo-assigned participants showed decreased fludeoxyglucose F 18 uptake in the parietotemporal, frontal, precuneus, and cuneus regions and insulin-minimized progression." The second placebo-controlled study of ViaNase delivered intranasal insulin administration consisted of 49 of 289 patients with mild cognitive impairment (MCI) or mild Alzheimer's disease (AD) who were randomized to receive either insulin or placebo daily for 12 months [70].[9] This was a phase 2/3 trial at 26 US sites and a change in cognitive function from baseline to 12 months served as the primary endpoint, with the primary outcome measuring the Alzheimer's

[8] In the olfactory system, the sites that are affected include the anterior olfactory nucleus, the uncus, and the medial group of amygdaloid nuclei—all receives fibers directly from the olfactory bulb ([69]:4534).

[9] Assessments were made at baseline and at 3-month intervals until the end of the study, when participants were offered open-label insulin treatment for another 6 months. The other 240 patients used a different device (Precisions Olfactory Delivery [POD]) which failed to produce any difference in outcome on the ADAS-Cog 12 measure at 12 months with the placebo group. Both POD and placebo groups increased by about 4 points on the ADAS-Cog 12 measure, indicating worsening. Nor were there any changes in any other Alzheimer-related biomarkers like amyloid-beta 40 and 42, total tau, or phosphorylated tau (Clinical Neurology News 12/4/18:2). The model is controlled for age, sex, genetic risk status, and investigation site. Patients were a mean of 71 years old, with a mean Mini Mental State Exam score of 25. Around 42% were positive for the high-risk apolipoprotein E epsilon-4 allele.

Disease Assessment Scale-Cognition measure (ADAS-Cog 12). The ViaNase delivered intranasal insulin *slowed the annual progress of cognitive decline by 50%*—or only a 2.5-point decline per patient on the ADAS-Cog12 versus the 5-point decline per patient of the placebo group. This significant "separation was evident at 3 months and continued to widen over the course of the [12 month] study" [71].

The finding in this chapter of the reduction of caregiver stress after the longer-term administration (3 plus years) of intranasal insulin is also evident from qualitative findings from an open-label study of 22 MCI and AD patients on the compassionate use of intranasal insulin.[10] These patients displayed, before ViaNase delivered treatment, significant symptoms of social and linguistic withdrawal, flattening of affect, and irritability, as well as moderate to high levels of family-reported caregiver stress [1–3, 60]. Several publications also extensively document treatment-mediated improvements in language, visuospatial, and, in particular, executive functioning test scores of patients at moderate AD and an early MCI patient (5) and a return of pragmatic competence in the areas of jokes, self-expression, and empathy in early and moderate AD and MCI patients [1, 60]. Over 90% of caregivers of the 22 compassionate use patients also reported moderate to very strong reductions in caregiver stress after 1 year of intranasal insulin administration to their family members [1, 60, 73, 74].

[10] These MCI and AD patients live in naturalistic settings (2011–present) and provide linguistic evidence on phenomena as they naturally occur, i.e., they provide conversational data for the case study methodology as used by sociologists for the purpose of theory development and building. Hamilton [72] found that it is only in such conversations that it is possible to describe the full range of communicative competence of a person with AD.

Author details

Sara Schatz
International Studies, The Ohio State University, Columbus, OH, USA

*Address all correspondence to: saraschatz@yahoo.com

References

[1] Schatz S, González-Rivera M. Pragmatic function impairment and Alzheimer's dementia. Pragmatics and Cognition. 2016;**23**:324-342

[2] Schatz S, González-Rivera M. Executive functioning, visuo-spatial and inter-personal skill preservation in Alzheimer's and mild cognitive impairment. In: Capone A, Carapezza M, Lo Piparo F, editors. Further Advances in Pragmatics and Philosophy: Part 2 Theories and Applications. Perspectives in Pragmatics, Philosophy and Psychology. Vol. 20. Cham: Springer; 2019. pp. 373-389

[3] Schatz S, González-Rivera M. Intranasal insulin in Alzheimer's disease: A pragmatic account. OBM Geriatrics. 2019;**3**(3):20. DOI: 10.21926/obm.geriatr.1903069

[4] Akintola AA, van Heemst D. Insulin, aging, and the brain: Mechanisms and implications. Frontiers in Endocrinology. 2015;**6**:13. DOI: 10.3389/fendo.2015.00013

[5] Hanson R, Frey WH. Intranasal delivery bypasses the blood-brain barrier to target therapeutic agents to the central nervous system and treat neurodegenerative disease. BMC Neuroscience. 2008;**9**:S5

[6] Chen Z, Zhang C. Decoding Alzheimer's disease from perturbed cerebral glucose metabolism: Implications for diagnostic and therapeutic strategies. Progress in Neurobiology. 2013;**108**:21-43. DOI: 10.1016/j.pneurobio.2013.06.004

[7] Craft S, Baker L, Montine T, et al. Intranasal insulin therapy for Alzheimer disease and amnestic mild cognitive impairment. Archives of Neurology. 2012;**69**(1):29-38

[8] Lindholm D, Carroll P, Tzimagiogis G, Thoenen H. Autocrine-paracrine regulation of hippocampal neuron survival by IGF-1 and the neurotrophins BDNF, NT-3 and NT-4. The European Journal of Neuroscience. 1996;**8**:1452-1460

[9] Bohannon NJ, Corp ES, Wilcox BJ, Figlewicz DP, Dorsa DM, Baskin DG. Localization of binding sites for insulin-like growth factor-1 (IGF-1) in the rat brain by quantitative autoradiography. Brain Research. 1988;**444**:205-213

[10] Akintola AA, van Opstal AM, Westendorp RG, Postmus I, van der Grond J, van Heemst D. Effect of intranasally administered insulin on cerebral blood flow and perfusion; a randomized experiment in young and older adults. Aging. 2017;**9**(3):790-802. DOI: 10.18632/aging.101192

[11] Attwell D, Iadecola C. The neural basis of functional brain imaging signals. Trends in Neurosciences. 2002;**25**:621-625

[12] Hughes TM, Craft S. The role of insulin in the vascular contributions to age-related dementia. Biochimica et Biophysica Acta. 2016;**1862**:983-991. DOI: 10.1016/j.bbadis.2015.11.013

[13] Hart J, Kraut M. Neural hybrid model of semantic object memory. In: Hart J, Kraut M, editors. Neural Basis of Semantic Memory. Cambridge, UK: Cambridge University Press; 2007. pp. 331-359

[14] Slotnick SD, Moo LR, Kraut MA, Lesser RP, Hart J Jr. Interactions between thalamic and cortical rhythms during semantic memory recall in human. Proceedings of the National Academy of Sciences of the United States of America. 2002;**99**(9):6440-6443

[15] Goldman-Rakic PS, Porrino LJ. The primate mediodorsal (MD) nucleus and its projection to the frontal lobe. Journal of Comparative Neurology. 1985;**242**:535-560

[16] Jones EG. The Thalamus. New York: Cambridge University Press; 2007

[17] Nadeau SE, Crosson B. Subcortical aphasia. Brain and Language. 1997;**58**:355-402; discussion 436-458

[18] Hebb AO, Ojemann GA. The thalamus and language revisited. Brain and Language. 2013;**126**(1):99-108

[19] Sherman SM, Guillery RW. Exploring the Thalamus and its Role in Cortical Function. Cambridge, MA: MIT Press; 2006

[20] Shipp S. The functional logic of cortico-pulvinar connections. Philosophical Transactions of the Royal Society B: Biological Sciences. 2003;**358**:1605-1624

[21] Saalmann YB, Kastner S. Cognitive and perceptual functions of the visual thalamus. Frontiers in Endocrinology. 2015;**6**(13):1-2. DOI: 10.3389/fendo.2015.00013

[22] Crosson B. Thalamic mechanisms in language: A reconsideration based on recent findings and concepts. Brain and Language. 2013;**126**(1):73-88

[23] Newman J. Thalamic contributions to attention and consciousness. Consciousness and Cognition. 1995;**4**:172-193

[24] Van der Werf YD, Witter MP, Uylings HB, Jolles J. Neuropsychology of infarctions in the thalamus: A review. Neuropsychologia. 2000;**38**:613-627

[25] Herrero MT, Barcia C, Navarro JM. Functional anatomy of thalamus and basal ganglia. Child's Nervous System. 2002;**18**:386-404

[26] de Jong LW, van der Hiele K, Veer IM, Houwing JJ, Westendorp RGJ, Bollen ELEM, et al. Strongly reduced volumes of putamen and thalamus in Alzheimer's disease: An MRI study. Brain. 2008;**131**(12):3277-3285. DOI: 10.1093/brain/awn278

[27] Cabeza R, Ciaramelli E, Olson IR, Moscovitch M. The parietal cortex and episodic memory: An attentional account. Nature Reviews Neuroscience. 2008;**9**(8):613-625

[28] Boyé M, Grabarb N, Tran M. Contrastive conversational analysis of language production by Alzheimer's and control people. Studies in Health Technology and Informatics. 2014;**205**:682-686

[29] Matsuzono K, Hishikawa N, Ohta Y, Yamashita T, Deguchi K, Nakano Y, et al. Combination therapy of cholinesterase inhibitor (donepezil or galantamine) plus memantine in the Okayama memantine study. Journal of Alzheimer's Disease. 2015;**45**(3):771-780

[30] Quental NB, Brucki SM, Bueno OF. Visuospatial function in early Alzheimer's disease—The use of the visual object and space perception (VOSP) battery. PLoS ONE. 2013;**8**(7):0068398

[31] Zhao Q, Zhou B, Ding D, Teramukai S, Guo Q, Fukushima M, et al. Cognitive decline in patients with Alzheimer's disease and its related factors in a memory clinic setting, Shanghai, China. PLoS ONE. 2014;**9**(4):e95755

[32] Avgerinos KI, Kalaitzidis G, Malli A, Kalaitzoglo D, Myserlis PG. Intranasal insulin in Alzheimer's dementia or mild cognitive impairment: A systematic review. Journal of Neurology. 2018;**265**(7):1497-1510

[33] Reger MA, Watson GS, Green PS, Baker LD, Cholerton B, Fishel MA, et al.

Intranasal insulin administration dose-dependently modulates verbal memory and plasma amyloid-beta in memory-impaired older adults. Journal of Alzheimer's Disease. 2008;**13**(3):323-331

[34] Claxton A, Baker L, Hanson A, Trittschuh E, Cholerton B, Morgan B, et al. Therapeutic effects of intranasal insulin and insulin analogues on cognition and MRI measures in mild cognitive impairment and Alzheimer's disease. Alzheimer's & Dementia. 2014;**10**(4):1-26

[35] Pasi M, Poggesi A, Pantoni L. The use of CT in dementia. International Psychogeriatrics. 2011;**23**(Suppl 2): S6-S12

[36] Wasim Dr. Neuroimaging of Alzheimer's disease and healthy aging. Slide Share, Dr. Wasim under the guidance of Dr. R. K. Solanki; 2017

[37] Bradley KM, Bydder GM, Budge MM, Hajnal JV, White SJ, Ripley BD. Serial brain MRI at 3-6-month intervals as a surrogate marker for Alzheimer's disease. The British Journal of Radiology. 2002;**75**:506-513

[38] Ferrarini L, Palm WM, Olofsen H, van Buchem MA, Reiber JH, Admiraal-Behloul F. Shape differences of the brain ventricles in Alzheimer's disease. NeuroImage. 2006;**32**:1060-1069

[39] Schott JM, Price SL, Frost C, Whitwell JL, Rossor MN, Fox NC. Measuring atrophy in Alzheimer disease: A serial MRI study over 6 and 12 months. Neurology. 2005;**65**:119-124

[40] Braak H, Braak E. Alzheimer's disease: Transiently developing dendritic changes in pyramidal cells of sector CA1 of the Ammon's horn. Acta Neuropathologica. 1997;**93**:323-325. DOI: 10.1007/s004010050622

[41] Braak H, Braak E. Neuropathological staging of Alzheimer-related changes. Acta Neuropathologica. 1991;**82**: 239-259. DOI: 10.1007/BF00308809

[42] Zhang H, Hao Y, Manor B, Novak P, Milberg W, Zhang J, et al. Intranasal insulin enhanced resting-state functional connectivity of hippocampal regions in type 2 diabetes. Diabetes. 2015;**64**:1025-1034

[43] Smith DA. Imaging the progression of Alzheimer pathology through the brain. Proceedings of the National Academy of Sciences of the United States of America. 2002;**99**(7):4135-4137. DOI: 10.1073/pnas.082107399

[44] Thorne RG, Frey WH. Delivery of neurotrophic factors to the central nervous system. Clinical Pharmacokinetics. 2001;**40**:907. DOI: 10.2165/00003088-200140120-0000

[45] Thorne RG, Pronk GJ, Padmanabhan V, Frey WH 2nd. Delivery of insulin-like growth factor-I to the rat brain and spinal cord along olfactory and trigeminal pathways following intranasal administration. Neuroscience. 2004;**127**:481-496

[46] Pearson RC, Esiri MM, Hiorns RW, Wilcock GK, Powell TP. Anatomical correlates of the distribution of the pathological changes in the neocortex in Alzheimer disease. In: Proceedings of the National Academy of Sciences of the USA; 1985;**82**(13):4531-4534. DOI:10.1073/pnas.82.13.4531

[47] Personal communication with patient's family. Patient Medical Record, 5/12; 10/16; 4/18

[48] Giesel FL, Hahn HK, Thomann PA, Widjaja E, Wignall E, von Tengg-Kobligk H. Temporal horn index and volume of medial temporal lobe atrophy using a new semiautomated method for rapid and precise assessment. American Journal of Neuroradiology. 2006;**27**:1454-1458

[49] Nestor SM, Rupsingh R, Borrie M, Smith M, Accomazzi V, Wells JL, et al. The Alzheimer's Disease Neuroimaging Initiative. Ventricular enlargement as a possible measure of Alzheimer's disease progression validated using the Alzheimer's disease neuroimaging initiative database. Brain. 2008;**131**(9): 2443-2454. DOI: 10.1093/brain/awn146

[50] Jack CR, Shiung MM, Gunter JL, O'Brien PC, Weigand SD, Knopman DS, et al. Comparison of different MRI brain atrophy rate measures with clinical disease progression in AD. Neurology. 2004;**62**:591-600

[51] Silbert LC, Quinn JF, Moore MM, Corbridge E, Ball MJ, Murdoch G. Changes in premorbid brain volume predict Alzheimer's disease pathology. Neurology. 2003;**61**:487-492

[52] Clark CN, Warren JD. The neurology of humor. Advances in Clinical Neuroscience & Rehabilitation. 2014;**13**:9-11

[53] de Leon MJ, George AE, Golomb J. Frequency of hippocampal formation atrophy in normal aging and Alzheimer's disease. Neurobiology of Aging. 1997;**18**:1-11

[54] Laakso MP, Soininen H, Partanen K. Volumes of hippocampus, amygdala and frontal lobes in the MRI-based diagnosis of early Alzheimer's disease: Correlation with memory functions. Journal of Neural Transmission - Parkinson's Disease and Dementia Section. 1995;**9**(1):73-86

[55] Schmidt H, Kern W, Giese R, Hallschmid M, Enders A. Intranasal insulin to improve developmental delay in children with 22q13 deletion syndrome: An exploratory clinical trial. Journal of Medical Genetics. 2009;**46**:217-222

[56] Sperling RA, Dickerson BC, Pihlajamaki M, Vannini P, LaViolette PS, Vitolo OV, et al. Functional alterations in memory networks in early Alzheimer's disease. Neuromolecular Medicine. 2010;**12**:27-43

[57] Benedict C, Grillo C. Insulin resistance as a therapeutic target in the treatment of Alzheimer's disease: A state-of-the-art review. Frontiers in Neuroscience. 2018;**12**:215. DOI: 10.3389/fnins.2018.00215

[58] Tappen R, Williams C, Barry C, DiSesa D. Conversation intervention with Alzheimer's patients: Increasing the relevance of communication. Clinical Gerontologist. 2002;**24**(3-4): 63-75. DOI: 10.1300/J018v24n03_06

[59] Wray A. Dementia and language. In: Chapell A, editor. The Encyclopedia of Applied Linguistics. Oxford: Blackwell; 2015

[60] Craft S. HBO, *The Connection* The Connection between Insulin and Alzheimer's; 2009. Available from: http://www.hbo.com/alzheimers/the-supplementary-series.html

[61] Ott V, Benedict C, Schultes B, Born J, Hallschmid M. Intranasal administration of insulin to the brain impacts cognitive function and peripheral metabolism. Diabetes, Obesity and Metabolism. 2011;**14**:214-221

[62] Herzog AG, Kemper TL. Amygdaloid changes in aging and dementia. Archives of Neurology. 1980;**37**:625-629

[63] Hurley D. Katherine P. Rankin, a Neuropsychologist, Studies Sarcasm—NYTimes.com. 2008. The New York Times [Retrieved: 03 November 2009]

[64] Minoshima S, Giordani B, Berent S, Frey KA, Foster NL, Kuhl DE. Metabolic reduction in the posterior cingulate cortex in very early Alzheimer's disease. Annals of Neurology. 1997;**42**:85-94

[65] Clark CN, Warren JD. The neurology of humor. ANCR. 2014;**13**(7):9-11

[66] Vrticka P, Black JM, Reiss AL. The neural basis of humour processing. Nature Reviews Neuroscience. 2013;**14**:860-868

[67] Patient Medical Records, 2012-2019. Records including CT scans provided to researcher from patient's family. Proceedings of the National Academy of Sciences USA. July 1985;**82**(13):4531-4534. DOI. 10.1073/pnas.82.13.4531

[68] Kapogiannis D, Boxer A, Schwartz JB, Abner EL, Biragyn A, Masharani U, et al. Dysfunctionally phosphorylated type 1 insulin receptor substrate in neural-derived blood exosomes of preclinical Alzheimer's disease. FASEB. 2015;**29**(2):589-596

[69] NonoSomiX. NanoSomiX, Inc. announces issuance of first US exosome patent. 2018. Available from: https://www.exosome-rna.com/nanosomix-inc-announces-issuance-of-first-us-exosome-patent/

[70] SNIF. The Study of Nasal Insulin in the Fight Against Forgetfulness (SNIF). 2018. Available from: www.clinicaltrials.gov, identifier–NCT01767909

[71] Sullivan MG. Latest intranasal insulin results for Alzheimer's muddied by malfunctioning inhaler. Clinical Neurology News. 2018. Available from: https://www.mdedge.com/clinicalneurologynews/article/190235/alzheimers-cognition/latest-intranasal-insulin-results. [Accessed: 04 December 2018]

[72] Hamilton H. Conversations with an Alzheimer's Patient: An Interactional Sociolinguistic Study. Cambridge: Cambridge University Press; 1994

[73] Giroux M. Personal Communication; 2017

[74] Michael T. Innovative Alzheimer's treatment. 2017. Available from: https://www.youtube.com/watch?v=FlJTN1XVBAw

Chapter 8

Deep Brain Stimulation in Non-motor Symptoms of Neurodegenerative Diseases

Vladimira Vuletic, Valentino Racki, Darko Chudy and Nenad Bogdanovic

Abstract

Deep brain stimulation (DBS) is a functional neuromodulatory technique that involves the use of a neurostimulator to deliver electrical impulses to the brain. It primarily alleviates the motor symptoms in neurodegenerative diseases; however, it has been found beneficial in a multitude of neurological and psychiatric diseases, such as dystonia, essential tremor, Tourette syndrome, intractable pain, epilepsy, treatment-resistant depression, and obsessive-compulsive disorder. Nonmotor symptoms, such as neurobehavioral disorders, autonomic dysfunction, sleep dysfunction, and somatosensory dysfunction, play an important role in neurodegenerative diseases and have a significant impact on the quality of life. The effects of deep brain stimulation on these symptoms are not yet apparent, although early results are promising and warrant future investigations. The main problem in interpretation is the lack of studies in this field, as most have methodological issues or small sample sizes, which limit the strength of the evidence. However, it is clear that DBS has a promising future in the treatment of neurodegenerative diseases in general and will have a vital role in personalized medicine as functional neuroimaging and our understanding of brain physiology improve.

Keywords: deep brain stimulation, nonmotor symptoms, neurodegenerative diseases, neuromodulation, neurostimulation

1. Introduction

Deep brain stimulation (DBS) is a functional neuromodulatory technique that involves the use of a neurostimulator to deliver electrical impulses to the brain [1]. It has been used for several decades, primarily in advanced Parkinson's disease (PD), to alleviate the motor symptoms of the disease [2]. The exact mechanisms of therapeutic efficacy are not yet precisely defined; however, DBS is beneficial in a multitude of neurological and psychiatric diseases, such as dystonia, essential tremor, Tourette syndrome, intractable pain, epilepsy, treatment-resistant depression, and obsessive-compulsive disorder [3]. It is generally used to target specific locations in the brain that will be discussed later in the chapter. Despite this, the effects of DBS can be considered as systemic, as it influences neuronal pathways in both an upstream and a downstream manner. In that sense, it can affect a plethora of symptoms, including nonmotor symptoms in neurodegenerative diseases [4]. It is becoming more apparent that neurostimulations will have an even more critical role in the future as our understanding of brain physiology and pathways improves with novel imaging techniques. This chapter includes the basics of how deep brain stimulation works, what are the nonmotor symptoms in neurodegenerative diseases, and what is the current evidence on the effects of DBS on nonmotor symptoms.

2. Deep brain stimulation

2.1 How does deep brain stimulation work?

The system for DBS consists of three key components: an electrode that is placed in specific cerebral structures, an implantable pulse generator (IPG), and an extension that connects the two. Even though the exact mechanism is not yet known, the current hypothesis is that DBS works via excitation and inhibition of neurons and axons that are in proximity of the placed electrode [5]. The desired effect is achieved by changing the frequency of stimulations, as low-frequency stimulations most often excite nearby neurons [1], while high-frequency stimulations reduce local neuronal activity. Details of the implantation procedure are beyond the scope of this chapter, although it is useful to know that it is implanted stereotactically. In most cases, the stimulation is bilateral, although it is possible to stimulate unilaterally as well. The targets for stimulation are deep brain structures, as well as deep white matter tracts. A key benefit of DBS is the ability to adjust stimulations wirelessly via handheld devices to improve symptom relief and reduce possible side effects [5].

Currently used method for DBS function is based on an open-loop system, which enables trained physicians to adjust various settings depending on the patient's condition [6]. This works adequately for most patients; however, changes in patient states bring challenges as modifying stimulations require a physician visit. A possible solution to this problem is the closed-loop or adaptive DBS that will enable real-time adjustment of the neurostimulations due to the continuous feedback signals. This will most likely be achieved with the help of various wearable sensors, neurochemical sensors, and electrophysiological recordings, which would all be interpreted with the Internet or mobile applications that will enable constant insight into the state of each patient [7]. Unfortunately, numerous challenges till the clinical application remain, but the prospects are bright, and hopefully such systems will be perfected in the near future.

The main and the most studied effect of DBS occurs via electrical potential generated by the neurostimulations. There was a prevailing thought that the effects of DBS are dominantly local in the areas that the electrodes were placed [8]. However, recent advances indicate that neuromodulation with DBS affects entire pathways, both afferently and efferently, and thus can influence more than just the stimulated structures [9]. Both animal and human studies in vivo show this, mainly through increased neurotransmitter release from axon functional magnetic resonance imaging (fMRI) studies [10]. In a practical sense, this means that targeting motor dysfunction, for example, in Parkinson's disease, has an added effect of changing the function of other neuronal pathways and not only the motoric dopamine pathways that are primarily disrupted in the disease. Therefore, choosing the right target is essential for adequate treatment response.

2.2 Targets for stimulation

The two most common targets for DBS are the globus pallidus internus (GPi) and the subthalamic nucleus (STN), which are a part of the cortico-basal-ganglia-thalamocortical circuit loop. They are most commonly used in Parkinson's disease for control of dopaminergic symptoms such as tremor, rigidity, and bradykinesia [5], although beneficial effects of GPi stimulation were found in dystonias as well [11]. Another possible target in PD is the ventral intermediate nucleus (VIM), an area of the thalamus, that if stimulated improves tremor-dominant variants of the disease and can also be used in patients suffering from essential tremor [12]. Furthermore, stimulating the anterior nucleus can help in medically refractory epilepsy, while benefits of thalamic stimulation were also seen in Tourette's syndrome, neuropathic pain, and traumatic brain injury as well.

Advancements in preclinical and neuroimaging research studies and neurosurgical experiences led to a discovery of several targets that could prove beneficial to numerous diseases. DBS in the ventral capsule, the ventral striatum, or nucleus accumbens (NA) has been shown to improve symptoms of obsessive-compulsive disorder [13], while NA stimulation has been shown to reduce the severity of obesity and anorexia [14]. Treating treatment-resistant depression is also possible with DBS; however it requires an individualized approach due to numerous possible targets [15]. Moreover, benefits of DBS are observed in dementia as well, with the possible targets being the fornix and the nucleus basalis of Meynert (NBM) in Alzheimer's disease [16]. In general, the most reliable evidence for DBS use comes from movement disorders, while other indications still require randomized, well-designed studies to prove efficacy. Different possible targets and adjustable nature of DBS put it at the forefront of personalized medicine in the future, especially as functional neuroimaging improves, as stimulations will be catered to each patient individually.

2.3 The mechanism of DBS

The neuromodulatory effects of DBS occur in various stages, while most of the focus in the early days of DBS was on the immediate effects. In time, it is becoming more apparent that short-term and long-term effects of DBS are just as significant, as those are opening new frontiers in therapy. All of the cells in the body function through changes in electric potential, but our neurons are special in the sense that they comprise a series of networks where this potential can be passed on to other neurons or cells [17]. This physiological basis creates the stage for neuromodulation with DBS, as different impulse settings create different effects on the cell bodies and axons of neurons. Even a single DBS pulse can influence neuronal activities for several milliseconds, while an increased frequency can prevent the cells from resetting to their base values [18]. In neurons, these pulses dissociate cell bodies of neurons from their axons and essentially "hijack" the signaling in both afferent and efferent directions [19]. Generally, the pulses inhibit cell body activity while creating action potentials in the axons [20]. The pulses also act on astrocytes and microglia in the area of stimulation, causing a change in glial activity and complete changes in ion concentrations such as potassium and calcium, which in turn influences the changes in action potentials of neurons [21]. Immediate effects of DBS are a consequence of the function of individual neurons that are stimulated in the vicinity of the placed electrode and vary greatly depending on the selected target.

In the neurochemical sense, the milieu of brain tissue is significantly changing as several changes occur in the concentration of neurotransmitters and neurotrophic factors. The values of crucial neurotransmitters (dopamine, noradrenaline, serotonin, and gamma-aminobutyric acid) are altered depending on the location of the modulation, which makes target selection key, as increasing serotonin [22] or noradrenaline by stimulating NA, for example, affects mood and can have an antidepressant effect [23]. However, even the presence of the electrode can significantly impact the neurochemical properties surrounding it. It is a foreign object that necessitates reaction from microglia and astrocytes that create an immediate inflammation and edema that subsides over the long term with the creation of a fibrotic membrane by astrocytes [24, 25].

Most programs for DBS are intended for long-term function, and all these changes that happen immediately or short term after initiating the therapy have a profound effect on the structure and function over extended periods. The physiological basis for this is a result of our brains' adaptive capacity, which we call synaptic and neural plasticity [26]. Constant stimulation on the same areas and the changes mentioned above in neuronal activity and extracellular milieu lead to changes in synaptic structure and density, neurogenesis, and neuroprotection, which in turn change the properties of neural networks [27]. This is most likely mediated by neurotrophic factors, such as the brain-derived neurotrophic factor (BDNF), similarly as in the physiological central nervous system conditions [28]. The changes in neuroplasticity and neuronal organization lead to functional improvements of various symptoms over time; this is especially pronounced in alleviating neuropathic pain, axial symptoms, obsessive-compulsive symptomatology, and several nonmotor symptoms as well [5].

Aside from the neurochemical changes, there are effects of DBS on brain oscillations present in numerous neuropsychiatric diseases. Current data points out that synchronous brain activity can be amplified in Parkinson's disease (beta oscillations in the basal ganglia [29]), Alzheimer's disease (gamma oscillations in the hippocampus [30]), and treatment-resistant depression (gamma and theta oscillations in the subcallosal cingulate gyrus [31]). Early data indicates that DBS can affect these oscillations and provide a balance to brain activity, reducing the amplification that is pathologically found [30–32]. Further research is required to detect various oscillation patterns in diseases to develop therapeutic goals for treatment, not only with DBS but with other neurostimulation techniques as well.

3. Nonmotor symptoms in neurodegenerative diseases

Nonmotor symptoms in neurodegenerative diseases are disturbances in neurobehavior, autonomic function, and sleep and sensory function that are not a consequence of motor symptoms [33]. Most of the studies are focused on nonmotor symptoms in Parkinson's disease, but they can be present in most other central nervous system disorders. The pathophysiology and incidence differ from one disease to another, although the spectrum of symptoms remains the same. In many cases, the first signs of neurodegeneration will be nonmotor disturbances as they often precede other symptoms [34]. It is important to point out that these symptoms are present as primary diseases as well, usually in the psychiatric spectrum of diseases. However, in the context of validated and approved DBS stimulation in the classical targets of stimulation, they can be considered as nonmotor symptoms in extrapyramidal diseases. It is clear that as the field matures, new nomenclature will be needed to accurately assess the effect of DBS on various neuropsychiatric symptoms, especially if those symptoms are primary targets (e.g., treatment-resistant depression or obsessive-compulsive disorder). We can divide the nonmotor symptoms into several key categories: neuropsychiatric symptoms, sleep disorders, autonomic symptoms, gastrointestinal symptoms, and sensory symptoms [33]. Nonmotor symptoms present a vital field of study as they can have a significant impact on the quality of life and are often overlooked in clinical practice.

Neurobehavioral symptoms frequently present in neurodegenerative disorders are excessive fatigue, depression, anxiety, apathy, and cognitive dysfunction.

Depression and anxiety both commonly occur at the same time in patients and often precede diagnosis with mild symptoms at the beginning, although more severe forms occur as the disease progresses [35]. On the other hand, apathy can be present as a separate symptom, mainly if there is a prominent degeneration of dopamine pathways in the limbic system [36]. Finally, cognitive dysfunction is considered as an inevitable consequence of long-term neurodegeneration. The extent of cognitive difficulties varies from mild to severe depending on the disease, with different cognitive domains affected as well [37].

Sleep dysfunction and sleep-related problems are common nonmotor symptoms in neurodegenerative diseases. The pathophysiological basis is likely the variation in physiological dopamine function, as changes in dopamine are known to impact wakefulness [38]. The physiological importance of sleep comes from enabling the regeneration of brain tissue and reestablishing homeostatic conditions. Therefore, sleep disorders can increase the severity of disease progression as a vicious circle forms that disables proper neural regeneration [39]. Sleep-onset insomnia is a frequent occurrence in neurodegenerative diseases, as the progression of the disease and chronic loss of neuronal function lead to neurotransmitter disbalance that in turn causes a sleep-wake disruption. This presents as a dysfunction of the circadian rhythm in Alzheimer's disease and Huntington's disease, while in Parkinson's disease the difficulties are mostly sleeping through the night and initiation of rapid eye movement phase during sleep [40]. Sleep quality can also be affected, as difficulties in nighttime mobility and excessive fragmentation of sleep are common, as well as problems in rapid eye movement (REM) phases of sleep [41]. Furthermore, difficulties with restless legs syndrome (RLS) and involuntary limb movements create sleep difficulties, although these symptoms are more frequently found in diseases that feature dopamine dysfunction and generally have a response to dopamine therapy [42].

Autonomic dysfunction develops as a consequence of progressive degeneration in neural pathways, mostly in diseases characterized by the accumulation of Lewy bodies or α-synuclein, and is much less pronounced in diseases such as Alzheimer's or frontotemporal lobar degeneration [43]. Three main symptoms of autonomic dysfunction are issues with bladder control, nocturia, and sexual dysfunction, all of which are linked to the dysfunction in the dopamine pathways and can somewhat improve with dopaminergic therapy [44]. Moreover, gastrointestinal symptoms fall in this category as well and are an interesting subset of symptoms as the dysfunction, which often presents as constipation or anorectal dysfunction, could be a consequence of both central and enteric nervous system degeneration [45]. Interestingly, these symptoms can be present in prodromal stages of many neurodegenerative diseases, which have made the gut-brain axis an attractive research target in recent times [46].

Finally, sensory symptoms have a significant role in the clinical course of neurodegenerative diseases, especially in the prodromal stages. Hyposmia, a reduced capacity for the sense of smell, is often seen in the early stages of Parkinson's and Alzheimer's disease [47, 48]. Recent neuroimaging studies reveal a decreased volume in the olfactory regions of the brain, while neuropathological studies found a high accumulation of α-synuclein, αβ amyloid, and Tau proteins in the olfactory bulb during the early stages of neurodegenerative diseases [47, 48]. Something similar can be seen in the optical pathways as well, as there is an increase of visual hallucinations, reduced color recognition, visual acuity problems, and double vision as neurodegeneration progresses [49]. Pain syndromes are frequent as well and are more likely of neuropathic origin. Unfortunately, the mechanisms for pain in neurodegeneration are varied, and managing pain requires an individualized approach, as specific types of pain require different medications. High prevalence of pain impacts the quality of life, as do all nonmotor symptoms in general, which makes proper measurement a necessity in the current clinical evaluation of neurodegenerative diseases.

3.1 How do we measure nonmotor symptoms?

Comprehensive measurements of all the symptoms mentioned present a challenge in everyday clinical practice. Naturally, objectifying the symptoms is crucial not only in the initial evaluation but also in the evaluation of the therapeutic effects as well. There is a wide variety of instruments available for a detailed assessment of each symptom, but this has proven to be inadequate in everyday use [50]. Best suited scales for rapid and accurate identification of nonmotor symptoms are multidomain instruments that cover most of the nonmotor symptomatology. Two scales were developed for use in Parkinson's disease; however, they are suitable for use in other neurodegenerative diseases as a quick screening of the prevalence of nonmotor symptoms.

First is the nonmotor symptom questionnaire (NMSQuest), a scale developed to provide a useful screening tool, as it contains 30 items that have yes and no questions covering various domains of nonmotor symptoms [51]. It is designed to be completed by patients themselves, and there is no grading of the severity of symptoms, just whether they exist or not. Nonetheless, it has proven to be an effective screening tool in further validation studies that can afterward lead to a more focused examination of reported symptoms [52]. On the other hand, the nonmotor symptom scale (NMSS) is developed to be rated by clinicians, and it incorporates the severity and impact of the symptoms on the daily life of the patients [53]. Similar to the NMSQuest, it has 30 items, spread across 9 domains, but the overlap is in 23 of the 30 items; therefore using both of them has clinical sense. It is crucial to point out that these scales have inevitable shortcomings as more nonmotor symptoms come into focus over time. Therefore, a modified NMSS is currently in active development that should improve its use in all neurodegenerative diseases. Furthermore, it is required to use the scales focused on each domain to precisely measure the severity of each symptom on its own, as only focused scales go into enough details to have a complete overview of the effect that each symptom has on the quality of life. In any case, as the focus of symptomatology studies turn toward nonmotor symptoms, it is to be expected that more comprehensive scales will be developed that are adequate for use in clinical and clinical trial settings.

4. Effects of DBS on nonmotor symptoms

The focus of clinical practice and research in DBS is on the effects it has for motor symptoms in advanced Parkinson's disease. As previously said, the nonmotor symptoms in neurodegenerative diseases are only recently coming into focus, as is the effect of DBS on them. Most robust studies come from the research done in Parkinson's disease and from patients whose targets for neuromodulation are STN and GPi; however, research from other diseases and stimulation targets will also be assessed in the coming paragraphs [54].

4.1 Neurobehavioral symptoms

Effects of DBS on neurobehavioral outcomes are a complex subject as there are possible advantages and disadvantages, depending on the initial patient selection and the deep brain target of neuromodulation. Cognitive dysfunction, as a frequent symptom in most neurodegenerative diseases, can have varying severity depending on the disease and between each patient individually [55]. In classical DBS targets, the STN and GPi, there are mixed results regarding the effect on cognition. Generally, stimulation of these areas will not improve cognitive function, and there is even a mild risk of cognitive decline, which has been found minor in more extensive trials and not clinically relevant [4]. There is a caveat to this, as DBS in patients with pronounced cognitive dysfunction tends to increase the severity of symptoms more than in those who do not have significant cognitive impairment [56]. The same can be observed in patients who had problems with depression or anxiety in the past before being diagnosed with a neurodegenerative condition [57]. STN stimulations, in particular, led to an increase in apathy and hallucinations, while there was a minor improvement in impulsive behavior (impulse buying, gambling, excessive sexual behavior) compared to the control groups [58–60]. Benefits of DBS were found in symptoms of depression as well but mostly in milder cases without pronounced symptoms [61].

On the other hand, phase I clinical studies in Alzheimer's disease with DBS targeting the fornix [62] or the NBM [63] show encouraging results on cognitive impairment in the early stages of the disease while being safe and well tolerated. There is currently a lack of studies in this field, but more are being conducted at the time of writing. Furthermore, early research shows that patients who suffer from depression could benefit from DBS, especially severe types that are resistant to therapy. Similar to Alzheimer's disease, there are promising early results, but proper targets and correct settings for stimulations are not yet clear, and larger, controlled studies are needed [15]. To summarize, the effects of DBS on neurobehavioral symptoms are significantly impacted by the target locations for stimulation, as both beneficial and harmful effects are present. Therefore, appropriate patient selection is critical, as the impact it can have on the quality of life depends much on an individual basis.

4.2 Autonomic dysfunction

Dysfunctions in the autonomous nervous system are the more frequent nonmotor symptoms in neurodegenerative diseases. Generally, there is a lack of extensive studies featuring a high number of patients, and studying the effects of DBS on autonomic dysfunction is usually not the main focus. Dysautonomia is more frequently found in movement disorders than other diseases in the neurodegeneration disease spectrum [43]. Early studies that focus on STN and GPi stimulation reveal that DBS has a beneficial effect on urinary symptoms, especially in reducing nocturia, frequency, and urgency [64]. The most likely mechanism, revealed by urodynamic evaluation, is through increased bladder capacity and reflex volume, and the effect seems to persist over time after initial surgery [65, 66]. Similarly, neuromodulation with DBS appears to be beneficial in gastrointestinal function as well, especially in the early phases after surgery. Significant improvement was found in constipation, salivation, and gastric emptying, as the contractions of the whole gastrointestinal tract improved [67–69]. However, studies show that there is no effect on dysphagia, possibly due to a different mechanism that causes it compared to problems with emptying the gastrointestinal tract [70]. Sexual dysfunction is not significantly impacted by DBS, with most patients reporting a slight improvement, especially in younger patients [71].

4.3 Sleep

Sleep disorders have a significant impact on the quality of life, as they lead to fatigue and daytime sleepiness. Sleep quality is often disrupted in neurodegenerative diseases and has been a subject of study after initiating DBS. Polysomnographic studies show that DBS in STN leads to an objective improvement sleep quality [72], which is seen in subjective-based studies as well [73, 74]. Improvement in sleep and pain was also observed in dystonia patients who were treated with STN DBS [75]. Interestingly, daytime sleepiness does not seem to be affected by DBS [76]. A possible reason for this could be a lacking effect on REM sleep, as DBS patients have an increased risk of developing REM sleep behavioral disorder in the case of STN stimulations [77]. The effect on restless legs syndrome appears to be positive in moderate to severe cases, but new cases of the syndrome can appear after initiating DBS [78, 79]. Overall, it seems that constant stimulations improve sleep quality over the long term by influencing nighttime mobility and sleep maintenance.

4.4 Sensory functions

Somatosensory dysfunction is often reported in neurodegenerative diseases and presents a significant burden in everyday life of the patients. Problems with the sense of smell and taste arise in the early phases of neurodegeneration. Subjective improvement in both smell and taste was reported in a recent prospective study [64]. It appears that the improvement in smell stems from improved odor information processing, as only odor discrimination and identification were improved, while the detection was not affected by DBS [80, 81]. There are improvements in visual function as well, mostly due to the effect on ocular smooth motor function and improving problems with saccade movement [82]; however, the amount of evidence in this field is severely limited and still inconclusive.

Fortunately, the DBS effects on pain are more apparent. Most studies suggest a beneficial effect of DBS on pain [83], especially in patients who suffer from pain in off periods [84]. There are varied types of pain that can be present in patients, but it appears that STN DBS has a substantial effect in curbing dystonic and musculoskeletal pain, while central and neuropathic pain are less affected [85]. However, severe neuropathic pain can be treated with DBS if the target for stimulations is the periaqueductal gray matter, possibility due to an increased release of endogenous opioids [86, 87]. There are promising results in chronic pain as well, with the anterior cingulate cortex showing potential, though it is too early to tell due to a lack of studies in this field [88]. This finding underlines the importance of selecting the right target for neuromodulation depending on the wanted results, which holds promise for the future of DBS.

5. Conclusion

Nonmotor symptoms represent a challenge in the treatment of neurodegenerative diseases and have a significant influence on the quality of life. DBS shows promise in alleviating these symptoms, depending significantly on the target of stimulation. The main problem is the lack of studies in this field, as most have methodological issues or small sample sizes, which limit the strength of the evidence. Likewise, only a handful of studies have nonmotor symptoms and primary end points. The number of approved indications for DBS is still small and mostly focused on extrapyramidal symptoms, and therefore, most studies are focused on the effects of DBS in STN or GPi. However, it is clear that DBS has a promising future in the treatment of neurodegenerative diseases in general and will have an important role in personalized medicine as functional neuroimaging and our understanding of brain physiology improves.

Conflict of interest

The authors declare no conflict of interest.

Appendices and nomenclature

DBS	deep brain stimulation
PD	Parkinson's disease
IPG	implantable pulse generator
fMRI	functional magnetic resonance imaging
GPi	globus pallidus internus
STN	subthalamic nucleus
VIM	ventral intermediate nucleus
NA	nucleus accumbens
NBM	nucleus basalis of Meynert
BDNF	brain-derived neurotrophic factor
REM	rapid eye movement
RLS	restless legs syndrome
NMSQuest	nonmotor symptom questionnaire
NMSS	nonmotor symptom scale

Author details

Vladimira Vuletic[1,2]*, Valentino Racki[1,2], Darko Chudy[3] and Nenad Bogdanovic[4]

1 Department of Neurology, Faculty of Medicine Rijeka, University of Rijeka, Rijeka, Croatia

2 Department of Neurology, University Hospital Centre Rijeka, Rijeka, Croatia

3 Department of Neurosurgery, University Hospital Dubrava, Zagreb, Croatia

4 Division of Clinical Geriatrics, Department for Neurobiology, Caring Science and Society, Karolinska Institutet, Stockholn, Sweden

*Address all correspondence to: vladimira.vuletic@gmail.com

References

[1] Pycroft L, Stein J, Aziz T. Deep brain stimulation: An overview of history, methods, and future developments. Brain and Neuroscience Advances. 2018;**2**:239821281881601. DOI: 10.1177/2398212818816017

[2] Hickey P, Stacy M. Deep brain stimulation: A paradigm shifting approach to treat Parkinson's disease. Frontiers in Neuroscience. 2016;**10**:173. DOI: 10.3389/fnins.2016.00173

[3] Ashkan K, Rogers P, Bergman H, Ughratdar I. Insights into the mechanisms of deep brain stimulation. Nature Reviews. Neurology. 2017;**13**:548-554. DOI: 10.1038/nrneurol.2017.105

[4] Kurtis MM, Rajah T, Delgado LF, Dafsari HS. The effect of deep brain stimulation on the non-motor symptoms of Parkinson's disease: A critical review of the current evidence. npj Parkinson's Disease. 2017;**3**:16024. DOI: 10.1038/npjparkd.2016.24

[5] Herrington TM, Cheng JJ, Eskandar EN. Mechanisms of deep brain stimulation. Journal of Neurophysiology. 2016;**115**:19-38. DOI: 10.1152/jn.00281.2015

[6] Ghasemi P, Sahraee T, Mohammadi A. Closed- and open-loop deep brain stimulation: Methods, challenges, current and future aspects. Journal of Biomedical Physics and Engineering. 2018;**8**:209-216

[7] Habets JGV, Heijmans M, Kuijf ML, Janssen MLF, Temel Y, Kubben PL. An update on adaptive deep brain stimulation in Parkinson's disease. Movement Disorders. 2018;**33**:1834-1843. DOI: 10.1002/mds.115

[8] Montgomery EB, Gale JT. Mechanisms of action of deep brain stimulation (DBS). Neuroscience and Biobehavioral Reviews. 2008;**32**:388-407. DOI: 10.1016/j.neubiorev.2007.06.003

[9] Lanotte MM, Rizzone M, Bergamasco B, Faccani G, Melcarne A, Lopiano L. Deep brain stimulation of the subthalamic nucleus: Anatomical, neurophysiological, and outcome correlations with the effects of stimulation. Journal of Neurology, Neurosurgery, and Psychiatry. 2002;**72**:53-58. DOI: 10.1136/jnnp.72.1.53

[10] Jech R, Urgosík D, Tintera J, Nebuzelský A, Krásenský J, Liscák R, et al. Functional magnetic resonance imaging during deep brain stimulation: A pilot study in four patients with Parkinson's disease. Movement Disorders. 2001;**16**:1126-1132

[11] Vuletic V, Chudy D, Almahariq F, Dobricic V, Kostic V, Bogdanovic N. Excellent outcome of pallidal deep brain stimulation in DYT6 dystonia: A case report. Journal of the Neurological Sciences. 2016;**366**:18-19. DOI: 10.1016/j.jns.2016.04.032

[12] Mitchell KT, Larson P, Starr PA, et al. Benefits and risks of unilateral and bilateral ventral intermediate nucleus deep brain stimulation for axial essential tremor symptoms. Parkinsonism & Related Disorders. 2019;**60**:126-132. DOI: 10.1016/J.PARKRELDIS.2018.09.004

[13] Borders C, Hsu F, Sweidan AJ, Matei ES, Bota RG. Deep brain stimulation for obsessive compulsive disorder: A review of results by anatomical target. Mental Illness. 2018;**10**:7900. DOI: 10.4081/mi.2018.7900

[14] Lee DJ, Elias GJB, Lozano AM. Neuromodulation for the treatment of eating disorders and obesity.

Therapeutic Advances in Psychopharmacology. 2018;**8**:73-92. DOI: 10.1177/2045125317743435

[15] Drobisz D, Damborská A. Deep brain stimulation targets for treating depression. Behavioural Brain Research. 2019;**359**:266-273. DOI: 10.1016/j.bbr.2018.11.004

[16] Hardenacke K, Kuhn J, Lenartz D, Maarouf M, Mai JK, Bartsch C, et al. Stimulate or degenerate: Deep brain stimulation of the nucleus basalis Meynert in Alzheimer dementia. World Neurosurgery. 2013;**80**:S27.e35-S27.e43. DOI: 10.1016/j.wneu.2012.12.005

[17] Kress GJ, Mennerick S. Action potential initiation and propagation: Upstream influences on neurotransmission. Neuroscience. 2009;**158**:211-222. DOI: 10.1016/j.neuroscience.2008.03.021

[18] Jakobs M, Fomenko A, Lozano AM, Kiening KL. Cellular, molecular, and clinical mechanisms of action of deep brain stimulation—A systematic review on established indications and outlook on future developments. EMBO Molecular Medicine. 2019;**11**:e9575. DOI: 10.15252/emmm.201809575

[19] Dostrovsky JO, Levy R, Wu JP, Hutchison WD, Tasker RR, Lozano AM. Microstimulation-induced inhibition of neuronal firing in human globus pallidus. Journal of Neurophysiology. 2000;**84**:570-574. DOI: 10.1152/jn.2000.84.1.570

[20] Degos B, Deniau J-M, Chavez M, Maurice N. Subthalamic nucleus high-frequency stimulation restores altered electrophysiological properties of cortical neurons in parkinsonian rat. PLoS One. 2013;**8**:e83608. DOI: 10.1371/journal.pone.0083608

[21] Sauleau P, Drapier S, Duprez J, et al. Weight gain following pallidal deep brain stimulation: A PET study. PLoS One. 2016;**11**:e0153438. DOI: 10.1371/journal.pone.0153438

[22] Bregman T, Nona C, Volle J, Diwan M, Raymond R, Fletcher PJ, et al. Deep brain stimulation induces antidepressant-like effects in serotonin transporter knockout mice. Brain Stimulation. 2018;**11**:423-425. DOI: 10.1016/j.brs.2017.11.008

[23] van Dijk A, Klompmakers AA, Feenstra MGP, Denys D. Deep brain stimulation of the accumbens increases dopamine, serotonin, and noradrenaline in the prefrontal cortex. Journal of Neurochemistry. 2012;**123**:897-903. DOI: 10.1111/jnc.12054

[24] Song S, Song S, Cao C, Lin X, Li K, Sava V, et al. Hippocampal neurogenesis and the brain repair response to brief stereotaxic insertion of a microneedle. Stem Cells International. 2013;**2013**:205878. DOI: 10.1155/2013/205878

[25] Reddy GD, Lozano AM. Postmortem studies of deep brain stimulation for Parkinson's disease: A systematic review of the literature. Cell and Tissue Research. 2018;**373**:287-295. DOI: 10.1007/s00441-017-2672-2

[26] Lu B, Nagappan G, Lu Y. BDNF and synaptic plasticity, cognitive function, and dysfunction. In: Lewin G, Carter B, editors. Neurotrophic Factors. Handbook of Experimental Pharmacology. Vol. 220. Berlin, Heidelberg: Springer; 2014. Available from: https://doi.org/10.1007/978-3-642-45106-5_9

[27] McIntyre CC, Hahn PJ. Network perspectives on the mechanisms of deep brain stimulation. Neurobiology of Disease. 2010;**38**:329-337. DOI: 10.1016/j.nbd.2009.09.022

[28] Fischer DL, Sortwell CE. BDNF provides many routes toward STN DBS-mediated disease modification. Movement Disorders. 2019;**34**:22-34. DOI: 10.1002/mds.27535

[29] Holt AB, Kormann E, Gulberti A, et al. Phase-dependent suppression of beta oscillations in Parkinson's disease patients. The Journal of Neuroscience. 2019;**39**:1119-1134. DOI: 10.1523/JNEUROSCI.1913-18.2018

[30] Mably AJ, Colgin LL. Gamma oscillations in cognitive disorders. Current Opinion in Neurobiology. 2018;**52**:182-187. DOI: 10.1016/J.CONB.2018.07.009

[31] Sun Y, Giacobbe P, Tang CW, Barr MS, Rajji T, Kennedy SH, et al. Deep brain stimulation modulates gamma oscillations and theta–gamma coupling in treatment resistant depression. Brain Stimulation. 2015;**8**:1033-1042. DOI: 10.1016/j.brs.2015.06.010

[32] Wang DD, de Hemptinne C, Miocinovic S, Ostrem JL, Galifianakis NB, San Luciano M, et al. Pallidal deep-brain stimulation disrupts pallidal beta oscillations and coherence with primary motor cortex in Parkinson's disease. The Journal of Neuroscience. 2018;**38**:4556-4568. DOI: 10.1523/JNEUROSCI.0431-18.2018

[33] Chaudhuri KR, Schapira AH. Non-motor symptoms of Parkinson's disease: Dopaminergic pathophysiology and treatment. Lancet Neurology. 2009;**8**:464-474. DOI: 10.1016/S1474-4422(09)70068-7

[34] Lee HM, Koh S-B. Many faces of Parkinson's disease: Non-motor symptoms of Parkinson's disease. Journal of Movement Disorders. 2015;**8**:92-97. DOI: 10.14802/jmd.15003

[35] Burn DJ. Beyond the iron mask: Towards better recognition and treatment of depression associated with Parkinson's disease. Movement Disorders. 2002;**17**:445-454. DOI: 10.1002/mds.10114

[36] Czernecki V, Schüpbach M, Yaici S, Lévy R, Bardinet E, Yelnik J, et al. Apathy following subthalamic stimulation in Parkinson disease: A dopamine responsive symptom. Movement Disorders. 2008;**23**:964-969. DOI: 10.1002/mds.21949

[37] Bland J. Mild cognitive impairment, neurodegeneration, and personalized lifestyle medicine. Integrative Medicine. 2016;**15**:12

[38] Dhawan V, Healy DG, Pal S, Chaudhuri KR. Sleep-related problems of Parkinson's disease. Age and Ageing. 2006;**35**:220-228. DOI: 10.1093/ageing/afj087

[39] Zielinski MR, McKenna JT, McCarley RW. Functions and mechanisms of sleep. AIMS Neuroscience. 2016;**3**:67-104. DOI: 10.3934/Neuroscience.2016.1.67

[40] Abbott SM, Videnovic A. Chronic sleep disturbance and neural injury: Links to neurodegenerative disease. Nature and Science of Sleep. 2016;**8**:55-61. DOI: 10.2147/NSS.S78947

[41] Iranzo A. Sleep in neurodegenerative diseases. Sleep Medicine Clinics. 2016;**11**:1-18. DOI: 10.1016/j.jsmc.2015.10.011

[42] Malhotra RK. Neurodegenerative disorders and sleep. Sleep Medicine Clinics. 2018;**13**:63-70. DOI: 10.1016/j.jsmc.2017.09.006

[43] Mendoza-Velásquez JJ, Flores-Vázquez JF, Barrón-Velázquez E, Sosa-Ortiz AL, Illigens B-MW, Siepmann T. Autonomic dysfunction in α-synucleinopathies. Frontiers in Neurology. 2019;**10**:363. DOI: 10.3389/fneur.2019.00363

[44] Chiaro G, Calandra-Buonaura G, Cecere A, Mignani F, Sambati L, Loddo G, et al. REM sleep behavior disorder, autonomic dysfunction and synuclein-related neurodegeneration: Where do we stand? Clinical Autonomic

Research. 2018;**28**:519-533. DOI: 10.1007/s10286-017-0460-4

[45] Jost WH. Gastrointestinal dysfunction in Parkinson's disease. Journal of the Neurological Sciences. 2010;**289**:69-73. DOI: 10.1016/J.JNS.2009.08.020

[46] Chalazonitis A, Rao M. Enteric nervous system manifestations of neurodegenerative disease. Brain Research. 2018;**1693**:207-213. DOI: 10.1016/j.brainres.2018.01.011

[47] Niu H, Shen L, Li T, et al. Alpha-synuclein overexpression in the olfactory bulb initiates prodromal symptoms and pathology of Parkinson's disease. Translational Neurodegeneration. 2018;7:25. DOI: 10.1186/s40035-018-0128-6

[48] Albers MW, Gilmore GC, Kaye J, et al. At the interface of sensory and motor dysfunctions and Alzheimer's disease. Alzheimers Dement. 2015;**11**:70-98. DOI: 10.1016/j.jalz.2014.04.514

[49] Doustar J, Torbati T, Black KL, Koronyo Y, Koronyo-Hamaoui M. Optical coherence tomography in Alzheimer's disease and other neurodegenerative diseases. Frontiers in Neurology. 2017;**8**:701. DOI: 10.3389/fneur.2017.00701

[50] Martinez-Martin P, Rodriguez-Blazquez C, Forjaz MJ, Kurtis MM, Skorvanek M. Measurement of nonmotor symptoms in clinical practice. International Review of Neurobiology. 2017;**133**:291-345

[51] Chaudhuri KR, Martinez-Martin P, Schapira AHV, et al. International multicenter pilot study of the first comprehensive self-completed nonmotor symptoms questionnaire for Parkinson's disease: The NMSQuest study. Movement Disorders. 2006;**21**:916-923. DOI: 10.1002/mds.20844

[52] Rios Romenets S, Wolfson C, Galatas C, Pelletier A, Altman R, Wadup L, et al. Validation of the non-motor symptoms questionnaire (NMS-quest). Parkinsonism & Related Disorders. 2012;**18**:54-58. DOI: 10.1016/j.parkreldis.2011.08.013

[53] Chaudhuri KR, Martinez-Martin P, Brown RG, et al. The metric properties of a novel non-motor symptoms scale for Parkinson's disease: Results from an international pilot study. Movement Disorders. 2007;**22**:1901-1911. DOI: 10.1002/mds.21596

[54] Hogg E, Wertheimer J, Graner S, Tagliati M. Deep brain stimulation and nonmotor symptoms. International Review of Neurobiology. 2017;**134**:1045-1089. DOI: 10.1016/BS.IRN.2017.05.022

[55] Trojsi F, Christidi F, Migliaccio R, Santamaría-García H, Santangelo G. Behavioural and cognitive changes in neurodegenerative diseases and brain injury. Behavioural Neurology. 2018;**2018**:4935915. DOI: 10.1155/2018/4935915

[56] Rothlind JC, York MK, Carlson K, Luo P, Marks WJ, Weaver FM, et al. Neuropsychological changes following deep brain stimulation surgery for Parkinson's disease: Comparisons of treatment at pallidal and subthalamic targets versus best medical therapy. Journal of Neurology, Neurosurgery, and Psychiatry. 2015;**86**:622-629. DOI: 10.1136/jnnp-2014-308119

[57] Houeto JL, Mesnage V, Mallet L, et al. Behavioural disorders, Parkinson's disease and subthalamic stimulation. Journal of Neurology, Neurosurgery, and Psychiatry. 2002;**72**:701-707. DOI: 10.1136/jnnp.72.6.701

[58] Kirsch-Darrow L, Zahodne LB, Marsiske M, Okun MS, Foote KD, Bowers D. The trajectory of apathy after deep brain stimulation: From

pre-surgery to 6 months post-surgery in Parkinson's disease. Parkinsonism & Related Disorders. 2011;**17**:182-188. DOI: 10.1016/j.parkreldis.2010.12.011

[59] Schupbach WMM, Chastan N, Welter ML, et al. Stimulation of the subthalamic nucleus in Parkinson's disease: A 5 year follow up. Journal of Neurology, Neurosurgery, and Psychiatry. 2005;**76**:1640-1644. DOI: 10.1136/jnnp.2005.063206

[60] Ardouin C, Voon V, Worbe Y, et al. Pathological gambling in Parkinson's disease improves on chronic subthalamic nucleus stimulation. Movement Disorders. 2006;**21**:1941-1946. DOI: 10.1002/mds.21098

[61] Combs HL, Folley BS, Berry DTR, Segerstrom SC, Han DY, Anderson-Mooney AJ, et al. Cognition and depression following deep brain stimulation of the subthalamic nucleus and globus pallidus pars internus in Parkinson's disease: A meta-analysis. Neuropsychology Review. 2015;**25**: 439-454. DOI: 10.1007/s11065-015-9302-0

[62] Laxton AW, Tang-Wai DF, McAndrews MP, et al. A phase I trial of deep brain stimulation of memory circuits in Alzheimer's disease. Annals of Neurology. 2010;**68**:521-534. DOI: 10.1002/ana.22089

[63] Kuhn J, Hardenacke K, Lenartz D, et al. Deep brain stimulation of the nucleus basalis of Meynert in Alzheimer's dementia. Molecular Psychiatry. 2015;**20**:353-360. DOI: 10.1038/mp.2014.32

[64] Dafsari HS, Reddy P, Herchenbach C, et al. Beneficial effects of bilateral subthalamic stimulation on non-motor symptoms in Parkinson's disease. Brain Stimulation. 2016;**9**:78-85. DOI: 10.1016/j.brs.2015.08.005

[65] Finazzi-Agrò E, Peppe A, D'Amico A, Petta F, Mazzone P, Stanzione P, et al. Effects of subthalamic nucleus stimulation on urodynamic findings in patients with Parkinson's disease. The Journal of Urology. 2003;**169**:1388-1391. DOI: 10.1097/01.ju.0000055520.88377.dc

[66] Seif C, Herzog J, van der Horst C, Schrader B, Volkmann J, Deuschl G, et al. Effect of subthalamic deep brain stimulation on the function of the urinary bladder. Annals of Neurology. 2004;**55**:118-120. DOI: 10.1002/ana.10806

[67] Arai E, Arai M, Uchiyama T, et al. Subthalamic deep brain stimulation can improve gastric emptying in Parkinson's disease. Brain. 2012;**135**:1478-1485. DOI: 10.1093/brain/aws086

[68] Jafari N, Pahwa R, Nazzaro JM, Arnold PM, Lyons KE. MDS-UPDRS to assess non-motor symptoms after STN DBS for Parkinson's disease. The International Journal of Neuroscience. 2016;**126**:25-29. DOI: 10.3109/00207454.2015.1065257

[69] Zibetti M, Torre E, Cinquepalmi A, Rosso M, Ducati A, Bergamasco B, et al. Motor and nonmotor symptom follow-up in parkinsonian patients after deep brain stimulation of the subthalamic nucleus. European Neurology. 2007;**58**:218-223. DOI: 10.1159/000107943

[70] Troche MS, Brandimore AE, Foote KD, Okun MS. Swallowing and deep brain stimulation in Parkinson's disease: A systematic review. Parkinsonism & Related Disorders. 2013;**19**:783-788. DOI: 10.1016/j.parkreldis.2013.05.001

[71] Castelli L, Perozzo P, Genesia ML, Torre E, Pesare M, Cinquepalmi A, et al. Sexual well being in parkinsonian patients after deep brain stimulation of the subthalamic nucleus. Journal of Neurology, Neurosurgery, and

Psychiatry. 2004;**75**:1260-1264. DOI: 10.1136/jnnp.2003.034579

[72] Iranzo A, Valldeoriola F, Santamaría J, Tolosa E, Rumià J. Sleep symptoms and polysomnographic architecture in advanced Parkinson's disease after chronic bilateral subthalamic stimulation. Journal of Neurology, Neurosurgery, and Psychiatry. 2002;**72**:661-664. DOI: 10.1136/jnnp.72.5.661

[73] Amara AW, Standaert DG, Guthrie S, Cutter G, Watts RL, Walker HC. Unilateral subthalamic nucleus deep brain stimulation improves sleep quality in Parkinson's disease. Parkinsonism & Related Disorders. 2012;**18**:63-68. DOI: 10.1016/j.parkreldis.2011.09.001

[74] Vuletic V, Chudy D. The effect of deep brain stimulation of the subthalamic nucleus on sleep in advanced Parkinson's disease. Journal of the Neurological Sciences. 2015;**357**:e292-e293. DOI: 10.1016/j.jns.2015.08.1017

[75] Vuletic V. Frequency of the pain and sleep problems in dystonia patients and influence of deep brain stimulation. Parkinsonism & Related Disorders. 2016;**22**:e136-e137. DOI: 10.1016/j.parkreldis.2015.10.331

[76] Kharkar S, Ellenbogen JR, Samuel M, Rizos A, Silverdale M, Chaudhuri KR, et al. Changes in Parkinson's disease sleep symptoms and daytime somnolence after bilateral subthalamic deep brain stimulation in Parkinson's disease. npj Parkinson's Disease. 2018;**4**:16. DOI: 10.1038/s41531-018-0053-5

[77] Kim YE, Jeon BS, Paek S-H, Yun JY, Yang H-J, Kim H-J, et al. Rapid eye movement sleep behavior disorder after bilateral subthalamic stimulation in Parkinson's disease. Journal of Clinical Neuroscience. 2015;**22**:315-319. DOI: 10.1016/j.jocn.2014.07.016

[78] Kedia S, Moro E, Tagliati M, Lang AE, Kumar R. Emergence of restless legs syndrome during subthalamic stimulation for Parkinson disease. Neurology. 2004;**63**:2410-2412. DOI: 10.1212/01.wnl.0000147288.26029.b8

[79] Klepitskaya O, Liu Y, Sharma S, Sillau SH, Tsai J, Walters AS. Deep brain stimulation improves restless legs syndrome in patients with Parkinson disease. Neurology. 2018;**91**:e1013-e1021. DOI: 10.1212/WNL.0000000000006162

[80] Cury RG, Carvalho M d J, Lasteros FJL, et al. Effects of subthalamic stimulation on olfactory function in Parkinson disease. World Neurosurgery. 2018;**114**:e559-e564. DOI: 10.1016/j.wneu.2018.03.033

[81] Guo X, Gao G, Wang X, Li L, Li W, Liang Q, et al. Effects of bilateral deep brain stimulation of the subthalamic nucleus on olfactory function in Parkinson's disease patients. Stereotactic and Functional Neurosurgery. 2008;**86**:237-244. DOI: 10.1159/000131662

[82] Shaikh AG, Antoniades C, Fitzgerald J, Ghasia FF. Effects of deep brain stimulation on eye movements and vestibular function. Frontiers in Neurology. 2018;**9**:444. DOI: 10.3389/fneur.2018.00444

[83] Kim H-J, Jeon BS, Lee J-Y, Paek SH, Kim DG. The benefit of subthalamic deep brain stimulation for pain in Parkinson disease. Neurosurgery. 2012;**70**:18-24. DOI: 10.1227/NEU.0b013e3182266664

[84] Juri C, Rodríguez-Oroz MC, Burguera JA, Guridi J, Obeso JA. Pain and dyskinesia in Parkinson's disease. Movement Disorders. 2010;**25**:130-132. DOI: 10.1002/mds.22874

[85] Cury RG, Galhardoni R, Fonoff ET, et al. Effects of deep brain stimulation

on pain and other nonmotor symptoms in Parkinson disease. Neurology. 2014;**83**:1403-1409. DOI: 10.1212/WNL.0000000000000887

[86] Pereira EAC, Aziz TZ. Neuropathic pain and deep brain stimulation. Neurotherapeutics. 2014;**11**:496-507. DOI: 10.1007/s13311-014-0278-x

[87] Sims-Williams H, Matthews JC, Talbot PS, Love-Jones S, Brooks JC, Patel NK, et al. Deep brain stimulation of the periaqueductal gray releases endogenous opioids in humans. NeuroImage. 2017;**146**:833-842. DOI: 10.1016/j.neuroimage.2016.08.038

[88] Farrell SM, Green A, Aziz T. The current state of deep brain stimulation for chronic pain and its context in other forms of neuromodulation. Brain Sciences. 20 Aug 2018;**8**(8):158. DOI: 10.3390/brainsci8080158

Section 4

Neurostimulation and Neuromodulation for Pain and Spinal Dysfunction

Chapter 9

Cerebellar Transcranial Direct Current Stimulation (ctDCS) Effect in Perception and Modulation of Pain

Tommaso Bocci, Roberta Ferrucci, Alberto Priori, Massimiliano Valeriani and Ferdinando Sartucci

Abstract

Transcranial direct stimulation (tDCS) in the treatment of intractable or marginally tractable pain is experiencing an increasing diffusion in many fields worldwide. Recently, new modality of tDCS application has been proposed and applied, as cerebellar transcranial direct current stimulation (ctDCS). Indeed, the cerebellum has been proved to play a role in pain processing and to be involved in a wide number of integrative functions. In this chapter, we encompass the history of the technique, analysis of principles, a general description, including the methodological procedures of ctDCS; then, main clinical applications and their main effects in perceptive threshold of pain and other sensation, pain intensity, and laser evoked potentials (LEPs) changes.

Keywords: cerebellum, tDCS, cerebellar stimulation, pain, phantom limb pain

1. Introduction

Pain still remains a challenge for clinicians and neuroscientists, and current pharmacological therapies are often ineffective for the prevention and treatment of chronic pain. In particular, chronization of pain represents a multi-step phenomenon, comprising spinal phenotypic switch in the expression of neuropeptides, as well as elusive brain mechanisms, ranging from the so-called "thalamo-cortical dysrhythmia" to a functional reorganization of sensorimotor maps (**Figure 1**) [1–4]. In this scenario, the putative relationship between pain and the cerebellum is particularly intriguing, as the cerebellum is anatomically located between the spinal cord and the brain, possibly interfering both with top-down and bottom-up mechanisms underlying pain control and ultimately responsible for central pain sensitization.

The cerebellum is involved in a wide range of integrative functions, ranging from motor adaptation to working memory and associative learning, but its role in nociceptive experience and pain processing remains debated [5–10].

Overall, the cerebellum likely belongs to a widespread network that mediates reactions stronger to negative external stimuli than to positive ones [11, 12]; recent

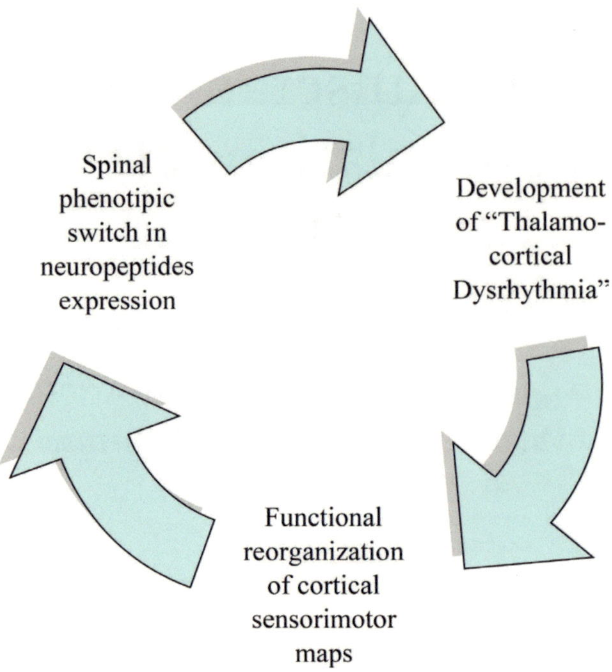

Figure 1.
"Red Flags" responsible for chronization of pain. Chronic pain is a multi-level and multi-step phenomenon, comprising changes at brain as well as spinal levels, and involves different neurotransmitters and neuronal pathways.

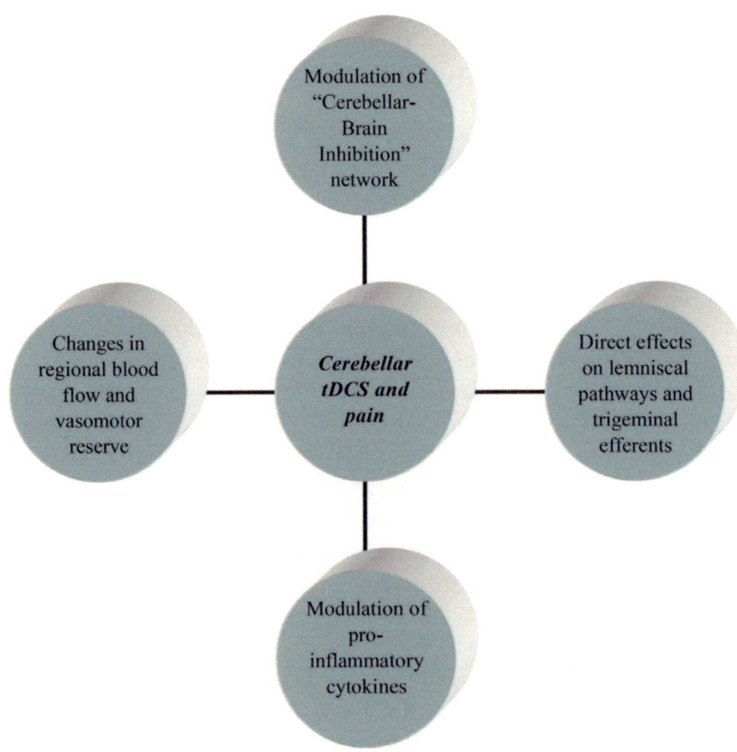

Figure 2.
Rationale for the use of cerebellar tDCS (tcDCS) for pain treatment: possible mechanisms of action and molecular pathways.

evidence has strengthened the hypothesis that plasticity subserving the storage and retention of unconditioned responses selectively occurs in the cerebellum [13–16]; recently we have proved a cerebellar role in learning of aversive reactions inside the peripersonal space [17], and studies in humans have highlighted a cerebellar engagement both in pain empathy and nocifensive withdrawal [18–20].

Nonetheless, some important questions remain open: (1) whether the cerebellum is engaged in the primary sensory-discriminative dimension of pain; (2) how it interacts with the cerebral cortex for pain processing; (3) whether it may be used as a putative target for non-pharmacological therapies, as non-invasive brain stimulation techniques (NIBS).

In this chapter, we encompass the current knowledge about the cerebellar role in pain processing, suggesting novel strategies for pain control and therapy in the emerging field of non-invasive neuromodulation (**Figure 2**).

2. Current pitfalls for the use of NIBS in pain treatment

Cerebellar direct current stimulation has been widely used for the treatment of several neuropsychiatric diseases, ranging from movement disorders [21–25] to autism and schizophrenia [26, 27], but only few evidence has been reached so far regarding pain therapy.

In general, transcranial direct current stimulation (tDCS) has been proposed for pain therapy, especially when applied over the primary motor area (M1) or the dorsolateral prefrontal cortex [28, 29]; nonetheless, the too small sample sizes and the extreme variability of stimulation parameters have limited its efficacy: as a result, pain improvement is often weak and brief, in line with the so-called "placebo-effect." There are also other possible explanations.

First, pain is a complex experience, involving phenomena at a sensory, affective-emotional and cognitive level: thus, clinical scales are often inappropriate to describe the whole phenomenon and follow putative effects of therapies over time.

Second, chronic pain involves different neurotransmitters and neuronal circuitries at a spinal and supra-spinal level: therefore, non-invasive stimulation applied over a limited brain target usually induces a transient pain improvement.

Third, only few groups have enough experience about the use of neurophysiological tools for pain assessment [30]; among these techniques, laser evoked potentials (LEPs) offer an unique opportunity to study the sensory-discriminative, as well as the affective-emotional dimension of pain, which are differently carried by medial and lateral spinal nociceptive systems and rely on the activation of distinct cortical areas [31–33].

3. Transcranial direct current stimulation (tDCS) and the cerebellum: an overview

3.1 Putative mechanisms of action of cerebellar tDCS and implications for pain treatment

Transcranial direct current stimulation (tDCS) has emerged in the past few years as a novel, noninvasive, inexpensive, and safe technique to modulate cortical excitability, both in health and disease. tDCS uses subthreshold currents (1.0–2.5 mA), too weak to induce neuronal activity independent from afferent input, but sufficient *per se* to alter both the excitability and spontaneous neuronal firing rate.

tDCS shows short- and long-term effects; the first ones outlast the end of stimulation for only a few minutes and involve non-synaptic mechanisms, comprising changes in membrane polarity, migration, and steric conformation of transmembrane proteins. Conversely, the long-term after-effects are mainly driven by synaptic modifications. In particular, anodal tDCS seems to have an overall excitatory effect, probably reducing intra-cortical GABA, whereas cathodal polarization dampens cortical excitability by reducing glutamate [34, 35]. Many studies reported the same polarity-specific effects for cerebellar tDCS, although they also depend on the position of the return electrode (namely, the "reference"), as well as on the size of electrodes and duration of the stimulation [36, 37].

Direct current polarization has both on-line and off-line effects on cerebellar excitability. This is in agreement with the effects elicited by tDCS in the cerebral cortex that are observable after both short-term and long-term delays and most likely interfering with long-term potentiation (LTP-like) phenomena [38]. From a cellular point of view, animal studies suggest that the electrical stimulation of Purkinje cells mediates on-line effects [39], whereas depolarization of Golgi inhibitory neurons is responsible for long-lasting changes [40]. Nonetheless, electrical fields induced by cerebellar tDCS in humans are much smaller than those used in animals, thus making it difficult to compare their mechanisms of action [41].

Purkinje cells represent the output from the cerebellar cortex, and their activation leads to the inhibition of cerebellar nuclei, ultimately dampening motor cortex excitability. Cerebellar tDCS (ctDCS) may interfere with this connectivity, influencing the so-called "Cerebellar-Brain Inhibition" (CBI); consequently, anodal ctDCS may reduce pain perception by increasing the inhibitory tone exerted by the cerebellum on different brain targets, whereas cathodal ctDCS could elicit opposite effects by inducing hyperalgesia. This tentative model has been recently confirmed by a clinical study of Ruscheweyh and co-workers [42], showing that patients with cerebellar infarctions have reduced pain thresholds, as concerns both placebo and offset analgesia.

Apart from non-synaptic and synaptic (neuroplastic) changes, tDCS may modulate pain experience and processing through different mechanisms. In recent years, a growing body of evidence has strengthen the importance of tDCS after-effects on regional blood flow and immune responses. In particular, animal studies have proved that tDCS elicits neural stem cells (NSCs) activation in vivo, thus influencing the development and the distribution of microglia in the adult brain [43]. In addition, tDCS likely modulates inflammatory response by regulating pro-inflammatory cytokines and increasing glutathione levels [44].

3.2 Cerebellar tDCS: setting parameters

Commonly, tDCS uses two electrodes, a cathode and an anode, but montages with multiple electrodes are possible. Their sizes vary among different studies and critically depend on the target; small electrodes (3 × 5 cm, 3 × 3 cm) are used for cerebellar polarization [36], whereas larger ones are commonly applied for direct spinal stimulation [45].

The return electrode (namely, the "reference") may be applied either over another cortical region or extra-cranially (e.g., the shoulder); the second choice should be preferred because cutaneous impedance is reduced and opposite effects of anodal and cathodal stimulation emerge more clearly.

Both electrodes are connected to a standard tDCS stimulator, delivering currents for 15–25 min, at an intensity ranging from 1 to 2 mA. This stimulation intensity

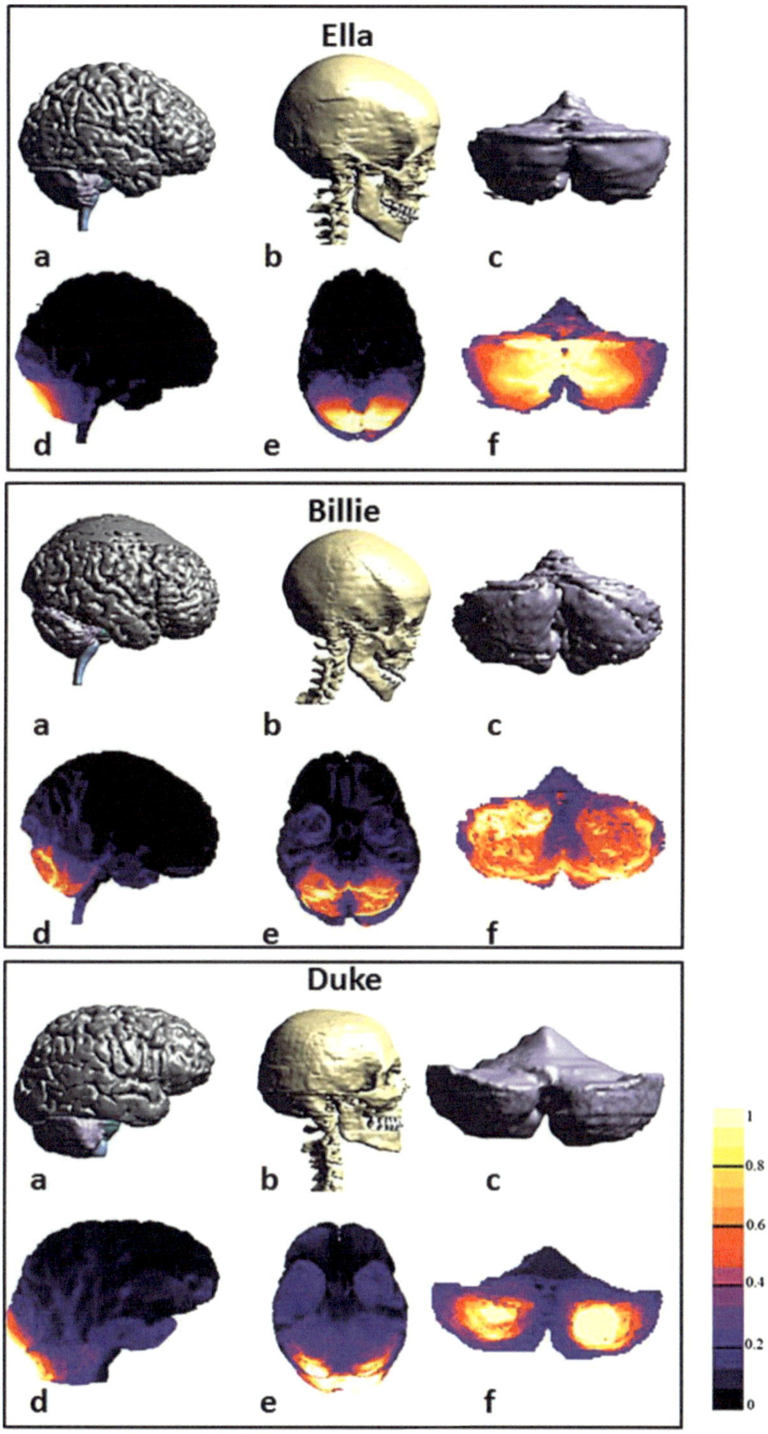

Figure 3.
Current density generated by cerebellar transcranial direct current stimulation (cerebellar tDCS) in humans. Examples of segmented tissues in two human realistic virtual family models (Ella and Duke) undergoing cerebellar tDCS. The spread of the current density (J) over the occipital cortex—quantified as the percentage of occipital volume where the amplitude of J-field is greater than 70% of the peak of J in the cerebellum—was only 4% for "Duke" and much less than 1% for "Ella" [modified from Parazzini et al. [49], with permission].

induces an electric field of the same order of magnitude as that influencing the cerebellar neuron activity in animal experiments [37].

3.3 Cerebellar tDCS: safety

When the procedure is correctly delivered, according to the safety guidelines, no adverse effects occur, except for a transient itching of tingling sensation.

In most subjects, cerebellar tDCS evokes no sensation likely because cutaneous nerves in the occipital region show a higher threshold than those located in the frontal trigeminal dermatomes [46].

Researchers and therapists should keep in mind only few exclusion criteria, such as the presence of metallic implants in the skull or in the brain [47], and subjects' skin should be lightly cleaned with a swab. Second, electrode sponges should be soaked with saline solution to reduce skin impedance. Finally, a current density limit of 0.029–0.142 mA/cm^2, corresponding to a maximum of charge density of about 40 μC/cm^2 at the stimulating electrode, has considered to be safe [48].

Notably, despite some inter-individual differences, recent modeling researches have revealed that the current spread to other structures outside the cerebellum is negligible and unlikely to produce functional effects (**Figure 3**) [49].

4. Cerebellar tDCS: emerging evidence for pain treatment

In previous papers from our laboratory, we have demonstrated for the first time that cerebellar tDCS modulates pain processing in healthy humans, probably by interfering with the CBI network [50–52]. In particular, ctDCS exerts polarity-specific effects on the amplitude of laser evoked potentials (LEPs), thus modifying the perception of experimentally induced pain in young volunteers: anodal stimulation leads to analgesia, whereas cathodal polarization increases pain perception.

This is in line with the theory that cerebellum exerts an overall inhibitory effect on pain processing at a cortical level, similar to that induced within motor pathways.

Because tDCS is effective on the modulation of both N1 and N2/P2 components of LEPs and these responses are generated by parallel and partially segregated spinal pathways reaching different cortical targets [32], we argue that the cerebellum is involved in pain processing by modulating the activity of both somatosensory and cingulate cortices. Indeed, from a functional point of view, the cerebellum is engaged in the sensory-discriminative, as well as in the emotional and cognitive dimension of pain [53, 54]: therefore, non-invasive cerebellar current stimulation may modulate pain experience and the associated cortical activities through different, not mutually exclusive mechanisms. Moreover, our results indicate, for the first time in humans, that the cerebellum is also engaged in the primary sensory-discriminative dimension of pain.

A recent paper by Pereira and co-workers [55] has confirmed our results, showing that anodal cerebellar tDCS reduces lower extremity pain perception in healthy humans.

However, in a previous study, Zunhammer and colleagues [56] failed to demonstrate analgesic effects of rTMS applied over the cerebellum; the discrepancy with our results, may be due to different factors: the authors evaluated changes in subjective pain thresholds, without any neurophysiological support, and used a different neuromodulation technique (rTMS vs. tDCS).

The efficacy of cerebellar tDCS on pain treatment has been recently confirmed also in patients suffered from "phantom limb pain" (PLP) [51].

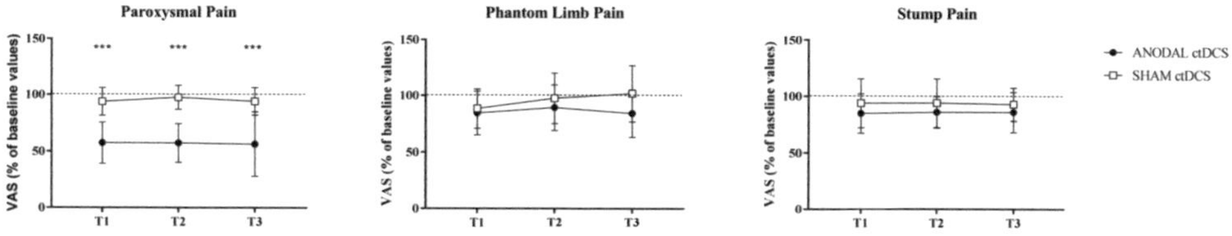

Figure 4.
*Painful (top row) phantom limb phenomena: changes in VAS scores overtime. Note that anodal ctDCS (black circles) significantly improved paroxysmal pain compared to the sham condition (white squares). Data are given as percentage of baseline value ±1 S.D. At each time interval, the statistical significance refers to the comparison between anodal (active) and sham (placebo) stimulation (***$p < 0.001$, Bonferroni post-hoc comparison; modified from [51], with permission).*

PLP remains a challenge for clinicians and neuroscientists. The short and long-term effectiveness of pharmacological interventions is unclear; most of the studies were limited by their small sample sizes and by different pharmacological effects on either painful and non-painful phenomena; also invasive spinal cord stimulation (SCS), probably due to its poor somatotopic specificity, failed to demonstrate significant and long-lasting effects specificity [57, 58].

Recent studies have shown that tDCS applied over the motor cortex represents a promising therapeutic tool in PLP, with effects likely arising from a transient restoration of the cortical representation of the phantom limb [59–62]. Based on this, we have recently shown that anodal ctDCS improves both paroxysmal pain and non-painful phantom limb sensations in subjects with upper limb amputations (**Figure 4**), as confirmed by changes observed in LEP amplitudes, with anodal tDCS significantly reducing the amplitude of both N1 and N2/P2 components [51]. We argue that, different from other brain targets and depending on the extent of anatomical connections between the cerebellum and the brain, ctDCS may reduce both painful and non-painful phantom limb sensations, which are induced by maladaptive changes in the sensorimotor network and posterior parietal cortex, respectively [59].

5. Laser evoked potentials (LEPs) as a valuable outcome measure: setting and method

Laser evoked potentials (LEPs) allow to evaluate both the lateral and the medial pain pathways, two different, parallel and partially segregated spinal "highways," targeting cortical areas differently involved in nociceptive experience and pain processing. In particular, the two main LEP components, formally named N1 and N2/P2 potentials, correspond, respectively, to the activation of the secondary somatosensory cortex (SII) and of the insular region; from a functional perspective, N1 reflects the sensory-discriminative, whereas N2/P2 complex the affective-emotional dimension of pain [32, 33].

A solid-state laser is commonly used in clinical trials (neodymium: yttrium-aluminum-perovskite, Nd: YAP; wavelength 1.04 mm, pulse duration 2–20 ms, maximum energy 7J: Stimul 1340VR, Electronical Engineering®, Florence, Italy). The laser beam was transmitted from the generator to the stimulating probe via a 10 m length optical fiber; signals were amplified, band pass filtered (0.1–200 Hz, time analysis 1000 ms) and fed to a computer for analysis [30, 63, 64]. Compared to CO_2 laser, Nd: YAP uses pulses with a shorter duration and lower wavelengths, thus resulting in a better synchronization of afferent inputs, reducing at the same time the possibility of tissue damage (**Figure 5**).

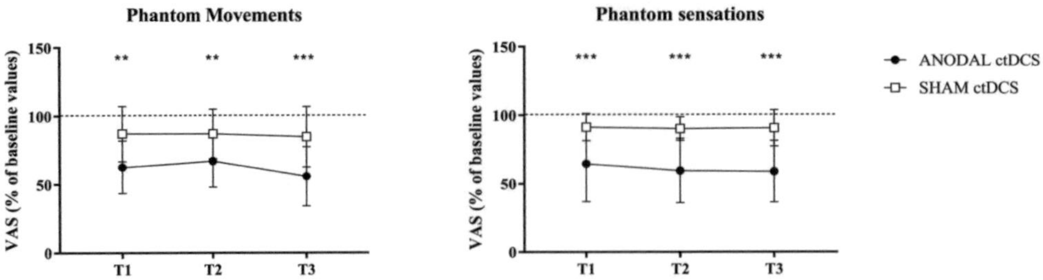

Figure 5.
*Non-painful (top row) phantom limb phenomena: changes in VAS scores overtime. Note that anodal ctDCS (black circles) significantly improved phantom movements and sensations compared to the sham condition (white squares). Data are given as percentage of baseline value ±1 S.D. At each time interval, the statistical significance refers to the comparison between anodal (active) and sham (placebo) stimulation (***p < 0.001, Bonferroni post-hoc comparison; modified from [51], with permission).*

In our paper [51], the stump was stimulated by laser pulses (individual variability: 15.75–24.91 J/cm^2) with short duration (5 ms) and small diameter spots (5 mm), inducing pinprick sensations. Twenty stimuli, whose intensity was established on the basis of the perceptive threshold of each patient, were delivered: we used a fixed intensity set at two times the individual sensory threshold, defined as the lower stimulus intensity that elicited a distinct painful pinprick sensation. In order to reduce both skin lesions and fatigue of peripheral nociceptors, the laser beam was shifted slightly by ~10 mm in a random direction between consecutive pulses [64]. Patients were reclined on a couch, wore protective goggles, and were instructed to keep their eyes open and gaze slightly downwards; they were requested to mentally count the number of stimuli, to keep their attention level constant. The interstimulus interval varied randomly between 15 and 30 s.

The main Aδ-LEP complex, N2/P2, and the earlier lateralized N1 component were recorded through standard disc, nonpolarizable Ag/AgCl surface electrodes (diameter 10 mm; BiomedVR, Florence, Italy). N2 and P2 components were recorded from the vertex (Cz), referenced to the earlobes; the N1 component was recorded from the contralateral temporal leads (T3 or T4), referenced to Fz [63]. The baseline-to-peak and the peak-to-peak amplitudes of N1 and N2/P2 components, respectively, were evaluated. Blinks and saccades were recorded with an EOG electrode placed on the supero-lateral right canthus connected to the system reference. Ground was placed on the mid-forehead.

Skin impedance was kept below 5 kΩ. An automatic artifact rejection system excluded all trials contaminated by transient signals exceeding the average value by ±65 μV on each recording channel, including the EOG.

6. Theoretical limitations to tDCS for cerebellar stimulation

Cerebellar tDCS has still some limitations. First, the variability in outcome measures as well as the applied stimulation parameters across studies prompts further research about montage, duration, intensity of stimulation, electrodes number, and placement.

Second, direct current stimulation may exert different, sometimes opposite, effects on motor and non-motor cerebellar functions; in this view, while studies exploring cognitive and emotional domains have used a classical monopolar configuration, others focusing on motor functions have adopted a different montage, in which the return electrode is positioned over the ipsilateral face. Only in the second case, tDCS has demonstrated long-lasting polarity-specific effects.

That could be critically depend also on the cerebellar somatotopy: the motor cerebellum is mainly represented within the anterior areas, whereas non-motor functions are likely located in the posterior regions. In this connection, only few studies have demonstrated to date the "reverse effect" between anodal and cathodal polarization [45, 52, 65].

Third, tDCS effects critically depend on the structure orientation relative to the electric field direction: neurons of the cerebellum are not identically orientated and follow complex anatomical distributions over folia. That might cause a hyperpolarization in some cells, while others are depolarized at the same time [66, 67].

7. Conclusions

Cerebellar current stimulation represents an emerging, safe, and effective neuromodulation strategy for pain treatment. The possibility to interfere with cerebellar activity is particularly fascinating in the field of chronic pain syndromes, given that the cerebellum itself regulates both ascending and descending pathways involved in pain processing and nociception. However, the exact mechanisms of action are not fully understood, and some stimulation parameters have to be clearly defined, comprising duration, intensity, and charge density. Moreover, more attention will be deserved to combine and integrate different NIBS techniques, as well as different targets at the same time; for instance, by using the same device, cerebellar tDCS may be associate to spinal direct current polarization, in order to improve the clinical outcome and possibly extend putative effects over time.

Author details

Tommaso Bocci[1,2], Roberta Ferrucci[1], Alberto Priori[1,2], Massimiliano Valeriani[3,4] and Ferdinando Sartucci[5]*

1 "Aldo Ravelli" Center for Neurotechnology and Experimental Brain Therapeutics, Department of Health Sciences, University of Milan and ASST Santi Paolo e Carlo, Milan, Italy

2 III Neurology Clinic, ASST Santi Paolo e Carlo, Milan, Italy

3 Division of Neurology, Ospedale Bambino Gesù, Rome, Italy

4 Center for Sensory-Motor Interaction, Aalborg University, Aalborg, Denmark

5 Section of Neurophysiopathology, Department of Clinical and Experimental Medicine, University of Pisa, Italy

*Address all correspondence to: ferdinando.sartucci@med.unipi.it

References

[1] Flor H. Maladaptive plasticity, memory for pain and phantom limb pain: Review and suggestions for new therapies. Expert Review of Neurotherapeutics. 2008;**8**:809-818

[2] Flor H, Nikolajsen L, Staehelin Jensen T. Phantom limb pain: A case of maladaptive CNS plasticity? Nature Reviews. Neuroscience. 2006;**7**:873-881

[3] Hsieh PC, Tseng MT, Chao CC, Lin YH, Tseng WY, Liu KH, et al. Imaging signatures of altered brain responses in small-fiber neuropathy: Reduced functional connectivity of the limbic system after peripheral nerve degeneration. Pain. 2015;**156**:904-916

[4] Lotze M, Flor H, Grodd W, Larbig W, Birbaumer N. Phantom movements and pain. An fMRI study in upper limb amputees. Brain. 2001;**124**:2268-2277

[5] Boehringer A, Macher K, Dukart J, Villringer A, Pleger B. Cerebellar transcranial direct current stimulation modulates verbal working memory. Brain Stimulation. 2013;**6**:649-653

[6] Ferrucci R, Marceglia S, Vergari M, Cogiamanian F, Mrakic-Sposta S, Mameli F, et al. Cerebellar transcranial direct current stimulation impairs the practice-dependent proficiency increase in working memory. Journal of Cognitive Neuroscience. 2008;**20**:1687-1697

[7] Galea JM, Vazquez A, Pasricha N, de Xivry JJ, Celnik P. Dissociating the roles of the cerebellum and motor cortex during adaptive learning: The motor cortex retains what the cerebellum learns. Cerebral Cortex. 2011;**21**:1761-1770

[8] Hardwick RM, Celnik PA. Cerebellar direct current stimulation enhances motor learning in older adults. Neurobiology of Aging. 2014;**35**:2217-2221

[9] Herzfeld DJ, Pastor D, Haith AM, Rossetti Y, Shadmehr R, O'Shea J. Contributions of the cerebellum and the motor cortex to acquisition and retention of motor memories. NeuroImage. 2014;**98**:147-158

[10] Mannarelli D, Pauletti C, De Lucia MC, Delle Chiaie R, Bersani FS, Spagnoli F, et al. Effects of cerebellar transcranial direct current stimulation on attentional processing of the stimulus: Evidence from an event-related potentials study. Neuropsychologia. 2016;**84**:127-135

[11] Ferrucci R, Giannicola G, Rosa M, Fumagalli M, Boggio PS, Hallett M, et al. Cerebellum and processing of negative facial emotions: Cerebellar transcranial DC stimulation specifically enhances the emotional recognition of facial anger and sadness. Cognition and Emotion. 2012;**26**:786-799

[12] Fox E, Lester V, Russo R, Bowles RJ, Pichler A, Dutton K. Facial expressions of emotion: Are angry faces detected more efficiently? Cognition and Emotion. 2000;**14**:61-92

[13] Bracha V, Kolb FP, Irwin KB, Bloedel JR. Inactivation of interposed nuclei in the cat: Classically conditioned withdrawal reflexes, voluntary limb movements and the action primitive hypothesis. Experimental Brain Research. 1999;**126**:77-92

[14] Bracha V, Zhao L, Irwin K, Bloedel JR. Intermediate cerebellum and conditioned eyeblinks. Parallel involvement in eyeblinks and tonic eyelid closure. Experimental Brain Research. 2001;**136**:41-49

[15] Thieme A, Thurling M, Galuba J, Burciu RG, Goricke S, Beck A, et al. Storage of a naturally acquired conditioned response is impaired in patients with cerebellar degeneration. Brain. 2013;**136**:2063-2076

[16] Timmann D, Baier PC, Diener HC, Kolb FP. Classically conditioned withdrawal reflex in cerebellar patients. 1. Impaired conditioned responses. Experimental Brain Research. 2000;**130**:453-470

[17] Bocci T, Ferrucci R, Barloscio D, Parenti L, Cortese F, Priori A, et al. Cerebellar direct current stimulation modulates hand blink reflex: Implications for defensive behavior in humans. Physiological Reports. 2018;**6**:e13471

[18] Borsook D, Moulton EA, Tully S, Schmahmann JD, Becerra L. Human cerebellar responses to brush and heat stimuli in healthy and neuropathic pain subjects. Cerebellum. 2008;**7**:252-272

[19] Dimitrova A, Kolb FP, Elles HG, Maschke M, Forsting M, Diener HC, et al. Cerebellar responses evoked by nociceptive leg withdrawal reflex as revealed by event-related FMRI. Journal of Neurophysiology. 2003;**90**:1877-1886

[20] Ploghaus A, Tracey I, Gati JS, Clare S, Menon RS, Matthews PM, et al. Dissociating pain from its anticipation in the human brain. Science. 1999;**284**:1979-1981

[21] Alizad V, Meinzer M, Frossard L, Polman R, Smith S, Kerr G. Effects of transcranial direct current stimulation on gait in people with Parkinson's disease: Study protocol for a randomized, controlled clinical trial. Trials. 2018;**19**:661

[22] Benussi A, Dell'Era V, Cantoni V, Ferrari C, Caratozzolo S, Rozzini L, et al. Discrimination of atypical parkinsonisms with transcranial magnetic stimulation. Brain Stimulation. 2018;**11**:366-373

[23] Benussi A, Dell'Era V, Cotelli MS, Turla M, Casali C, Padovani A, et al. Long term clinical and neurophysiological effects of cerebellar transcranial direct current stimulation in patients with neurodegenerative ataxia. Brain Stimulation. 2017;**10**:242-250

[24] Ferrucci R, Cortese F, Bianchi M, Pittera D, Turrone R, Bocci T, et al. Cerebellar and motor cortical Transcranial stimulation decrease levodopa-induced Dyskinesias in Parkinson's disease. Cerebellum. 2016;**15**:43-47

[25] Grimaldi G, Oulad Ben Taib N, Manto M, Bodranghien F. Marked reduction of cerebellar deficits in upper limbs following transcranial cerebello-cerebral DC stimulation: Tremor reduction and re-programming of the timing of antagonist commands. Frontiers in Systems Neuroscience. 2014;**8**:9

[26] Gupta T, Dean DJ, Kelley NJ, Bernard JA, Ristanovic I, Mittal VA. Cerebellar transcranial direct current stimulation improves procedural learning in nonclinical psychosis: A double-blind crossover study. Schizophrenia Bulletin. 2018;**44**:1373-1380

[27] Martin DM, Chan HN, Alonzo A, Green MJ, Mitchell PB, Loo CK. Transcranial direct current stimulation to enhance cognition in euthymic bipolar disorder. Bipolar Disorders. 2015;**17**:849-858

[28] Lefaucheur JP. A comprehensive database of published tDCS clinical trials (2005-2016). Neurophysiologie Clinique. 2016;**46**:319-398

[29] Lefaucheur JP, Antal A, Ayache SS, Benninger DH, Brunelin J,

Cogiamanian F, et al. Evidence-based guidelines on the therapeutic use of transcranial direct current stimulation (tDCS). Clinical Neurophysiology. 2017;**128**:56-92

[30] Truini A, Panuccio G, Galeotti F, Maluccio MR, Sartucci F, Avoli M, et al. Laser-evoked potentials as a tool for assessing the efficacy of antinociceptive drugs. European Journal of Pain. 2010;**14**:222-225

[31] Garcia-Larrea L, Frot M, Valeriani M. Brain generators of laser-evoked potentials: From dipoles to functional significance. Neurophysiologie Clinique. 2003;**33**:279-292

[32] Valeriani M, Le Pera D, Restuccia D, de Armas L, Miliucci R, Betti V, et al. Parallel spinal pathways generate the middle-latency N1 and the late P2 components of the laser evoked potentials. Clinical Neurophysiology. 2007;**118**:1097-1104

[33] Valeriani M, Pazzaglia C, Cruccu G, Truini A. Clinical usefulness of laser evoked potentials. Neurophysiologie Clinique. 2012;**42**:345-353

[34] Rango M, Cogiamanian F, Marceglia S, Barberis B, Arighi A, Biondetti P, et al. Myoinositol content in the human brain is modified by transcranial direct current stimulation in a matter of minutes: A 1H-MRS study. Magnetic Resonance in Medicine. 2008;**60**:782-789

[35] Stagg CJ, Best JG, Stephenson MC, O'Shea J, Wylezinska M, Kincses ZT, et al. Polarity-sensitive modulation of cortical neurotransmitters by transcranial stimulation. The Journal of Neuroscience. 2009;**29**:5202-5206

[36] Ferrucci R, Cortese F, Priori A. Cerebellar tDCS: How to do it. Cerebellum. 2015;**14**:27-30

[37] Priori A, Ciocca M, Parazzini M, Vergari M, Ferrucci R. Transcranial cerebellar direct current stimulation and transcutaneous spinal cord direct current stimulation as innovative tools for neuroscientists. The Journal of Physiology. 2014;**592**:3345-3369

[38] Hamada M, Strigaro G, Murase N, Sadnicka A, Galea JM, Edwards MJ, et al. Cerebellar modulation of human associative plasticity. The Journal of Physiology. 2012;**590**:2365-2374

[39] Chan CY, Nicholson C. Modulation by applied electric fields of Purkinje and stellate cell activity in the isolated turtle cerebellum. The Journal of Physiology. 1986;**371**:89-114

[40] Hull CA, Chu Y, Thanawala M, Regehr WG. Hyperpolarization induces a long-term increase in the spontaneous firing rate of cerebellar Golgi cells. The Journal of Neuroscience. 2013;**33**:5895-5902

[41] Parazzini M, Rossi E, Ferrucci R, Fiocchi S, Liorni I, Priori A, et al. Computational model of cerebellar transcranial direct current stimulation. Conference Proceedings: Annual International Conference of the IEEE Engineering in Medicine and Biology Society. 2013;**2013**:237-240

[42] Ruscheweyh R, Kuhnel M, Filippopulos F, Blum B, Eggert T, Straube A. Altered experimental pain perception after cerebellar infarction. Pain. 2014;**155**:1303-1312

[43] Rueger MA, Keuters MH, Walberer M, Braun R, Klein R, Sparing R, et al. Multi-session transcranial direct current stimulation (tDCS) elicits inflammatory and regenerative processes in the rat brain. PLoS One. 2012;7:e43776

[44] Leffa DT, Bellaver B, Salvi AA, de Oliveira C, Caumo W, Grevet EH, et al. Transcranial direct current stimulation

improves long-term memory deficits in an animal model of attention-deficit/hyperactivity disorder and modulates oxidative and inflammatory parameters. Brain Stimulation. 2018;**11**:743-751

[45] Bocci T, Marceglia S, Vergari M, Cognetto V, Cogiamanian F, Sartucci F, et al. Transcutaneous spinal direct current stimulation modulates human corticospinal system excitability. Journal of Neurophysiology. 2015;**114**:440-446

[46] Mehrabyan A, Guest S, Essick G, McGlone F. Tactile and thermal detection thresholds of the scalp skin. Somatosensory & Motor Research. 2011;**28**:31-47

[47] Utz KS, Dimova V, Oppenlander K, Kerkhoff G. Electrified minds: Transcranial direct current stimulation (tDCS) and galvanic vestibular stimulation (GVS) as methods of non-invasive brain stimulation in neuropsychology—A review of current data and future implications. Neuropsychologia. 2010;**48**:2789-2810

[48] Poreisz C, Boros K, Antal A, Paulus W. Safety aspects of transcranial direct current stimulation concerning healthy subjects and patients. Brain Research Bulletin. 2007;**72**:208-214

[49] Parazzini M, Rossi E, Ferrucci R, Liorni I, Priori A, Ravazzani P. Modelling the electric field and the current density generated by cerebellar transcranial DC stimulation in humans. Clinical Neurophysiology. 2014;**125**:577-584

[50] Bocci T, Barloscio D, Parenti L, Sartucci F, Carli G, Santarcangelo EL. High hypnotizability impairs the cerebellar control of pain. Cerebellum. 2017;**16**:55-61

[51] Bocci T, De Carolis G, Ferrucci R, Paroli M, Mansani F, Priori A, et al. Cerebellar Transcranial direct current stimulation (ctDCS) ameliorates phantom limb pain and non-painful phantom limb sensations. Cerebellum. 2019;**18**:527-535

[52] Bocci T, Santarcangelo E, Vannini B, Torzini A, Carli G, Ferrucci R, et al. Cerebellar direct current stimulation modulates pain perception in humans. Restorative Neurology and Neuroscience. 2015;**33**:597-609

[53] Moriguchi Y, Decety J, Ohnishi T, Maeda M, Mori T, Nemoto K, et al. Empathy and judging other's pain: An fMRI study of alexithymia. Cerebral Cortex. 2007;**17**:2223-2234

[54] Singer T, Seymour B, O'Doherty J, Kaube H, Dolan RJ, Frith CD. Empathy for pain involves the affective but not sensory components of pain. Science. 2004;**303**:1157-1162

[55] Pereira M, Rafiq B, Chowdhury E, Babayev J, Boo H, Metwaly R, et al. Anodal cerebellar tDCS modulates lower extremity pain perception. NeuroRehabilitation. 2017;**40**:195-200

[56] Zunhammer M, Busch V, Griesbach F, Landgrebe M, Hajak G, Langguth B. rTMS over the cerebellum modulates temperature detection and pain thresholds through peripheral mechanisms. Brain Stimulation. 2011;**4**(210-7):e1

[57] Aiyer R, Barkin RL, Bhatia A, Gungor S. A systematic review on the treatment of phantom limb pain with spinal cord stimulation. Pain Management. 2017;7:59-69

[58] McAuley J, van Groningen R, Green C. Spinal cord stimulation for intractable pain following limb amputation. Neuromodulation. 2013;**16**:530-536; discussion 36

[59] Bolognini N, Olgiati E, Maravita A, Ferraro F, Fregni F. Motor and parietal

cortex stimulation for phantom limb pain and sensations. Pain. 2013;**154**:1274-1280

[60] Bolognini N, Spandri V, Ferraro F, Salmaggi A, Molinari AC, Fregni F, et al. Immediate and sustained effects of 5-day transcranial direct current stimulation of the motor cortex in phantom limb pain. The Journal of Pain. 2015;**16**:657-665

[61] Bolognini N, Spandri V, Olgiati E, Fregni F, Ferraro F, Maravita A. Long-term analgesic effects of transcranial direct current stimulation of the motor cortex on phantom limb and stump pain: A case report. Journal of Pain and Symptom Management. 2013;**46**:e1-e4

[62] Pinto CB, Saleh Velez FG, Bolognini N, Crandell D, Merabet LB, Fregni F. Optimizing rehabilitation for phantom limb pain using mirror therapy and transcranial direct current stimulation: A randomized, double-blind clinical trial study protocol. JMIR Research Protocols. 2016;**5**:e138

[63] Cruccu G, Aminoff MJ, Curio G, Guerit JM, Kakigi R, Mauguiere F, et al. Recommendations for the clinical use of somatosensory-evoked potentials. Clinical Neurophysiology. 2008;**119**:1705-1719

[64] Truini A, Galeotti F, Romaniello A, Virtuoso M, Iannetti GD, Cruccu G. Laser-evoked potentials: Normative values. Clinical Neurophysiology. 2005;**116**:821-826

[65] Panouillères MT, Miall RC, Jenkinson N. The role of the posterior cerebellum in saccadic adaptation: A transcranial direct current stimulation study. Journal of Neuroscience. 2015;**35**(14):5471-5479

[66] Bikson M, Inoue M, Akiyama H, Deans JK, Fox JE, Miyakawa H, et al. Effects of uniform extracellular DC electric fields on excitability in rat hippocampal slices in vitro. The Journal of Physiology. 2004;**557**(Pt 1):175-190

[67] Manola L, Roelofsen BH, Holsheimer J, Marani E, Geelen J. Modelling motor cortex stimulation for chronic pain control: Electrical potential field, activating functions and responses of simple nerve fibre models. Medical & Biological Engineering & Computing. 2005;**43**(3):335-343

Chapter 10

From Mechanisms to Analgesia: Towards the Use of Non-Invasive Neuromodulation for Pain Relief in the Clinic

Alice G. Witney

Abstract

The use of electricity for analgesic effects has a long history and yet currently neuromodulation devices based on electrical stimulation are typically restricted to being a last resort intervention for pain patients after the failure of pharmacological treatments. Whilst spinal cord stimulation is an established intervention for intractable neuropathic pain, the use of neuromodulation for other forms of pain and targeting different aspects of pain processing is less well established. Non-invasive neuromodulation as part of a standard intervention for pain relief would be ideal for the long term treatment of a chronic pain condition as it would avoid the inevitable side effects associated with long term use of pharmacological interventions or interactions between different drug treatments. This is particularly relevant as chronic pain can be associated with diseases that would require pharmacological treatment for the primary condition. However, there is currently both a deficit in understanding the mechanisms of the different non-invasive devices and also in how these devices may facilitate pain relief for specific conditions. This review will focus on the application of electric currents non-invasively to different sites for pain relief and outline the future potential of these technologies.

Keywords: pain, electric current stimulation, non-invasive neuromodulation, transcutaneous stimulation, tDCS, tACS, ta-VNS

1. What is neuromodulation? Why is pain a challenge?

Neuromodulation has been defined by the International Neuromodulation Society (INS) as "the alteration of nerve activity through targeted delivery of a stimulus, such as electrical stimulation or chemical agents, to specific neurological sites in the body" [1, 2]. Neuromodulation has a wide range of possible clinical applications from the enhancement of vision, auditory function and the control of musculature, but the application to alleviate pain is perhaps one of the most challenging for the field. Whilst the efficacy of neuromodulation interventions, for instance for movement disorders, can be easily measured due to the many ways in which successful movement execution can be characterized, and improvements in vision and audition measured via sensory detection thresholds, the efficacy of a potential neuromodulation intervention to alleviate pain is far harder to determine. Currently there is not an established biomarker for pain, and objective measurement of an individual's pain levels either before or after an intervention is difficult due to the subjectivity inherent in the pain experience.

Pain involves multiple processing regions from the periphery through to the brain and therefore, successful neuromodulation for pain relief has a number of possible targets. A clear premise of clinical neuromodulation is that pathological alterations in neuronal function are targeted, but for chronic pain these alterations can occur due to dysfunctions at a number of different sites within the multiple interconnected pain processing pathways. Additionally the mechanisms underlying the persistence of pain long after the initial injury, and the formation of a chronic pain state, still remain elusive. Pain, particularly chronic pain, is typically regarded as a human phenomenon, with other animals simply experiencing nociception; a stimuli that generates a reflexive response but without key aspects that encompass pain; that is without cognitive and emotional evaluative aspects.

Neuromodulation, particularly non-invasive neuromodulation, is a rapidly emerging field for therapeutic interventions and although the effects of stimulation are evident, many questions remain open; what patient groups will this technique be effective for?; what stimulation parameters should be used for optimum efficacy?; what is the most efficacious target for pain relief? Furthermore the mechanisms underlying neuromodulation has not been completely established. Therefore, taken together, the design of optimum neuromodulation protocols and targets for pain relief is an area that still requires development.

2. Importance of developing neuromodulation for pain relief

Chronic pain is a global health problem with both a high economic cost in addition to its substantial detrimental impact on quality of life [3]. Remarkably lifetime prevalence of chronic pain has been put as high as 50% of the global population [4, 5]. Chronic pain is the most common co-morbidity for a disease, with pain as the most frequent reason for seeking healthcare. Recently chronic pain has been recognized by the World Health Organization as a disease and included in the international classification of diseases (ICD-11) [6]. However, treatment interventions are lacking; pharmacological interventions providing inadequate pain relief with the mismanagement of opioids well documented as both increasing mortality and exacerbating pain. For neuromodulation to be an effective alternative for analgesia, an understanding of the mechanisms leading to pain conditions and the networks that enhance pain or inhibit pain is essential. For therapeutic benefit, neurostimulation techniques should modulate the nervous system in a non-destructive way with reversible effects that can be applied long term and have specificity to a targeted network. Further the intervention should be controlled dependent on individual patient requirements [7]. Recently a number of new non-invasive techniques have emerged; weak electric currents applied transcranially to cortical or sub-cortical site are proposed as interventions for a number of diseases that are associated with pathological alterations in neuronal excitability [8, 9], including chronic pain. Further the recent development of transcutaneous vagal nerve stimulation also offers therapeutic potential for some pain patients. Although these novel non-invasive interventions offer promise, there remain areas of uncertainty with regards to how to optimize stimulation protocols and standardize their efficacy across individuals.

3. The anatomical substrates for pain: potential targets for neuromodulation

The sensation of acute pain originates from stimulation of nociceptors. Nociceptive input has different modalities; thermal, chemical or mechanical; that are all capable of causing pain. Receptor types and ion channels will differ dependent on the stimulus and intensity, but with free nerve endings transmitting the noxious information to Aδ and C afferents. The TRP channels for transduction of noxious temperature sensation are well characterized [10, 11], with less known about mechanical pain [12]. Myelinated, high velocity (20 m/s) Aδ fibers and un-myelinated, low velocity (2 m/s) and C fibers transmit nociceptive information from the periphery to the dorsal horn. Both Aδ and C afferent fibers terminate in the dorsal horn of the spinal cord, where afferent input is organized in the rexed laminae; finer diameter fibers terminate more laterally, and larger fibers more medially. Large diameter Aβ fibers conveying innocuous touch can modulate nociception transmission as formulated by the gate-control theory of pain. This theory represented a ground breaking advance in the understanding of the peripheral and spinal processing of nociceptive inputs that led to the development of therapeutic neuromodulation interventions [13]. There is transmission from the spinal cord via multiple ascending pathways; spinothalamic, spinoreticular, spinomesencephalic, and spinocervical pathways [14]. The thalamus is an important site of nociceptive transmission to different brain regions known to be involved in pain processing and interpretation. Additionally significant modulation of afferent input occurs at the thalamus that has led to the region being one of the first supraspinal areas targeted in neuromodulation interventions. The multiple cortical and sub-cortical regions of the brain that are involved in pain processing and modulation have become known as the pain neuromatrix [15], or the pain connectome [16]. Particularly critical to the modulation of pain is the descending pain pathways providing endogenous inhibitory control of nociceptive input.

Chronic pain typically is defined as pain that lasts 3-6 months, with the pain experienced no longer associated with a tissue injury. Chronic pain can result from defects in different sites of the pain processing pathways [17] and is often associated with both peripheral and central sensitization [18]. The pain processing network is known to be complex and distributed. In the brain, painful stimuli is known to lead to activation in diverse brain regions; including the frontal lobe, anterior cingulate cortex (ACC), primary motor cortex (M1), primary sensory cortex (S1), secondary sensory cortex (S2), insular; hypothalamus; nucleus cuneiformis; periaqueductal grey; rostral ventromedial medulla; as observed via fMRI studies [19]. The development of chronic pain is thought not just to involve neural changes but also alterations in glia [20]. These glial changes are thought to partly underlie alterations in pain transmission and the formation of chronic pain circuitry. Imaging studies show that chronic pain leads to structural and functional changes in multiple brain regions [21]. Chronic pain has also been reported to be associated with dysregulation of both the sympathetic and parasympathetic nervous systems [22]. Therefore, the potential targets for non-invasive neuromodulation for pain relief are diverse and could be within the central or peripheral nervous systems.

3.1 Primary motor cortex

Electrical stimulation of the primary motor cortex (M1) is long established as an effective treatment for pain. Originally this intervention was limited to invasive epidural electrode implantation, and so associated with the risk of surgery [23]. More recently non-invasive cortical stimulation has emerged as an interesting, effective, and promising modality in the investigation of novel approaches for pain relief [24]. The motor cortex represents a cortical region with high intra-cortical connectivity as well as connectivity to sub-cortical regions. There are a number of explanations for the efficacy of M1 stimulation [25]. M1- thalamic connectivity is thought to be particularly significant in neuromodulation effects [26]. Efficacy of M1 neuromodulation is also proposed to be due to inhibitory effects via the limbic, cortical and subcortical brain areas involved in descending modulatory pain control. Further M1 tDCS has been shown to reduce secondary hyperalgesia and enhances descending modulatory control [27].

3.1.1 Monitoring the efficacy of M1 stimulation

The measurement of pain in a clinical setting has been typically through visual analogue scales (VAS) and numerical rating scales (NRS). However many studies now include pain threshold testing via standardized quantitative sensory testing (QST) which involves testing across different modalities of nociceptive stimuli so that a pain modulation profile can be monitored pre and post treatment intervention [28]. MRI studies have examined resting-state functional connectivity alterations in pain patients before and after intervention with tDCS and found alterations in connectivity within pain processing areas that correlate with a reduction in pain in these patients [29].

Neurophysiological techniques have also been used to monitor changes in cortical excitability after the application of electric currents so that these changes may be correlated with pain measures. Increased excitability of the corticospinal tract (CST) as measured by the standard neurophysiological technique of motor evoked potentials (MEPs) have shown that increased CST excitability is associated with analgesic effects [30] and beneficial outcomes for patients [31]. Other neurophysiological measures that have been shown to have value include intracortical disinhibition. A number of studies have observed that there is a reduction in intracortical inhibition and an increase in intracortical facilitation, suggesting that motor cortex inhibition is dysregulated in chronic pain patients [32] and so providing a neurophysiological basis for monitoring efficacy of neuromodulation protocols.

3.2 Endogenous descending control of pain

It is well known that once a nociceptive stimuli has been identified, the typical response across all animals is rapid reflexive movement away from the source of the noxious stimulus combined with an autonomic response which acts to optimize the animal's ability to escape from threats. The periaqueductal gray (PAG) has a critical role in the response to threatening stimuli, both aversion and the autonomic response [33, 34]. The PAG is also a key component of the endogenous descending pain pathway [35]. It receives nociceptive input from spinal, subcortical and cortical inputs, and projects to the rostral ventromedial medulla (RVM) and also to cortical areas and the spinal cord. The initial rodent studies of PAG stimulation demonstrated a large analgesic effect subsequent to stimulation [36]. Subsequently, PAG stimulation has shown anti-nociceptive effects from rodents to man and is now known as an essential circuit for opioid based analgesia. However, it is also established that the PAG and descending pathways play a complex role in pain and can facilitate as well as inhibit pain. Importantly, these endogenous descending pain pathways are thought to be defective in some patients, leading to chronic pain. To improve and develop neuromodulatory interventions it would be ideal to first characterize the integrity of the patient's descending modulatory pathway and subsequently monitor the effect of an intervention on this pathway. Two experimental observations using psychophysical methods are thought to enable important insights in the endogenous descending modulatory control and have generated interest in pain research. These are offset analgesia (OA) [37] and conditioned pain modulation (CPM) [38]. It would be useful if these methods could monitor the efficacy of neurostimulation protocols aimed at enhancing inhibitory pain pathways.

3.2.1 Offset analgesia

Offset analgesia (OA) is a phenomenon observed in both experimental and clinical studies [39]. OA is defined as a disproportionate reduction in pain after a very slight decrease in experimental pain stimulus intensity. The size of the OA effect is very large, with the effect thought to be over 250% when compared with equivalent increases in pain intensity [39].

The physiological mechanism and function of this phenomenon is not completely understood, but there is substantial interest in OA due to the apparent analgesia that it can convey in the presence of a previously painful heat stimulus. Additionally deficits in OA has been demonstrated in a number of different clinical group of chronic pain patients, and therefore a psychophysical OA protocol could be incorporated as part of a diagnostic protocol for chronic pain patients [40]. However, there is debate over whether OA could be used as a means to monitor the success of pharmacological interventions [41, 42] and suggests that this protocol requires reliability testing prior to use for the assessment of intervention efficacy. fMRI evidence has suggested that the PAG is activated during OA suggesting that the descending control pain pathway is important in the experience of this phenomenon [43].

3.2.2 Conditioned pain modulation

Conditioned pain modulation (CPM) represents the phenomenon of 'pain inhibits pain' and is thought to be the human counterpart to descending noxious inhibitory control (DNIC) that has strong electrophysiological evidence in rodent pain models [44]. Although DNIC was observed in rats in the 1970s, the human counterpart as observed through psychophysical methods is much more recent [38]. While there is increasing evidence that deficits in CPM can predict the development of chronic pain the reliability of the response has been questioned and there are a number of alternative protocols in the literature [38].

Patients with knee osteoarthritis have also been found to have defects in the descending pain control that can be characterized by defects in CPM. Further CPM paradigms have been used to monitor the effect of neuromodulation interventions on the endogenous inhibitory pathways in experimental pain in healthy participants [45] and clinical pain in Fibromyalgia patients [46]. As well as M1 stimulation influencing descending pain pathways it is possible that prefrontal stimulation may also modulate PAG due to the known connectivity [47]. Prefrontal tDCS is a common target for tDCS for pain modulation [25, 48], but not currently assessed in the context of descending pain pathways as monitored via CPM protocols. However patient studies using tDCS of the left dorsolateral prefrontal cortex have suggested efficacy is achieved via enhancement of descending pain modulation as well as known cognitive effects of this stimulation [49]. The link between PAG and cerebellar circuitry [50] may suggest that cerebellar tDCS could also influence PAG. Experimental pain studies have explored the use of cerebellar tDCS as a target for modulating pain thresholds [51], but there are currently only a few studies.

3.3 Vagal nerve stimulation

The vagus nerve is a large tract originating at the brainstem and is known for its widespread innervation, targeting every major thoracic and abdominal organ [52, 53]. Vagal nerve stimulation (VNS) has similarly been shown to provide multi-systems effects, and thus useful for a wide range of disease interventions. The recent development of non-invasive vagal nerve stimulation; via transcutaneous auricular vagus nerve stimulation (ta-VNS); rather than the traditional cervical implantation; increases therapeutic potential of the intervention as it removes the need for surgery [54]. Due to the novelty of ta-VNS there is currently a lack of consensus over the optimal stimulation protocol [55]. Stimulation is typically of low amplitude current (~5 mA) with pulses of 250–500 μs with a frequency of between 10 and 25 Hz [54]. Recently a number of studies have made efforts to individualize the stimulation level based on perceptual threshold using sequential testing protocols.

There is increasing evidence that VNS has anti-nociceptive effects [56, 57]. Analgesia is thought to occur through both the inhibition of spinal nociceptive reflexes and ascending transmission. There is evidence VNS and ta-VNS also modulates ascending inputs in the brain by altered activity in pain processing regions as observed via fMRI [55, 58]. Further a recent study examined the brainstem fMRI response to a respiratory gated ta-VNS protocol (known as RAVANS). Interestingly this study found that stimulation led to greater blood oxygen level dependent (BOLD) responses in the PAG [59]. Further this study explored the use of different stimulation frequencies, with a frequency of 100 Hz showing increased responsiveness of PAG. This alteration to a key site for endogenous pain modulation provides additional support for the potential of VNS for pain relief. Opioid receptor antagonists are found to reduce the efficacy of VNS, indicating that there is an opioid based mechanism for analgesia. Further VNS is also widely thought to have anti-inflammatory effects [56]. These anti-inflammatory effects are proposed to be due to neural-immune interaction at the peripheral nerves [60], with electric stimulation of the vagus nerve triggering a neural-immune reflex via cholinergic anti-inflammatory pathways that dampen the inflammatory response to infection or tissue injury and suppress the release of pro-inflammatory cytokines.

4. Translation for patient pain relief?

Early studies using tDCS in patient studies have had variable success and lack strong evidence of treatment efficacy [61]. Initial randomized controlled trials of anodal tDCS to primary motor cortex (M1) as an intervention for neuropathic pain found the intervention to be ineffective [62]. However, recent studies provide support for tDCS of M1 as a treatment intervention for knee osteoarthritis [63], fibromyalgia [64] and inflammatory bowel disease [29]. There have also been randomized clinical trials using prefrontal tDCS demonstrating tDCS to be effective in pain reduction in patients with multiple sclerosis [65] and fibromyalgia [49] and also reduce post-surgical opioid use [66]. A recent meta-analysis of selected randomized controlled trials of tDCS for non-cancer pain included predominantly M1 tDCS but also left dorsolateral prefrontal tDCS [48]. The meta-analysis showed active stimulation was consistently better than sham stimulation with stronger evidence for the efficacy of anodal M1 tDCS [48]. However, overall there remain shortcomings in the current literature on tDCS in patient groups; the study numbers are small; the tDCS protocols differ across studies; the patient groups are heterogeneous making meta-analysis challenging; and the study designs used inconsistent, with some studies favoring a cross-over design to a control group. For tDCS to become an established treatment intervention, large multi-centre randomized controlled trials with standardized protocols and patient cohorts are necessary.

Studies using VNS in patient groups report beneficial effects of this form of stimulation in patients with pain associated with inflammatory conditions, for instance rheumatoid arthritis or migraine. Indeed recent studies have provided strong support for the use of vagal nerve stimulation in arthritis patients [56]. The combination of anti-inflammatory effects of VNS [67] with the previously mentioned analgesic effects via the endogenous opioid system may explain the potential for this technique in these patient groups. In fibromyalgia, although the disease etiology is uncertain, patients are known to experience systemic inflammation and neuroinflammation, and so may be a patient group that particularly benefits from this intervention.

5. Methodology for translation of electric current stimulation to the clinic

Evidence for the efficacy of non-invasive application of electric currents in humans for neuromodulatory effects has been rapidly increasing, with many proposed applications, including pain. The potential applications explored have been extensive as the technique is easy to implement, cheap and well tolerated by participants. Additionally an interesting potential development of non-invasive neuromodulation interventions suggests the method is a viable technique for patients to use in their homes with remote monitoring [68]. However there is not currently a consensus on the optimal protocols and variability in effects across individuals have been widely reported. For translation to the clinic, systematic study into the effect of altering the amplitude and duration of the applied electrical current is essential. These parameters include; electrode montage when targeting a given area; size of the electrodes; magnitude of stimulation and duration of stimulation [69]. As with many therapeutic interventions key questions are; how can neurostimulation dose be determined?; how can treatment fidelity be ensured?; how can individual variability be controlled when determining dose?

5.1 Electrode montage in tDCS

In tDCS the stimulation electrodes are typically two saline soaked sponge electrodes; an anode and a cathode; that range from 25 to 35 cm^2 placed above the region of interest and the reference electrode is positioned at another cortical region [70]. Early studies with tDCS used a very simple electrode montage, with two electrodes of the same size often with the assumption that the effect of the active electrode would be independent of the placement and size of the second, reference electrode. For motor cortex stimulation the typical electrode montage is to have the reference electrode placed over the contralateral orbit. It has been suggested that anodal stimulation protocols can be optimized by having the cathodal reference electrode as a larger size, thus rendering it functionally inert [71]. Another montage option has been the selection of an extracephalic reference electrode; typically the deltoid or buccinator muscles. Regardless of site used the montage of the two electrodes will inevitably impact on the regions where brain modulation will occur due to stimulation. Further the different forms of electrodes now available will also influence the applied stimulation as it is known that the electrode-skin interface has variable impedance that will be dependent on a number of factors that lead to variability in the delivered current. Modern stimulators are current controlled, but some earlier studies are voltage controlled leading to the current that reaches the scalp being dependent on differences in impedance thus leading to greater variability and difficulty in making comparisons across studies.

5.2 Modeling current flow in tDCS

One limitation of tDCS is that the sites of stimulation are typically identified based on the cranial landmarks of the 10-20 system for EEG electrode placement. However individual differences in brain anatomy will result in electrode placement that may not correspond exactly to the intended target site of stimulation. M1 stimulation can be improved by identifying the individual's motor hotspot via transcranial magnetic stimulation (TMS) before electrode placement, but currently this is not typically included in the protocols for tDCS studies for pain relief. Recently current flow diagrams have been developed and are regarded as critical to the optimal administration of tDCS [72]. Ideally these predictions of the current flow are adapted to the specific anatomy as recorded via magnetic resonance imaging (MRI). Implementing tDCS in this way may help to control for some of the observed inconsistency in the effects of tDCS across populations [73]. This may be particularly important in some patient populations; recent work has further suggested that brain atrophy may also impact of the flow of current [74]. Given the observation of structural changes in the brain of chronic pain patients this may be problematic [22]. This may to some extent be ameliorated by individualized electric field models that can optimize tDCS dosage for patients [75, 76]. Current flow modeling also enables tailoring the dose to electrodes of different sizes, including high-definition transcranial direct stimulation protocols with smaller electrodes arranged in more complex montages to facilitate more focused effects [77, 78]. Additionally the current flow modeling may be able to facilitate the use of non-invasive neurostimulation techniques to deeper brain structures [77], so that novel targets in the pain neuromatrix could be stimulated.

5.3 What is the optimum magnitude of the applied electric current?

The effects of electric stimulation of the brain have long been studied in animal models [79, 80]. When applied to the brain, the current is thought to alter underlying neuronal excitability but is also thought to affect functionally connected distant cortical and sub-cortical regions. However many animal studies apply direct current stimulation onto the cortical area (DCS). Therefore the current reaching the cortex is typically much greater than with transcranial application. The magnitude of electric current may be critical for the observed effects so the two methodologies could differ substantially. Similarly the trans-cutaneous application of electric currents to nerves is also emerging as a useful non-invasive intervention, and again the existing animal and human studies are often based on observations from invasive methods.

tDCS and tACS studies typically apply low currents (typically 1–3 mA) with 1.5–2 mA being the most usual stimulation levels. Recent studies have experimented with the use of higher currents (up to 4 mA) [81]. Studies have varied substantially in the protocols used, but all would lead to charge densities that would be far lower than that required to elicit an action potential. The charge density used in a study varies dependent on the size of the electrodes used, and is calculated by the size of the electrical current applied divided by the electrode area. The duration of the applied electrical stimulation has also been variable across studies but is typically within the range of 10–30 minutes. To enhance intervention comparisons studies could compare the total charge administered over stimulation period, so taking into account the duration electrical stimulation is applied in the intervention period.

Future work exploring the appropriate current, as well as how this can be adjusted for different individuals is essential. It already known that lower currents are sufficient to lead to membrane polarization and have potential therapeutic benefits. Indeed the lower stimulation levels applied to primary motor cortex were in fact more effective in increasing motor cortical excitability [82], and may avoid the problematic finding of non-linear tDCS effects that have recently been reported when increasing current, with a reversal of effects observed in the mid-range of applied current (2 mA) [83]. This observation has been paralleled in animal models but pharmacological studies are required to discern the effect of the current on specific ion channels. Since it has been reported that there is non-linear effect in the stimulation magnitude, individual differences in cortical excitability; determined by differences in motor evoked potentials when primary motor cortex is the target; could become critical for appropriately setting therapeutic dose.

A further tDCS effect that has not undergone much investigation and yet is important for implementation in a patient population is the duration of any tDCS therapeutic effects, and the impact of protocols involving repetitive stimulation is applied. Recent research has explored the short and long stimulation durations and compared these with those where short duration protocols are repeated with intervals. There is some evidence that repeated stimulation is more efficacious than continual longer duration stimulation protocols [84].

5.4 Interaction with individual patient characteristics

There are multiple parameters that can be altered in the administration of tDCS stimulation [48]. There will also be alterations of the effect of tDCS due to differing characteristics of the patient. There will be environmental factors that will impact on tDCS effects that could include the patient's current cognitive state and fatigue levels. Increasingly studies have explored the interaction between tDCS and pharmacological interventions, but it must also be considered that other medications taken by the participant could impact on the effect of neurostimulation. Many of the conditions that tDCS has been proposed to treat would mean that the patient would be taking medication [85]. This is particularly critical when considering the use of tDCS for pain relief, as chronic pain is a frequent comorbidity. Hormonal influences have been suggested to impact both on the perception of pain but also on the effects of tDCS. The effect of the interaction of tDCS with estrogen has only recently been explored [86]. This is particularly important when considering pain interventions as many conditions associated with chronic pain have a higher prevalence in women than men.

5.5 Mechanisms of tDCS

The effect of tDCS has been shown to be polarity-dependent [87]. Application of the anodal electrode (a-tDCS) over the target area increases neuronal excitability whereas a cathodal electrode (c-tDCS) decreases neuronal excitability [70, 88]. The underlying mechanisms of tDCS effects are unclear but tDCS is thought to alter neuronal membrane potential and so impact on the action potential threshold [89]. These studies suggest that anodal stimulation induced neuronal excitability results from neuronal membrane subthreshold depolarization and cathodal inhibitory effects are produced by membrane hyperpolarization. It was originally proposed that the polarization was from the somatic membrane where there is a higher density of sodium channels. Following from this, the short term effect of tDCS have been suggested to be related to increasing permeability to sodium. Additionally the neuronal excitability that occurs during anodal tDCS can be removed by pharmacologically inhibiting calcium channels and voltage-dependent sodium channels [90].

Human spectroscopy studies have demonstrated that anodal tDCS causes a local gamma aminobutyric acid (GABA) reduction [91] whereas cathodal stimulation leads to decreased glutamatergic neuronal activity. Currently the suggested mechanism of tDCS is thought to include presynaptic modulation of neurons, with the stimulation effects related to synaptic inputs rather than solely action potential generation [92, 93]. Evidence from animal studies of DCS also suggests presynaptic effects, with cathodal stimulation reducing the probability of glutamate release and anodal stimulation increasing glutamate release probability.

To explain the longer term effects of tDCS, anodal tDCS had been initially assumed to induce long term potentiation (LTP)-like effects whereas cathodal tDCS thought to induce long term depression (LDP)-like effects. However this is now thought to be overly simplistic. Some of the variability in effects of anodal and cathodal stimulation has been explained by mechanisms of homeostatic plasticity [94] formalized in the Bienenstock-Cooper-Munro (BCM) rule of bidirectional synaptic plasticity [95]. These mechanisms are proposed to occur within neural networks to prevent hyperactivity or hypoactivity [95].

Importantly recently it has also been highlighted that polarization of the cell membrane must be dependent on the orientation of the neuron to the extracellular current vector [96]. Further evidence of the importance of axonal orientation has been provided by animal studies with evidence from rat hippocampus suggests that effects of electrical current vary dependent on the orientation of axons [97]. The significance of axonal orientation in the effects of DCS could have wider implications as to how develop tDCS methods. Diffusion magnetic resonance imaging (dMRI) enables an assessment of the structural connectivity and integrity of tracts. It has been suggested that tractography achieved from dMRI may be beneficial for optimal electrode positioning in clinical instances where there has been disruption in fibre tracts due to disease [98] or that dMRI may aid understanding of the effects of neuromodulation at a cellular level [99]. Imaging techniques may also offer a means of individualizing interventions, but they would have the disadvantage of a substantial cost increase for an otherwise cheap intervention.

5.6 tACS

Transcranial alternating current (tACS) of the primary motor cortex (M1) has been shown in the past to be effective in modulating sensory thresholds for tactile sensation and visual phenomena [100] and offers potential for pain modulation [101]. tACS involves weak alternating currents being applied through the skull via electrodes on the scalp with montages similar to those used with tDCS. tACS can be applied in a wide frequency range, with the effect of each frequency range still to be explored. There is evidence of gamma and alpha oscillations being associated with pain processing and perception. Despite its potential only a limited number of studies have used tACS although alpha range stimulation has been found beneficial for pain relief [102]. Studies combining tACS with fMRI, neurophysiology or QST may help address the optimum tACS frequency for pain relief. The mechanistic effects of tACS are less well understood than tDCS and interestingly there has been the suggestion that tACS effects could be a result of stimulation of peripheral nerves trans-cutaneously rather than effects on cortical neurons [103].

5.7 Less explored effects of electric currents and future research avenues

Imposed electric fields may have a wider biological effects. For instance tDCS could influence glia [89, 104]. Future work should consider these largely unexplored effects so as to provide a more comprehensive mechanistic basis for weak electric currents dependent on targeted pain processing region. Further some consequences of weak electric currents are not widely monitored. Recent studies have begun to explore the possible consequences of tDCS on immune responses, which is particularly relevant when considering tDCS and ta-VNS for analgesia. However, thus far this has been in animal models [105, 106]. Imaging techniques such as proton magnetic resonance spectroscopy (H-MRS) could provide a useful methodology for monitoring changes in metabolites in response to patient tDCS or ta-VNS interventions. For instance, choline and myo-inositol are thought to be altered in chronic pain patients and are associated with neuroinflammation [21].

6. Conclusion

Pain is a complex sensation associated with the activity of multiple cortical and sub-cortical regions in the brain. The overall pain percept must result from the interplay between multiple ascending pathways that convey nociceptive input from the peripheral with descending pathways that act to modulate nociceptive input. The mechanisms for the formation of chronic pain are uncertain; though it is known that there are both peripheral, spinal cord and central mechanisms underlying the formation of chronic pain. Non-invasive neuromodulation through tDCS presents a particularly interesting treatment intervention for pain as recent evidence also suggests that its mechanism of action is not only the modulation of neuronal activity but that the technique also influences the neuro-immune response. However, for appropriate translation of tDCS to a clinical setting there remains the need for research for both increased mechanistic understanding as well as studies how the level of electric stimulation applied can be accurately targeted and tailored to individuals and different disease groups.

Author details

Alice G. Witney
Department of Physiology, Trinity Centre for Biomedical Engineering, Trinity College Institute of Neurosciences, Dublin, Ireland

*Address all correspondence to: awitney@tcd.ie

References

[1] International Neuromodulation Society. International Neuromodulation Society Webpage. 2017. Available from: http://www.neuromodulation.com/

[2] Krames ES, Rezai AR, Peckham PH. Defining neuromodulation. In: Krames ES, Rezai AR, Peckham PH, editors. Neuromodulation. Comprehensive Tectbook of Principles, Technologies, and Therapies. Vol. 1. London: Academic Press; 2018. pp. 1-13

[3] Eccleston C, Wells C, Morlion B. European Pain Management. Oxford: Oxford University Press; 2018

[4] Breivik H, Collett B, Ventafrida V, Cohen R, Gallacher D. Survey or chronic pain in Europe: Prevalence, impact on daily life and treatment. European Journal of Pain. 2006;**10**(4):287-333

[5] Harstall C, Ospina M. How prevalent is chronic pain? PAIN: Clinical Updates. 2003;**11**:1-4

[6] Treede RD et al. A classification of chronic pain for ICD-11. Pain. 2015;**156**(6):1003-1007

[7] Deer TR, Jain S, Hunter C, Chakravarthy K. Neurostimulation for intractable chronic pain. Brain Sciences. 2019;**9**(23):1-20

[8] To WT, De Ridder D, Hart J, Vanneste S. Changing brain networks through non-invasive neuromodulation. Frontiers in Human Neuroscience. 2018;**12**:128

[9] Zaghi S et al. Inhibition of motor cortex excitability with 15 Hz transcranial alternating current stimulation (tACS). Neuroscience Letters. 2010;**479**:211-214

[10] Cortright DN, Krause JE, Broom DC. TRP channels and pain. Biochimica et Biophysica Acta. 2007;**1772**:978-988

[11] Jardin I et al. TRPs in pain sensation. Frontiers in Physiology. 2017;**8**(392):1-10

[12] Piers C, Seal RP. Neural circuits for pain: Recent advances and current views. Science. 2016;**354**(6312):578-584

[13] Melzack R, Wall PD. Pain mechanisms: A new theory. Science. 1965;**150**(3699):971-979

[14] Almeida QF, Frank JS, Roy EA, Jenkins ME, Spaulding S, Patla AE. An evaluation of sensorimotor integration during locomotion toward a target in Parkinson's disease. Neuroscience. 2005;**134**(1):283-293

[15] Melzack R. From the gate to the neuromatrix. Pain. 1999;(suppl 6)

[16] Kucyi A, Davies KD. The dynamic pain connectome. Trends in Neurosciences. 2015;**38**(2):86-95

[17] Kuner R. Central mechanisms of pathological pain. Nature Medicine. 2010;**16**(11):1258-1266

[18] Costigan M, Scholz J, Woolf CJ. Neuropathic pain: A maladaptive response of the nervous system to damage. Annual Review of Neuroscience. 2009;**32**:1-32

[19] Tracy LM, Ioannou L, Baker KS, Gibson SJ, Georgiou-Karistianis N, Giummarra MJ. Meta-analytic evidence for decreased heart rate variability in chronic pain implicating parasympathetic nervous system dysregulation. Pain. 2016;**157**(1):7-29

[20] Tracey I, Mantyth PW. The cerebral signature for pain perception and its modulation. Neuron. 2007;**55**:377-391

[21] Jung C et al. Magnetic resonance imaging of neuroinflammation in chronic pain: A role for astrogliosis? Pain. 2020;**161**(7):1555-1564

[22] Kuchinad A, Schweinhardt P, Seminowicz DA, Wood PB, Chizh BA, Bushnell MC. Accelerated brain gray matter loss in fibromyalgia patients: Premature aging of the brain? Journal of Neuroscience. 2007;**27**(15):4004-4007

[23] Monsalve GA. Motor cortex stimulation for facial chronic neuropathic pain: A review of the literature. Surgical Neurology International. 2012;**3**:S290-S311

[24] Zaghi S, Heine N, Fregni F. Brain stimulation for the treatment of pain: A review of costs, clinical effects and mechanisms of treatment for three different central neuromodulatory approaches. Journal of Pain Management. 2009;**2**:339-352

[25] Witney AG. Neurostimulation techniques for the modulation of pain. In: Ustohal L, editor. Transcranial Magnetic Stimulation in Neuropsychiatry. London: Intech Open; 2018. pp. 103-121

[26] Polania R, Paulus W, Nitsche MA. Modulating cortico-striatal and thalamo-cortical functional connectivity with transcanial direct current stimulation. Human Brain Mapping. 2012;**33**:2499-2508

[27] Meeker TJ, Keaser ML, Khan SA, Gullapalli RP, Seminowicz DA, Greenspan JD. Non-invasive motor cortex neuromodulation reduces secondary hyperalgesia and enhances activation of the descending pain modulatory network. Frontiers in Neuroscience. 2019;**13**(467):1-18

[28] Giannoni-Luza S et al. Non-invasive motor cortex stimulation effects on quantitative sensory testing (QST) in healthy and chronic pain subjects: A systematic review and meta-analysis. Pain. 2020. (In Press)

[29] Neeb L et al. Transcranial direct current stimulation in inflammatory bowel disease patients modifies resting-state functional connectivity: A RCT. Brain Stimulation. 2019;**12**(4):978-980

[30] Moloney TM, Witney AG. Pressure pain thresholds increase after preconditioning 1 Hz repetitive transcranial magnetic stimulation with transcranial direct current stimulation. PLoS One. 2014;**9**:e92540

[31] Granovsky Y, Sprecher E, Sinai A. Motor corticospinal excitability: A novel facet of pain modulation? PAIN Reports. 2019;**4**(e725):1-7

[32] Thibaut A, Zeng D, Caumo W, Liu J, Fregni F. Corticospinal excitability as a biomarker of myofascial pain syndrome. PAIN Reports. 2017;**2**(e594):1-8

[33] Faull OK, Subramanian HH, Ezra M, Pattinson KTS. The midbrain periaqueductal gray as an integrative and interoceptive neural structure for breathing. Neuroscience & Biobehavioral Reviews. 2019;**98**:135-144

[34] Faull OK, Jenkinson M, Ezra M, Pattinson KTS. Conditioned respiratory threat in the subdivisions of the human periaqueductal gray. eLife. 2016;**5**:e12047

[35] Ossipov MH. The perception and endogenous modulation of pain. Scientifica (*Cairo*). 2012;**561761**:1-25

[36] Reynolds DV. Surgery in the rate during electrial analgesia induced by focal brain stimulation. Science. 1969;**164**:3878

[37] Nilsson M, Nissen TD, Graversen C, Gazerani P, Drewes AM, Brock C. Offset analgesia: A reproducibility study. Scandinavian Journal of Pain. 2012;**3**:192

[38] Kennedy DL, Kemp HI, Ridout D, Yarnitsky D, Rice ASC. Reliability of conditioned pain modulation:

A systematic review. Pain. 2016;**157**(11):2410-2419

[39] Grill JD, Coghill RC. Transient analgesia evoked by noxious stimulus offset. Journal of Neurophysiology. 2002;**87**:2205-2208

[40] Oudejans LCJ, Smit JH, van Velzen M, Dahan A, Niesters M. The influence of offset analgesia on the onset and offset of pain in patients with fibromyalgia. Pain. 2015;**156**:2521-2527

[41] Niesters M, Hoitsma E, Sarton E, Aarts L, Dahan A. Offset analgesia in neuropathic pain patients and effect of treatment with morphine and ketamine. Anesthesiology. 2011;**115**:1063-1071

[42] Olesen AE et al. Offset analgesia and the impact of treatment with oxycodone and venlafaxine: A placebo-controlled, randomized trial in healthy volunteers. Basic & Clinical Pharmacology & Toxicology. 2018;**123**(6):727-731

[43] Derbyshire SWG, Osborn J. Offset analgesia is mediated by activation in the region of the periaqueductal grey and rostral ventromedial medulla. NeuroImage. 2009;**47**:1002-1006

[44] Le Bars D, Dickenson AH, Besson JM. Diffuse noxious inhibitory controls (DNIC) 1 effects on dorsal horn convergent neurones in the rat. Pain. 1979;**6**:283-304

[45] Serrano GB et al. Comparison of hypnotic suggestion and transcranial direct-current stimulation effects on pain perception and the descending pain modulating system: A crossover randomized clinical trial. Frontiers in Neuroscience. 2019;**13**:662

[46] Castelo-Branco L et al. Optimised transcranial direct current stimulation (tDCS) for fibromyalgia-targeting the endogenous pain control system: A randomized, double-blind factorial clinical trial protocol. BMJ Open. 2019;**9**(10):e032710

[47] Ong W-Y, Stohler CS, Herr DR. Role of the prefrontal cortex in pain processing. Molecular Neurobiology. 2018;**56**:1137-1166

[48] Zortea M et al. Transcranial direct current stimulation to improve the dysfunction of descending pain modulatory system related to opioids in chronic non-cancer pain: An integrative review of neurobiology and meta-analysis. Frontiers in Neuroscience. 2019;**13**:1218

[49] Silva AF et al. Anodal transcranial direct current stimulation over the left dorsolateral prefrontal cortex modulates attention and pain in fibromyalgia: Randomized clinical trial. Scientific Reports. 2017;**7**:135

[50] Koutsikou S et al. Neural substrates underlying fear-evoked freezing: The periaqueductal grey-cerebellar link. Journal of Physiology. 2014;**592**:2197-2213

[51] Bocci T et al. Cerebellar direct current stimulation modulates pain perception in humans. Restorative Neurology and Neuroscience. 2015;**33**:597-609

[52] Johnson RL, Wilson CG. A review of vagus nerve stimulation as a therapeutic intervention. Journal of Inflammation Research. 2018;**11**:203-213

[53] Vonck KEJ, Larsen LE. Vagus nerve stimulation: Mechanisms of action. In: Krames ES, Peckham PH, Rezai AR, editors. Neuromodulation. Comprehensive Textbook of Principles, Technologies, and Therapies. Vol. 1. London: Academic Press; 2018. pp. 211-220

[54] Badran BW et al. Laboratory administration of transcutaneous

auricular vagus nerve stimulation (taVNS): Technique, targeting and considerations. Journal of Visualized Experiments. 2020;**143**

[55] Badran BW et al. Neurophysiologic effects of transcutaneous auricular vagus nerve stimulation (taVNS) via electrical stimulation of the tragus: A concurrent taVNS/fMRI study and review. Brain Stimulation. 2018;**11**(3):492-500

[56] Koopman FA, Schuurman PR, Vervoordeldonk MJ, Tak PP. Vagus nerve stimulation: A new bioelectronics approach to treat rheumatoid arthritis. Best Practice & Research. Clinical Rheumatology. 2014;**28**:625-635

[57] Addorisio ME et al. Investigational treatment of rheumatoid arthritis with a vibrotactile device applied to the external ear. Bioelectronic Medicine. 2019;**5**(4)

[58] Narayanan JT, Watts R, Haddad N, Labar DR, Li MP, Filippi CG. Cerebral activation during vagus nerve stimulation: A functional MR study. Epilepsia. 2002;**43**(12):1509-1514

[59] Sclocco R et al. Stimulus frequency modulates brainstem response to respiratory-gated transcutaneous auricular vagus nerve stimulation. Brain Stimulation. 2020;**13**:970-978

[60] Chiu IM, von Hehn CA, Woolf CJ. Neurogenic inflammation - the peripheral nervous system's role in host defense and immunopathology. Nature Neuroscience. 2013;**15**(8):1063-1067

[61] O'Connell NE, Wand BM, Marston L, Spencer S, Desouza LH. Non-invasive brain stimulation techniques for chronic pain. Cochrane Database of Systematic Reviews. 2014;**4**:CD008204

[62] Wrigley PJ, Gustin SM, McIndoe LN, Chakiath RJ, Henderson LA, Siddall PJ. Longstanding neuropathic pain after spinal cord injury is refractory to transcranial direct current stimulation: A randomized controlled trial. Pain. 2013;**15**:2178-2184

[63] Ahn H et al. Efficacy of transcranial direct current stimulation over primary motor cortex (anode) and contralateral supraorbital area (cathode) on clinical pain severity and mobility performance in persons with knee osteoarthritis: An experimenter- and participant - blinded randomized, sham-controlled pilot clinical study. Brain Stimulation. 2017;**10**:902-909

[64] Khedr EM et al. Effects of transcranial direct current stimulation on pain, mood and serum endorphin level in the treatment of fibromyalgia: A double blinded, randomized clinical trial. Brain Stimulation. 2017;**10**:893-901

[65] Ayache SS et al. Prefrontal tDCS decreases pain in patients with multiple sclerosis. Frontiers in Neuroscience. 2016;**10**:147

[66] Borckardt JJ et al. Prefrontal versus motor cortex transcranial direct current stimulation (tDCS) effects on post-surgical opioid use. Brain Stimulation. 2017;**10**(6):1096-1101

[67] Caravaca AS et al. An effective method for acute vagus nerve stimulation in experimental inflammation. Frontiers in Neuroscience. 2019;**13**:877

[68] Charvet LE, Shaw MT, Bikson M, Woods AJ, Knotkova H. Supervised transcranial direct current stimulation (tDCS) at home: A guide for clinical research and practice. Brain Stimulation. 2020;**13**:686-693

[69] Peterchev AV et al. Fundamentals of transcranial electric and magnetic stimulation dose: Definition, selection and reporting practices. Brain Stimulation. 2012;**5**(4):435-453

[70] Nitsche MA, Liebetanz D, Antal A, Lang N, Tergau F, Paulus W. Modulation of cortical excitability by weak direct durrent stimulation - technical, safety and functional aspects. Supplements to Clinical Neurophysiology. 2003;**56**:255-276

[71] Nitsche MA et al. Shaping the effects of transcranial direct current stimulation of the human motor cortex. Journal of Neurophysiology. 2007;**97**:3109-3117

[72] Mikkonen M, Laakso I, Tanaka S, Hirata A. Cost of focality in TDCS: Interindividual variability in electric fields. Brain Stimulation. 2020;**13**:117-124

[73] Datta A, Truong D, Minhas P, Parra LC, Bikson M. Inter-individual variation during transcranial direct current stimulation and normalisation of dose using MRI-derived computational models. Frontiers in Psychiatry. 2012;**3**(91):1-8

[74] Unal G et al. Impact of brain atrophy on tDCS and HD-tDCS current flow: A modeeling study in three variants of primary progressive aphasia. Neurological Sciences. 2020;**41**:1781-1789

[75] Evans C, Bachmann C, Lee JSA, Gregoriou E, Ward N. Dose-controlled tDCS reduces electric field intensity variability at a cortical target site. Brain Stimulation. 2020;**13**(1):125-136

[76] Caulfield KA et al. Transcranial electrical stimulation motor threshold can estimate individualised tDCS dosage from reverse calculation electric-field modeling. Brain Stimulation. 2020;**13**:961-969

[77] Datta A, Bansal V, Diaz J, Patel J, Reato D, Bikson M. Gyri-precise head model of transcranial direct current stimulation: Improved spatial focality using a ring electrode versus conventional rectangular pad. Brain Stimulation. 2009;**2**:201-207

[78] Kuo H-I et al. Comparing cortical plasticity induced by conventional and high definition 4X1 ring tDCS: A neurophysiological study. Brain Stimulation. 2013;**6**:644-648

[79] Bindman LJ, Lippold OC, Redfearn JW. The action of brief polarizing currents on the cerebral cortex of the rat (1) during current flow and (2) in the production of long-lasting after-effects. Journal of Physiology. 1964;**172**:369-382

[80] Bikson M, Lian J, Hahn PJ, Stacey WC, Sciortino C, Durand DM. Suppression of epileptiform activity by high frequency sinusoidal fields in rat hippocampal slices. Journal of Physiology. 2001;**531**(1):181-191

[81] Khadka N et al. Adaptive current tDCS up to 4mA. Brain Stimulation. 2020;**13**:69-79

[82] Jamil A et al. Systematic evaluation of the impact of stimulation intensity on neuroplastic after-effects induced by transcranial direct current stimulation. Journal of Physiology. 2017;**595**(4):1273-1288

[83] Esmaeilpour Z et al. Incomplete evidence that increasing current intensity of tDCS boosts outcomes. Brain Stimulation. 2018;**11**(2):310-321

[84] Samani MM, Agboada D, Kuo M-F, Nitsche MA. Probing the relevance of repeated cathodal transcranial direct current stimulation over the primary motor cortex for prolongation of after-effects. Journal of Physiology. 2020;**598**(4):805-816

[85] McLaren ME, Nissim NR, Woods AJ. The effects of medication use in transcranial direct current stimulation: A brief review. Brain Stimulation. 2018;**11**:52-58

[86] Chung SW, et al. The influence of endogenous estrogen on high-frequency prefrontal transcranial magnetic stimulation. Brain Stimulation. 2019;**12**(5):1271-1279

[87] Galea JM, Jayaram G, Ajagbe L, Celnik P. Modulation of cerebellar excitability by polarity-specific noninvasive direct current stimulation. Journal of Neuroscience. 2009;**29**:9115-9122

[88] Nitsche MA et al. Transcranial direct current stimulation: State of the art 2008. Brain Stimulation. 2008;**1**:206-223

[89] Pelletier SJ, Cicchetti F. Cellular and molecular mechanisms of action of transcranial direct current stimulation: Evidence from in vitro and in vivo models. International Journal of Neuropsychopharmacology. 2015;**18**(2):1-13

[90] Nitsche M, Liebetanz D, Lang N, Antal A, Tergau F, Paulus W. Safety criteria for transcranial direct current stimulation (tDCS) in humans. Clinical Neurophysiology. 2003;**114**:2220-2222

[91] Stagg CJ et al. Polarity sensitive modulation of cortical neurotransmitters by transcranial stimulation. Journal of Neuroscience. 2009;**29**:5202-5206

[92] Kronberg G, Bridi M, Abel T, Bikson M, Parra LC. Direct current stimulation modulates LTP and LTD: Activity dependence and dendritic effects. Brain Stimulation. 2017;**10**:51-57

[93] Kronberg G, Rahman A, Sharma M, Bikson M, Parra LC. Direct current stimulation boosts hebbian plasticity in vitro. Brain Stimulation. 2020;**13**:287-301

[94] Turrigiano G. Too many cooks? Intrinsic and synaptic homeostatic mechanisms in cortical circuit refinement. Annual Review of Neuroscience. 2011;**34**:89-103

[95] Bienenstock EL, Cooper LN, Munro PW. Theory for the development of neuron selectivity: Orientation specificity and binocular interaction in visual cortex. The Journal of Neuroscience. 1982;**2**(1):32-48

[96] Bikson M et al. Effects of uniform extracellular DC electric fields on excitability in rat hippocampal slices in vitro. Journal of Physiology (London). 2004;**557**:175-190

[97] Kabakov AY, Muller PA, Pascual-Leone A, Jensen FE, Rotenberg A. Contribution of axonal orientation to pathway-dependent modulation of excitatory transmission by direct current stimulation in isolated rat hippocampus. Journal of Neurophysiology. 2012;**107**:1881-1889

[98] Lin RL, Douaud G, Filippini N, Okell TW, Stagg CJ, Tracey I. Structural connectivity variances underlie functional and behavioural changes during pain relief induced by neuromodulation. Scientific Reports. 2017;**7**:41603

[99] Shahid SS, Bikson M, Salman H, Wen P, Ahfock T. The value and cost of complexity in predictive modelling: Role of tissue anisotropic conductivity and fibre tracts in neuromodulation. Journal of Neural Engineering. 2014;**11**:036003

[100] Clancy JA, Johnson R, Raw R, Deuchars SA, Deuchars J. Transcranial direct current stimulation (tDCS)/ Transcranial alternating current stimulation (tACS): Anodal Transcranial direct current stimulation (tDCS) over the motor cortex increases sympathetic nerve activity. Brain Stimulation. 2014;**7**:97-104

[101] Hohn VD, May ES, Ploner M. From correlation towards causality:

Modulating brain rhythms using transcranial alternating current stimulation. PAIN Reports. 2019;**4**:e723

[102] Prim JH, Ahn S, Alexander ML, McCulloch KL, Frohlich F. Targeting the autonomic nervous system balance in patients with chronic low back pain using transcranial alternating current stimulation: A randomized, crossover double-blind, placebo-controlled pilot study. Journal of Pain Research. 2019;**12**:3265-3277

[103] Asamoah B, Khatoun A, McLaughlin M. tACS motor system effects can be caused by transcutaneous stimulation of peripheral nerves. Nature Communications. 2019;**10**(1):1-16

[104] Ruohonen J, Karhu J. tDCS possibly stimulates glial cells. Clinical Neurophysiology. 2012;**123**:2006-2009

[105] Cioato SG et al. Long-lasting effect of transcranial direct current stimulation in the reversal of hyperalgesia and cytokine alterations induced by the neuropathic pain model. Brain Stimulation. 2016;**9**(2):209-217

[106] Lopes BC et al. Transcranial direct current stimulation combined with exercise modulates the inflammatory profile and hyperalgesic response in rats subjected to a neuropathic pain model: Long term effects. Brain Stimulation. 2020;**13**:774-782

Chapter 11

Neuromodulation in Urology: Current Trends and Future Applications

Said M. Yaiesh, Abdullatif E. Al-Terki and Tariq F. Al-Shaiji

Abstract

Urological applications of neuromodulation and neurostimulation are among the most evolving fields for these technologies. First approved for management of refractory urge incontinence, different modalities of neuromodulation and stimulation have been tested, applied and verified for a vast spectrum of voiding and pelvic floor dysfunction disorders. The modalities of delivering this treatment have also evolved in the last three decades, with a focus on sacral neuromodulation. The experimental and established "off-label" applications of neuromodulation have also encompassed chronic pelvic pain disorders, including chronic prostatitis and bladder pain syndrome, among others. In this chapter, we discuss all the hypothesized theories suggested on how this technology provides therapeutic potential for a number of chronic and debilitating urological conditions, the modes of delivery be it anterior, sacral, and posterior tibial to name a few, and the evolving and future applications.

Keywords: neuromodulation, sacral neuromodulation, posterior tibial nerve stimulation, lower urinary tract dysfunction

1. Introduction

Neuromodulation in urological practice is not a novel concept, but certainly one that has lagged in dissemination. The first reports of the use of neuromodulation to stimulate bladder emptying date back to as early as the 1970s, although the results back then were disappointing [1]. It was not until 1988 that Schmidt and Tanagho restarted the discussion on applications of neuromodulation and electrical stimulation of the sacral nerve in urology, and since then reports on different novel techniques and applications ensued [2, 3]. The term "neurostimulation" was recoined later to "neuromodulation," as experts in the neuro-urology field argued that electrical currents do not only stimulate but rather modulate the messages carried by different nerves involved in the micturition reflex and the lower urinary tract [4].

1.1 Review of lower urinary tract innervation and processes of storage and micturition

The urinary bladder has both afferent and efferent innervation. Efferent innervation is both sympathetic and parasympathetic. The hypogastric nerve carries postganglionic sympathetic fibers innervated at the inferior mesenteric ganglion

IntechOpen

by preganglionic fibers arising from T11-L2. Their main function is inhibition of bladder wall contraction and excitation of the internal urethral sphincter, both necessary to maintain continence and facilitate urinary storage. Parasympathetic efferents which originate preganglionically from the sacral spinal cord through the S2 to S4 spinal nerve roots reach postganglionic fibers in the pelvic plexus and bladder wall and through stimulation of release of acetylcholine act on muscarinic receptors to produce bladder wall contraction.

Afferent innervation from the bladder consists of small myelinated Aδ fibers, which relay information via the pelvic and pudendal nerves to the sacral spinal cord at S2 to S4 about the properties of a bladder contraction, and synapse with spinal interneurons and autonomic fibers constituting what is known as the micturition reflex arc. The interneurons also relay information to higher centers, namely the periaqueductal gray and pontine micturition centers, as well as the hypothalamus, thalamus, prefrontal cortex and angulate gyrus in the cerebrum, among other areas. These centers have a modulatory voluntary control over bladder function and what is perceived by us from somatic sensation in the bladder and pelvic floor, such as sensation of bladder fullness. Bladder afferents also consist of unmyelinated C-fibers which are inactive in normal circumstances but are responsible for transmission of noxious stimuli such as bladder pain and are involved in the development of neurologic lower urinary tract dysfunction [1].

During the phase of urinary storage, information about increasing bladder volume and pressure is carried by afferent discharges that stimulate both the sympathetic and parasympathetic preganglionic fibers. While the stimulated parasympathetic fibers would elicit a bladder contraction, their activity is inhibited by sympathetic discharges at the postganglionic level, which also maintain contraction of the internal urethral sphincter at the level of the bladder neck and contraction of the pelvic floor in response to bladder filling. This coordination of afferent and efferent pathways ensures stable bladder filling and urinary storage and subsequently continence. Beyond a certain threshold of bladder filling, afferent discharges trigger the micturition reflex at the pontine level. This reflex results in inhibition of sympathetic and efferent continence signals and allowance of parasympathetic mediated bladder contractions to facilitate bladder emptying, preceded by relaxation of the urinary sphincters and pelvic floor.

Any interruption at the gross or microcellular level of these neural circuits would result in voiding dysfunction, be it by increased bladder sensation resulting in urinary frequency as is the case in overactive bladder and urgency-frequency disorders, loss of continence as in urgency urinary incontinence, loss of bladder sensation or inability to generate a voiding pressure as in non-obstructive urinary retention, or formation or upregulation of pathological neural circuits for reflex bladder activity or transmission of noxious stimuli such as is neurogenic bladder or pelvic pain disorders.

1.2 Mechanisms of action of neuromodulation of lower urinary tract

Neuromodulation of the lower urinary tract aims to restore lost or dysfunctional neural functions to fulfill the two main functions of the bladder, storage and voiding. Artificial stimulators directly or indirectly apply electrical stimulation that achieves this purpose. Through continuous or intermittent electrical stimuli at different nerves and sites, neuromodulation treats both bladder over- and under-activity, as well as pelvic and bladder pain [5].

The modes by which these electrical stimulations achieve such restoration differ from one type of neuromodulation to the other, and this will be further discussed in each section.

1.3 General indications

Neuromodulation in urology is aimed at control of uninhibited bladder contractions to eliminate sensation of urgency and provide appropriate urinary continence. This is the scenario for overactive bladder disease and neurogenic bladder overactivity. Inability to void resulting in urinary retention is also corrected by neuromodulation, though the literature has been less evident for neurogenic causes of retention versus the established restorative effects on voiding in idiopathic non-obstructive urinary retention (NOUR). Other effects through action on shared nerves between the lower urinary tract and the pelvic floor musculature are less reported on and are yet to be approved, but results have shown consistent alleviation of pelvic pain and sexual dysfunction parameters.

2. Neuromodulation modalities in urology

The spectrum of neuromodulation modalities in urology has evolved yet focuses around two manners that correspond to our understanding of the innervation of the lower urinary tract and pelvic floor muscles: sacral neuromodulation, by sacral anterior root stimulation, sacral nerve modulation and recently pudendal nerve stimulation (PNS) and its derivatives, and less invasive neuromodulators and peripheral nerve stimulators, the most studied of which is posterior tibial nerve stimulation.

2.1 Sacral anterior root stimulation

Though this mode of urological neuromodulation is almost of historical interest in the face of current advances in the field and the dominance of sacral neuromodulation, it yet deserves honorable mention as it paved the way to utilize the sacral region for restoration of bladder function. Through stimulation of the anterior sacral nerve, both bladder parasympathetic efferents and somatic motor fibers to the external urethral sphincter are activated. This ventral activation facilitates intermittent bladder emptying [1].

Brindley in 1976 implanted intradurally and bilaterally on the ventral roots from S2 to S5 subcutaneous cables that were externally powered and would provide on-demand electromagnetic stimulation to facilitate voiding [5–7]. He later modified his procedure by performing posterior rhizotomy at the S2–S3 level during implantation of the stimulator to improve the continence outcome by eliminating the effect C-fiber bladder afferents had on amplifying the micturition reflex. This is what was later named the Brindley procedure, and its popularity phased out years later as more studies and reports demonstrated debilitating and unacceptable complications such as sacral dermatome hyperalgesia, cerebrospinal fluid leak, and damage to the anterior nerve root. The procedure, however, remains indicated for patients with complete spinal cord injury (SCI) with maintained bladder reflexes [1, 7–9].

2.2 Sacral neuromodulation

The first reports describing the application of sacral neuromodulation were by Schmidt and Tanagho, the latter concentrating on its application in neurogenic lower urinary tract dysfunction [2, 3]. Since then, both experimental and approved applications and research aiming to understand the mechanism of action by which sacral neurostimulation, or more appropriately now termed sacral neuromodulation (SNM), affects and rehabilitates the functions of the lower urinary tract, both in facilitating bladder storage and voiding, has expanded. Researchers also embarked on assessing its efficacy, particularly cost-effectiveness, when compared to other modes of treatment for its indications. SNM is, perhaps, the best studied mode of neuromodulation in urology [5].

Compared to the Brindley procedure, SNM posed numerous advantages and technical differences. The SNM procedure involves extradural electrode implantation usually in one of the paired S3 foramens. It does not require posterior rhizotomy either. This minimized the risks of nerve root injury or cerebrospinal fluid leakage. It provides continuous electrical stimulation to the nerves in its proximity and is controlled remotely without the need for subcutaneous cables as it has a built in-battery and antenna. It also modulates for restoration of normal micturition and suppresses bladder overactivity, which made it applicable to non-neurogenic voiding dysfunctions as well [1, 3].

The first SNM device made commercially available was the Interstim® (Medtronic Neuromodulation, Minneapolis USA). It was first approved in 1997 by the US Food & Drug Administration (FDA) for use in refractory urge incontinence, and later in 1999 its approval was expanded to include significant urgency, frequency, and idiopathic urinary retention. The US market was the most enthusiastic to adopt it, and back then and by the year 2004 15,000 units were implanted, the majority of which were in the USA [10, 11]. Since then, the rates of SNM implantations increased by at least 10 to 20-folds [12, 13].

Sacral neuromodulation is dedicated to the S3 foramen, targeting the S3 nerve root which is identified as the most relevant home for impulses, containing sensory fibers from the pelvic floor and parasympathetic neural fibers affecting the detrusor muscle of the bladder. This differs from the target of other neuromodulation modalities, and provides a distinct pattern of identification during implantation, which will be discussed later [14, 15].

2.2.1 Mechanism of action

The goal of SNM is to modulate abnormal bladder sensations the patient may have, as well as involuntary uncontrollable reflexes in the lower urinary tract to restore the patient's voluntary control and facilitate normal function [16]. The theories on how it actually achieves these goals are vast, and expanding to date, and remain complex. This is perhaps in part due to the sophisticated interaction of higher central voiding centers in the brain and spinal cord and the peripheral nervous system in facilitating the functions of the lower urinary tract.

Investigators have assessed a multitude of concepts, from the molecular neurophysiological level to broader neurocirculatory behaviors in the brain and spine, in both animal models and human studies. Yet to date, no single theorem has been solely agreed upon. Some studies have even shown dual or multiple mechanisms through different channels by which SNM exerts its modulatory effect on the lower urinary tract, partly by studying its different effects in many neuro-urological conditions ranging from bladder overactivity to chronic pelvic pain.

SNM therapeutic effects are speculated to arise through electric stimulation of both afferent and efferent neural circuits in the pelvic viscera and connections with spinal interneurons. The stimulator produces an electrical charge in close proximity to the sacral root nerves, regenerating propagational axonal action potentials in the region. This in turn stimulates somatic afferents which modulate higher center control of micturition including the prefrontal cortex and insula, by restoring normal bladder function and perhaps suppressing reflex bladder activity such as that seen in overactive bladder (OAB). This indirect effect both on the bladder and the urinary sphincter is achieved through adaptive neural plasticity, and thus, an intact neural system, at least distally, is a neural requirement for SNM to successfully restore bladder function [15–21]. The SNM device can provide different levels of stimulation, which may further modulate efferents to the bladder-sphincter complex; however, it does not have any direct effect on urethral resistance [16, 22].

Several studies have proved that SNM has modulatory effects in the brain. Earlier work has demonstrated stimulatory and inhibitory effects in specific brain regions including those responsible for alertness, sensation of bladder filling, and timing of micturition [23, 24]. Utilizing positron emission tomography (PET) and functional magnetic resonance imaging (fMRI) of the brain, researchers were able to identify decreased function after SNM in areas like the orbitofrontal cortex, angulate gyrus, and thalamus, while stimulating the dorsolateral prefrontal cortex, and the therapeutic effect of SNM corresponded to pre-implantation increased activity in the angulate and inferior frontal gyri, insula and thalamus. Such patterns of activity in the brain were shown to predict response to SNM treatment in females with OAB. Furthermore, investigators were able to show that different SNM stimulus intensities had varied brain responses, which may have differential therapeutic implications [23–27].

On the neurophysiological level, much has been investigated to understand which neural receptors and neurotransmitters may be affected by neuromodulation, SNM in particular. Opiod receptors are shown to be inhibited by SNM, and this inhibitory effect is augmented by tramadol and other opiod receptor agonists [28]. From animal models, blockade of opiod receptors with naloxone significantly reduced bladder capacity during sacral neuromodulation for reflex bladder activity. Blockade of beta-2 receptors, however, showed the opposite response during SNM [29]. Also mediated by opiod receptors are the SNM inhibitory effects of bladder overactivity mediated by supraspinal $GABA_A$ receptors [30].

2.2.2 Indications and contraindications

2.2.2.1 FDA approved indications

The US Food and Drug Administration has approved four main indications for SNM application, three of which are urological: refractory urinary urgency and frequency, urge urinary incontinence (UUI), non-obstructive urinary retention (NOUR), and lastly, fecal incontinence. This has been agreed upon and resounded by multiple authorities including the International Continence Society in their best practice statements, among other bodies [4]. However, FDA approval does not indicate level of recommendation, and authoritarians and experts in the field have built on this approval to debate and set the grade and the line of therapy at which SNM serves for a number of conditions, as well as argue for and against other indications or applications the FDA has not seen the benefit of SNM for eye-to-eye with available literature and results. There are, moreover, conditions that must be met prior to justifying an implantation regardless of the aforementioned indications and contraindications that must be observed.

The International Continence Society (ICS) assessed the evidence available for SNM in different pathological genitourinary conditions and published its recommendations based on available literature. In summary, the ICS panel found grade A evidence to support the efficacy of SNM in overactive bladder and non-obstructive urinary retention including Fowler's syndrome and voiding dysfunction; however, this high level evidence did not change their recommendation of maintaining SNM as a second or third-line mode of therapy in these disorders. For other conditions including interstitial cystitis/bladder pain syndrome (IC/BPS) and neurogenic lower urinary tract symptoms, SNM remained an option based on lower levels of evidence (grade C evidence/level III recommendations) [4, 31].

2.2.2.2 Off-label uses

Although the FDA has not recognized or approved these applications of SNM, there is a growing body of evidence that demonstrates its effectiveness in other genitourinary pathological conditions. In particular are chronic pelvic pain disorders including both IC/BPS and non-IC chronic pelvic pain syndrome (CPPS). Despite lack of availability of high-level evidence, the off-label application of SNM in these conditions continues with variable results in improving associated urinary symptoms and quality of life parameters.

Other non-approved applications of SNM include its use in special populations such as those with neurogenic lower urinary tract symptoms, pediatrics and adolescents, and even in contraindicated situations including continued SNM in pregnancy for women with urological conditions. Most of these applications carry hypothetical risks, a spectrum of which have been refuted in small case series and reports in literature, but bigger studies are needed to elucidate and clarify the role of SNM in these situations.

2.2.2.3 Contraindications

Authorities have agreed on certain absolute and relative contraindications for SNM [4], with exceptions and points up for debate to date in the literature.

Absolute contraindications of SNM are:

1. An inadequate clinical response—this is dictated by the universally accepted cut-off of more than 50% improvement during the test phase of SNM.

2. The patient's inability to operate the SNM device, or lack of caregiver support thereof who could assist in doing so.

3. Pregnancy, and this remains a point of debate across literature, as will be discussed further next.

The *relative contraindications* for SNM therapy, as outlined by many guidelines including the ICS best practice statements, do not preclude use of SNM, but must be vigilantly observed and discussed with the patient prior to embarking on treatment. These include:

1. Severe and/or rapidly progressive neurologic disease with urinary symptoms—in such a state, the patient's foreseeable benefit from treatment, even based on a successful test phase, would be challenged by the changing neurological status or development and progression of the disease.

2. Complete SCI, which would hinder the modulatory effect of SNM in higher nervous centers as discussed earlier.

3. The ongoing recognized or observed need for magnetic resonance imaging (MRI) examination, particularly in patients with established neurological disorders like multiple sclerosis (MS) that may need continued MRI assessment or patients undergoing work-up for other conditions that may need it, particularly non-head MRI examination, which will be discussed further in a separate segment as growing reports continue to argue MRI safety with implanted SNM devices.

4. Abnormal sacral anatomy is a sensible contraindication in which such deformities would hinder the identification of the correct sacral foramens required for optimum effect and implantation.

2.2.2.4 Magnetic resonance imaging

With the exception of head MRI examination, the ongoing or anticipated need for MRI examination for patients is a relative contraindication for SNM implantation [4, 32]. The potential effect of non-head MRI examinations on an implantable metallic device such as SNM have debilitated practitioners and potential patients alike with one series reporting that 23% of device explantations at their center were due to the need of the patient to undergo this examination. This has absurd financial and clinical implications in the face of an effective implantation [33].

In the same series, two thirds of the explanted patients required a change in management post-explantation, including intradetrusor botulinum injections, or to resort to self-intermittent urinary catheterization or even require in one case cystectomy and urinary diversion. Thus, explantation has dire consequences that must be outweighed against the potential need and risks of undergoing MRI especially when over 20% of the patients that were explanted prior to MRI examination ended up not undergoing the imaging test and just over 50% of those MRI results influenced non-genitourinary treatment decision making [33]. Additionally, one cannot help but wonder the number of patients who may have benefitted from SNM therapy had they not been excluded due to prospective need for MRI with better and alternative planning.

2.2.2.5 Pregnancy

It is difficult to design trials to test for the effects of SNM, or any form of neuromodulation or therapy for that matter, when there is a hypothesis of potential teratogenic effect on the fetus, or risk of abortion or premature delivery. Apart from the overridden potential for damage to the SNM system when it was historically being implanted in the anterior abdominal wall, completely posterior SNM implants or their predecessors have not been shown in a number of series and reviews to be associated with any fetal malformations or early deliveries or a higher rate of cesarean sections. These reports are based on pregnant women who against recommendation and electively opted to maintain their SNM devices on during their pregnancies fully or at certain periods and trimesters [34, 35].

Thus, the decision to continue neuromodulation, or to proceed with implantation for a woman who has not completed her family or is actively trying to conceive, remains a debatable and individualized decision, but in accordance with manufacturer recommendations and societal guidelines and until more compelling evidence arises, pregnancy will remain a contraindication for SNM, though more relatedly relevant than absolute [34].

2.2.2.6 Other considerations

Potential interference of SNM devices with other implantable electrostimulators such as cardiac pacemakers has long been speculated. A series of three patients who have cardiac pacemakers and underwent SNM implantation has reported that no interference was observed on the part of either of the implanted devices by the other [36].

2.2.3 Predictors of effect

One of the hallmarks of diagnosis of urinary and voiding dysfunction disorders is the utility of urodynamic testing (UDS). Of different types and modes, this diagnostic test aims at reproducing patient symptoms and correlating them to net intradetrusor pressure, among other parameters, in simulated bladder filling and voiding phases. Much has been disputed about the need for UDS testing to diagnose straightforward and clinically apparent conditions such as overactive bladder, and whether UDS findings could help predict outcomes of therapy including SNM prior to its implantation. However, evidence suggests that no single UDS parameter or finding can predict SNM success [37].

In its best practice statement, the ICS did not find sufficient evidence to support that urodynamic studies can predict outcomes of treatment for SNM, while it supported based on higher level of evidence a stronger recommendation for performing SNM trial phases as the "single most valuable tool" to predict outcome of SNM [4].

Attention has been given to difference in SNM effects between certain patient populations. Gender differences have been long hypothesized, with attention focusing on SNM effects on pelvic floor rehabilitation and its close relatedness to urinary and chronic pelvic disorders in females as a potential modality of effect. In a matched pair analysis, a group of researchers reported on 80 patients who received SNM implants for urge urinary incontinence and found that more women tended to receive implants than men. While urinary frequency and symptom scores improved in both groups, over 3 years, the number of urge incontinence episodes per day improved in men more than women, while the severity of the incontinence improved in women more than men [38]. This gender discrepancy may be explained in part by SNM effect, but perhaps is also due to anatomical difference of the distal urinary tract in men and women.

Another patient population suspected to be at a lesser advantage from SNM efficacy are older patients and those with certain comorbidities such as obesity. Interestingly, one study did not only find no difference in response among older patients but further identified that age correlated with a lower rate of surgical revisions of the implantation—3% lower odds per year. In the same study, BMI did not influence explantation rates [39].

It is undeniable that there are identifiable structural changes in the bladder muscle and wall that incur from long standing overactive bladder and non-obstructive urinary retention, and hypotheses suggest this may affect the therapeutic outcomes of SNM as the symptom duration increases. However, even symptoms extending for more than 10 years have not been shown to have any significant effect on the success of SNM [40].

2.2.4 Results of SNM and its efficacy

SNM has proven an efficacious modality of treatment of different genitourinary disorders, with durable success rates between 70 to 80% in certain conditions such as refractory OAB [11, 31, 41, 42]. In one survey of SNM patients, satisfaction rates were reported to be over 95% with SNM therapy and were not affected by patient age or any complications or program type, a testament to the efficacy of this treatment [43]. The multitude of data in the literature also attests to the general safety of SNM [44].

History of prior back surgery may be deemed a challenging patient condition for SNM implantation, but a review of 500 patients has shown that such a history did not negatively affect SNM outcomes [45]. Even in patients with prior anti-incontinence surgery and history of pelvic organ prolapse surgery, the efficacy of SNM has been established. Surgeries of the bladder and pelvic floor may slightly affect the outcomes of SNM, however, these remain generally good and acceptable [46].

2.2.5 Cost-effectiveness

The debate continues on what is the cost-effectiveness of SNM compared to other available treatments for refractory voiding conditions be it OAB or UUI or others. These include in general combination medication, intradetrusor botulinum injections (repeated as the effect of one injection wears out necessitating periodic repeat injections), and more definite bladder or anti-incontinence surgeries.

The long term outcomes of SNM compared to the need for maximal medical therapy or repeated botulinum injections poses a cost-effective benefit superior to the aforementioned counterparts, with some authors even arguing that from a patient's perspective it may well be considered an appropriate primary therapy rather than a second or third line alternative [47]. Compared to botulinum injections in particular, SNM was shown in one study to be cost-effective from the third year of application onwards, with a clear dominance should treatment be continued for 10 years [48]. However, results from the ROSETTA randomized trial which compared SNM and botulinum bladder injections for refractory UUI showed SNM as a less cost-effective alternative [49].

Perhaps the arguments for and against the cost-effectiveness of SNM versus other treatments lay not just in the treatments it is being compared to but in terms of what condition these treatments are being utilized for. In a focus article on safety and cost of SNM compared to botulinum injections for OAB, although SNM was costlier, it was safer than intradetrusor botulinum injections. The latter carries a substantial side effect profile including urinary tract infections, hematuria, urinary retention, and more frequent emergency room visits, all not common occurrences, but may tip the scale in favor of SNM [50].

2.2.6 Preoperative assessment and counseling

As with any surgical procedure, preoperative assessment and counseling are of paramount importance. It has been identified that such counseling should include discussions on possible expected side effects and adverse events of SNM therapy, such as implant site pain, infection, paresthesia, and leg and buttock pain. Moreover, the patient must understand that within the spectrum of approved devices in clinical practice, currently the Interstim® device in its two generations, there may arise a need for surgical revision of the implant or ongoing reprogramming atop an eminent and eventual need for replacement of the implantable pulse generator (IPG) once the battery wears out should treatment extend beyond an expected life-expectancy of 3 to 5 years on average. Additionally, and based on ICS recommendations, urodynamic testing is not mandatory, but phase testing is highly recommended prior to embarking on surgical implantation of the SNM IPG [4, 51].

One side effect profile that has been raised in the literature has been the psychological aspects of SNM therapy, though some authors have argued that a reverse pathology is possible with patients with chronic genitourinary and pelvic pain disorders who are potential candidates for SNM are pre-operatively burdened or have pre-existing psychological ailments. As is the limited evidence from some case reports and series, some patients encounter behavioral changes or exacerbation of preexisting psychological conditions such as depression, which has led to the argument of need for psychological assessment of certain traits that may affect SNM outcomes [52]. However, this has yet to be reflected in the guidelines and societal recommendations and a causality has not been established. On the other hand, other researchers have shown no influence of psychological and psychiatric factors on SNM outcomes [53].

2.2.6.1 General considerations

SNM implantation requires, most commonly, fluoroscopic guidance in the lead placement stage of the procedure to correctly identify the S3 foramen and the depth of lead placement and direction and correlate it with the reflex responses of the patient. Though of ongoing concern, studies have shown that radiation during SNM implantation, be it staged or office-based percutaneous nerve evaluation (PNE), is safe and within the recommended limits set by the International Commission on Radiological Protection [54]. That, however, did not alter an ongoing debate on whether "fluoro-guidance" can be replaced by a less radioactive imaging modality, the ultrasound. Apart from having a far lower radiation exposure profile, if any, ultrasound-guided lead placement was found in one study to lower the number of needle punctures needed to identify the most suitable S3 foramen for patient response; however, that had minimal effects on total operative time [55].

Preoperative antibiotic administration is also advocated in both stages of implantation. The recommended antibiotic regimens should target common skin flora pathogens. Guidelines published by the French Association of Urology suggest the use of amoxycillin or broad-spectrum cephalosporins, and in case of hypersensitivity to these antibiotics, an alternative combination of vancomycin and clindamycin is suitable [56].

2.2.7 Technical aspects and techniques

2.2.7.1 The device: lead and implantable pulse generator

The SNM device consists of a tinned lead, connected to a stimulator, the implantable pulse generator (IPG), by insulated cords. Improvements have been made between the initial and current Interstim II device available on the market, including the tinned lead technology, deflected lead tip, and increased capacity of storage of programming and patient data, among others.

The tines allow for anchorage of the lead and prevent displacement. The quadripolar lead contains four electrical stimulation contact regions or electrodes, which are used to designate four different programmable charges on each region to provide an endless number of possible combinations of modulatory programs for patients for a variety of symptoms and effects. These are under the control of an external programming remote that allows the surgeon or programmer to store certain programs to the system of the patient. The patient can then use their own remote to initiate or shutdown certain programs at different times, or switch off the device all together, as well as control the intensity of the stimulation. An illustration of the quadripolar tinned lead can be seen in **Figure 1**.

The IPG is a battery-dependent neuromodulator that delivers electrical stimulation transmitted via the lead. It has an embedded antenna that receives signals from the operator remote controllers [42].

2.2.7.2 Office-based percutaneous nerve evaluation

This modality of lead testing or screening for possible responses is done in the office setting under local anesthesia and allows assessment of both sensory and motor responses of the patient to stimulation. It can be done under fluoroscopy or ultrasound guidance. It is deemed a less invasive and less resource-intensive testing phase prior to implantation. However, it is more uncomfortable to the patient since

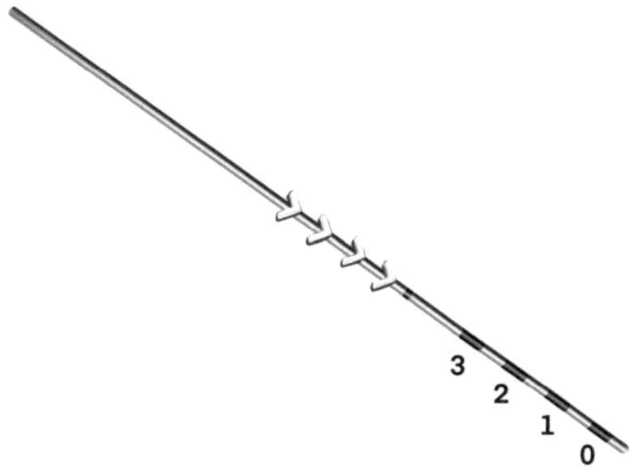

Figure 1.
Quadripolar tinned lead utilized in SNM. Labeled are the electrode positions, "0" being most distal and "3" most proximal. An optimum insertion is eliciting a response on all electrodes at low voltage.

only local anesthesia is being used [57]. As a matter of fact, single-staged implantation after PNE could save US $1500–5000 depending on how high the success rate of the implantation is, an argument well utilized on part of advocates at both ends of the debate of whether to stage or not [58].

Local anesthesia is applied subcutaneously to the mid-sacral region where testing will be performed. In the prone position, a needle harboring a single-electrode lead is advanced to correctly identify the S3 foramen. The S3 foramen can be identified fluoroscopically, or approximated anatomically as evident from cadaveric studies that showed the mean distance of the superior aspect of the S3 foramen is approximately 9 cm from the coccyx, and laterally it is 2 cm from the middle of the sacral back region, while vertical interforamenal spaces are around 1.5 cm in length [59].

The patient is asked to report any sensations felt in the perineal region or the foot, and motor responses are also examined in the buttock region and the ipsilateral foot. Stimulation is then performed at different voltages and the area is marked. Successful office-based PNE is followed by one-stage surgical tinned 4-electrode lead placement and IPG implantation. Motor responses are rechecked during implantation, and location and laterality may be modified to obtain the most appropriate response. This is probably one of the most important disadvantages and arguments against PNE in favor of staged implantation: bypassing a longer assessment or testing period that would reveal more information about the prospective efficacy of the chosen S3 foramen and SNM implant.

The ideal patient for PNE is a cooperative and apprehensive one who can remain relaxed during the procedure. Patients who cannot lay prone for any reason or medical condition, and those who may need more deeper stimulation such as those morbidly obese or anyone with anatomical variations or previous sacral scars may preclude office-based PNE [57]. However, in one study by Gonssen and colleagues, the need for general anesthesia was substituted by a complete permanent SNM implantation under local anesthesia, and was reported to be both safe and tolerable with successful outcomes [60].

Focus has been given in current research and modifications of leads to replace current PNE leads with more functional multipolar leads that would allow a more idealistic response and minimal manipulation of the lead [57].

2.2.7.3 Stage I testing of two-stage implantation

Under sedation or general anesthesia should the patient require it if they cannot maintain an airway in the prone position, staged SNM implantation depends on a primary stage I of testing done in the operative theater where the tinned lead is eventually implanted after eliciting the best motor response and insulated cord cables are tracked to the contralateral side and eventually out of the skin to be connected to a temporary pulse generator for the testing phase. These cables are later re-tunneled back the ipsilateral side where the tinned leads have been implanted and are connected to the implantable IPG.

This is the method utilized at our center, where we deem it and it has been proven to be more comfortable for the patient in a controlled setting where even sedation can be switched to anesthesia should the patient become restless. Nevertheless, muscle relaxation is not administered to maintain the ability to assess motor response on lead placement and testing. One particular population of patients which are ideal candidates for this mode of testing are morbidly obese patients where local anesthesia administered subcutaneously may not be sufficient for the deep layer manipulation necessary to deliver the lead to the sacral foramens [57].

Some researchers have continuously advocated staged testing and implantation despite PNE being a more resourceful alternative. Arguments included the increased comfort of the patient allows for better identification of ideal patients for therapy and less likely to result in a misleading positive screening but unsuccessful subsequent implantation. It also allows the employment of a longer testing trial period and has the added potential of fine-tuning stimulation parameters. It has been advocated as the ideal modality of screening for responses in patients with NOUR, sensory urgency and CPPS [57].

The two-stage implantation technique depends on a 2–4 weeks arbitrary period of testing for improved responses in patients planned for implantation. This period has been contested in literature, as are the arguments in favor of office-based PNE. The range of reported successful test phases is around 60% [61]. However, the length of this period has been also up for debate. One group of researchers studied a group of patients who underwent stage I SNM implantation test phase and found that the mean time needed to identify potential successful outcomes of the test was 3 days, ranging from 1 to 9 days in total. This was not different between patients implanted for OAB and those for NOUR, and thus they concluded that a test stage I period of two or more weeks may not be necessary [61].

The importance of such an argument lays in the potential morbidities of a prolonged test period, with partially exposed external leads liable for displacement and a possible route for infection, though the literature does not report on either. The length of stage I has been suspected to be a risk factor for SNM implant infections, but the evidence is lacking, and the identifiable association if any may be the result of improper antibiotic regimens or assessment of small sample sizes of patients [62].

Disadvantages of staged screening and implantation include that only motor responses are assessed during lead placement. Sensory responses cannot be assessed in the presence of even light sedation. However, two formal studies have found that motor responses more importantly surpass sensory responses in predicting SNM successful outcomes [57]. These are in addition to the logical added financial and time requirements for testing in the operation theater and the need for anesthesia.

2.2.7.4 Lead placement

In SNM, the lead is placed in the S3 foramen, either on the right or left side, and rarely bilateral lead placement is undertaken. The S3 foramen has been identified to be relevant to the target nerve fibers required to achieve the effect of SNM [15]. Patients exhibit and experience typical motor and sensory responses to lead placement in the S3 foramen, depending on the setting of lead placement under local or general anesthesia. This is further summarized in **Table 1**, along with responses

Foramen	Sensory response	Motor response
S2	Buttock sensation Leg sensation	Foot: plantar flexion, foot rotation Anal sphincter "clamp movement"
S3	Perineal paresthesia or pulling sensation in rectum, scrotum or vagina	Anal bellows "winking" Great toe dorsiflexion
S4	Pulling sensation in rectum only	Anal bellows only without leg or foot movement
Hubsher et al. [63] and Thompson et al. [64].		

Table 1.
Expected responses from SNM at different sacral levels.

of adjacent S2 and S4 foramens, which surgeons utilize to correctly identify the S3 foramen and avoid the formers [63, 64].

The placement of the actual tinned lead is preceded by testing or screening using a conductive long needle that is introduced first in the correct foramen, and a conductor is used to elicit the best response possible on the most number of electrodes (optimum being four-out-of-four positive electrodes at the lowest stimulatory voltage possible). Once finalized, a small skin incision around the needle facilitates for the introduction of the tinned lead in the chosen foramen. This tracking is aided by an introducer stylet [42, 63, 65, 66]. **Figures 2–5** show an illustration of the steps on the introduction of the tinned lead and implantation of the IPG, while **Figure 6** shows how the inserted tinned lead looks like and is confirmed to be correctly placed on fluoroscopy.

There is no agreed upon definition of optimal lead placement, and many factors have been speculated to alter placement and SNM outcomes, including position and depth of lead, angle, and deflection (straight, lateral or medial related to the foramen), but none shown to have any relation to SNM outcome. Lateral deflection is the only factor found to be associated with identifying more active electrodes, although the number of active electrodes itself has not been shown to correlate with a better motor response. Thus, the concentration during lead placement especially under general anesthesia should be on identifying the best motor response rather than on anatomical details [67].

In the quest for optimal lead positioning and how to facilitate this process, some researchers have advocated for the use of a curved stylet during the introduction of

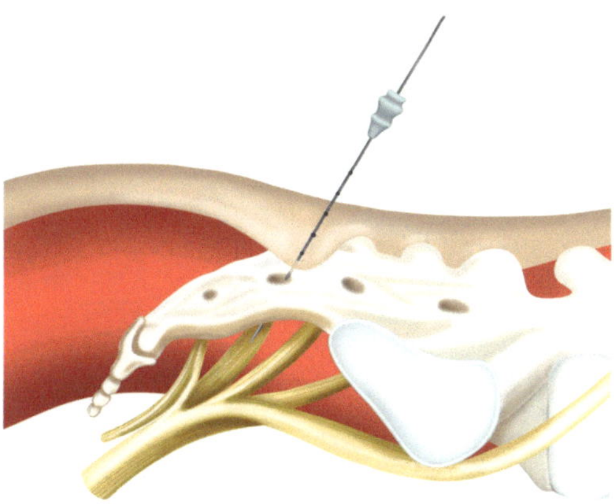

Figure 2.
Test needle insertion into the S3 foramen. The needle position is confirmed fluoroscopically or by ultrasound. An electrostimulation probe is then used in contact with the distal end of the needle to test for appropriate motor responses.

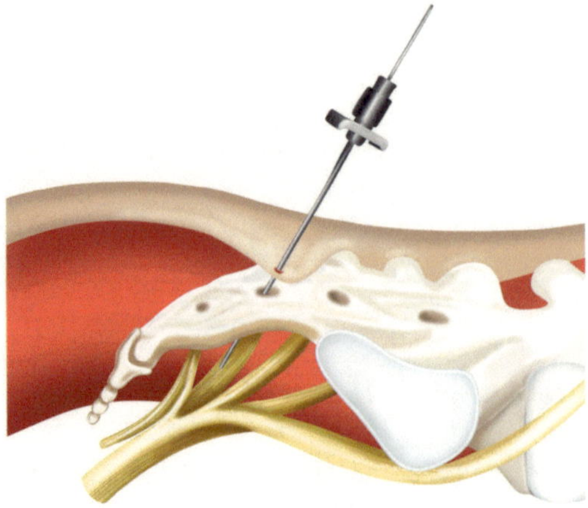

Figure 3.
Introductory stylet inserted in chosen S3 foramen. The stylet guides enclosed lead. Once removed, tines allow for anchorage of lead in proper position.

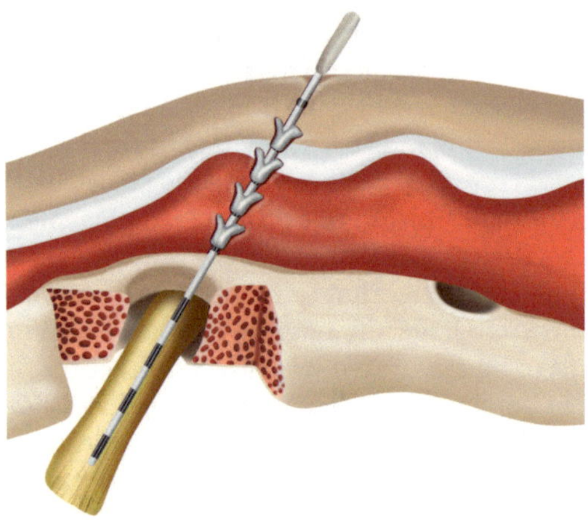

Figure 4.
Tined lead position after removing of stylet and introductory sheath. Note position of electrodes deep to foramen and in proximity to nerve root.

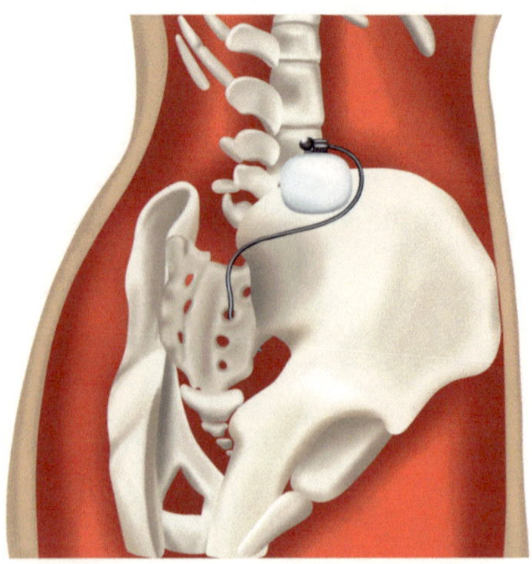

Figure 5.
Final position of implanted pulse generator (IPG) and connections.

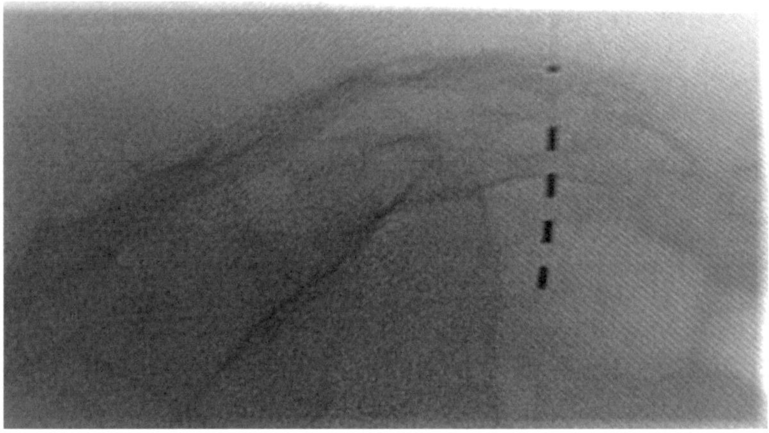

Figure 6.
Fluoroscopic confirmation of position of lead and electrodes in relation to sacral spine.

the tinned lead into the foramen. The tip of this stylet has an 18° bend that allows it to follow the natural pathway of the sacral root nerve. This is thought to allow for identification of an ideal response on all 4 electrodes at low voltage, subsequently providing greater flexibility with programming [68].

During lead placement and testing, the requirement is not only limited to correct identification of the S3 foramen, but also to eliciting the best response from the patient on stimulation at the lowest voltage possible. Researchers have argued for years for unilateral or bilateral lead testing. What is evident from studies to date is that the side that tests with the best motor response (or sensory response if patient can relay it) does not necessarily translate into the best outcome for therapy on the long-term. However, bilateral testing has the advantage of allowing patients to choose the side that they find more beneficial or comfortable [57].

2.2.7.5 Implantation of internal pulse generator/stage II procedure

Implantation of the internal or implantable pulse generator (IPG) can be in the setting of a single-stage along with lead placement following successful PNE testing, or the second stage of a staged implantation after a successful trial period following stage I lead implantation. Regardless of the staging, the IPG is implanted in a subcutaneous pocket on the same side the tinned lead has been placed in the S3 foramen. Sterility of the IPG device must be maintained to avoid acute or chronic infections.

After skin preparation and administration of necessary local anesthesia, a subcutaneous pocket is created under the skin in the patient's buttock. This pocket should be high enough away from the seating area of the patient, and deep enough to avoid superficial sensation of the IPG by the patient as well. Preoperative marking is helpful in such scenarios, keeping in mind distance from the employed S3 foramen as well to avoid tension on the connection between the tinned lead and the IPG. The cord is tunneled from the lead to the IPG subcutaneously and the connections are made. Before wound closure, wash with a sterile water-based antibiotic solution has been described by some authors. It is important to avoid saline-based solutions that may cause electronic malfunction of the device [41, 42, 63, 65, 69].

2.2.8 Post-implantation programming and troubleshooting

Programming is done after IPG implantation when the patient is fully awake and conscious to provide feedback on different modes and programs as they are being tested and tried out and allows them to choose their preferred settings. At our center this is done on the next day postoperatively and ensues removal of the urinary catheter placed during the procedure to allow for trials of voiding [41, 70]. Patient follow-up is periodic thereafter, during which voiding and stimulation parameters are checked and patient compliance is evaluated [42].

Good communication between the patient, surgeon and the programmer are necessary to obtain the optimum results and efficacy of SNM. In cases where any unforeseeable event occurs, such as sudden loss of efficacy or any of the adverse events that will be discussed as follows, proper testing of the programs and circuit impedance, as well as efforts at reprogramming operational electrodes should be utilized extensively before reaching the morbid decision of revision or explantation [42, 71, 72].

2.2.9 Adverse events and complications

Adverse events associated with SNM are numerous and well-documented. The majority of such events are anticipated and even counseled for preoperatively, with a documented range of 16–30% between the test and final implantation stages. Unanticipated or unexpected adverse events and complications are rare and are limited to isolated case reports and limited series [73].

2.2.9.1 Pain

Implant site pain is pain perceived at the site of the IPG. This could be the result of many reasons. A too-superficial implant may be cutaneously felt and pose a source of discomfort especially if implanted at a lower gluteal point and as such would be "sat on" by the patient. In one review, the most commonly cited reason for explantation was site pain [74]. Another series reported this to occur in 7% of implants, with the majority presenting beyond 30 days of implantation and some associated with trauma.

Another cause of pain could be stimulation program related. Turning off the IPG can differentiate between IPG-related and program-related pain, the latter usually requiring changes in stimulator settings by the programmer [42]. In the most debilitating cases, and often, this complaint would require surgical revision of the pocket or implant [73].

Pain could also be felt at the site where the stimulatory sensation is perceived, and this too, could often be differentiated by turning off the stimulator, and subsequently altering the settings [42].

2.2.9.2 Undesirable change in stimulation

Perhaps one of the most unfortunate adverse events is an undesirable change in stimulation that leads to loss of a successful SNM effect or subjective dissatisfaction with an objectively successful implant. In one series, researchers reported this to occur in 12% of their surveyed adverse events in SNM implants for OAB. The majority of such incidences can be corrected with simple or sometimes more complex reprogramming of the neuromodulator, and rarely requires revision or explantation [73]. However, decrease in efficacy of stimulation is a major reason for reoperation and explantation should reprogramming in absence of lead migration fail to correct the deficiency [42, 75].

Checking the impedance can be useful to assess for any possible lead breakage or dislodgement which would show high impedance, but if the impedance is less than 50 ohms, this may indicate a short circuit that could be due to a wet connection.

Reprogramming electrodes with acceptable impedances could provide a temporary or alternative solution, but lead revision is often necessary [71].

2.2.9.3 Implant infection

In a multicenter retrospective case–control assessment of risk factors for explantation of the SNM device due to infection, researchers reported on an almost 2–3% incidence of infection and identified that hematoma formation and IPG pocket depth of greater than 3 cm were independently associated with development of infection, while implant infection was the leading cause of device explantation at 1 year follow-up in another large trial [68, 73, 76]. The most common pathogen reported on cultures obtained from these explants was the skin flora resident *S. aureus*. Infection is probable both early in the postoperative period within 30 days of implantation, or later beyond 30 days and sometimes up to 10 months post-implantation [73, 76].

Risk factors associated with SNM implantation infection have been studied, and some have been refuted. The choice of preoperative antibiotic regimen is of importance in both stage I and final IPG implant, and the antibiotic administered should target potential and common skin organisms such as *S. aureus* [62].

Prevention of such infections has also been reviewed. One group of researchers reported on the use of an antibiotic-coated collagen layer placed over the IPG before wound closure with noticeable results. Skin preparation is also important, particularly with chlorhexidine-based solutions per international recommendations [62, 68]. And although many surgeons still do administer certain courses of post-implantation antibiotics, this is not supported by any clinical evidence of benefit, though further research may better define its role as is the case with other prosthetic or implantable devices [62].

2.2.9.4 Lead fracture and displacement

Lead fracture, migration or dislodgement are a rare occurrence reported at around 1% of adverse events and eminent needs for device and lead replacements. The introduction of the tinned leads has aided in lowering the incidence of lead migration [41].

Patients may have, against better judgment and counseling, engaged electively in physically demanding exercises, or it may be the result of sudden acute movements or trauma. The result is a sudden loss of or major change in stimulation. On testing, high impedance (>4000 ohms) is found on all 4 electrodes [73]. Additionally, sacral x-ray imaging can help determine if any lead displacement or dislodgement is present. If evident, especially in the presence of complete loss of efficacy and all other alternative reprogramming efforts have been extorted, replacement of the lead is necessary, and sometimes contralateral placement or even bilateral stimulation may be needed, though the latter may not always prove successful [42, 71, 77].

2.2.9.5 Unanticipated adverse events and complications

It is important to understand that although rare, complications are an important predictor of SNM reoperation and may result in severe morbidity [75, 78]. Rare complications of lead placement and implantation have been reported in separate case reports and limited series, including one case of retroperitoneal hemorrhage after SNM implanted for urge incontinence [79]. Another case of lead migration into the sigmoid colon during implantation was complicated by and presented as a colocutaneous fistula [80].

2.3 Direct PNS

As our understanding grew of the neurological contribution and circuits from the sacral nerve roots, new-found focus has been on stimulation of the whole pudendal nerve as it originates from its S2, S3 and S4 nerve roots, and not just the S3 nerve root as with SNM. Theoretically, this should provide a more inclusive sacral nerve stimulation than targeting S3 alone, resulting in inhibition of the micturition reflex and controlling uninhibited detrusor contractions while increasing bladder capacity [14]. This was the hypothesis of the early work on PNS, proposing it would particularly benefit neurogenic bladder patients who fared less successfully with SNM [5].

By placement of both a sacral and pudendal tinned leads in Alcock's canal either tranperineally or through a posterior approach, continuous electrical stimulation similar to SNM is delivered to both nerves [5]. One group of researchers demonstrated comparable improvements in voiding parameters between the PNS and SNM groups, but subjective superiority for PNS reported by patients [81]. PNS was not only found to improve continence but increase bladder capacity in neurogenic bladder patients [5]. Another variation of pudendal PNS is dorsal genital nerve stimulation (DGN), the pudendal nerve's most anterior branch, and this may be the next therapeutic alternative [5, 82].

2.4 Peripheral, cutaneous and minimally invasive neuromodulation modalities

Bypassing the need for formal implantation of any device, these varied modalities of neuromodulation employ concepts on transmitted electrical stimulatory signals from the skin to the nerve vicinity or from peripheral nerves to more central sacral nerve roots and in turn, resulting in a modulatory effect and control on reflex bladder activity particularly bladder hyperactivity, neurogenic or non.

2.4.1 Posterior tibial nerve stimulation

2.4.1.1 Mode of effect

Posterior tibial nerve stimulation (PTNS) provides indirect and retrograde electrical stimulation to the posterior tibial nerve as it passes posteriorly to the medial malleolus of the ankle; the posterior tibial nerve is a mixed nerve with roots from L4 to S3, and as such, provides its modulatory effects on sacral complex roots involved in the lower urinary tract through activation of somatic fibers and inhibiting bladder contractions [1, 15, 83].

PTNS is performed by placement of a needle superoposteriorly to the medial malleolus and a grounding pad placed on the sole of the foot laterally (**Figure** 7). The needle is connected to the stimulator device, and low-voltage stimulation is applied: correct placement is confirmed when flexion of the greater toe is observed and the patient reports sensations from the sole of the foot [84]. Treatment sessions are repeated weekly for a period of 12 weeks and in 30-minute sessions. Repeat session cycles are possible [85].

One of the advantages of PTNS is a "carryover" effect. This has been described as continued symptomatic improvement not necessarily just during the nerve stimulation sessions, which is in contrast to the loss of efficacy when the SNM device is switched off. Many studies have examined the carryover effect and what implications it may have in devising PTNS regimens and schedules, with variable success [84, 86, 87].

Another advantage of PTNS is the fact it can be administered by any healthcare provider or the patient themselves after appropriate training. As a matter of fact,

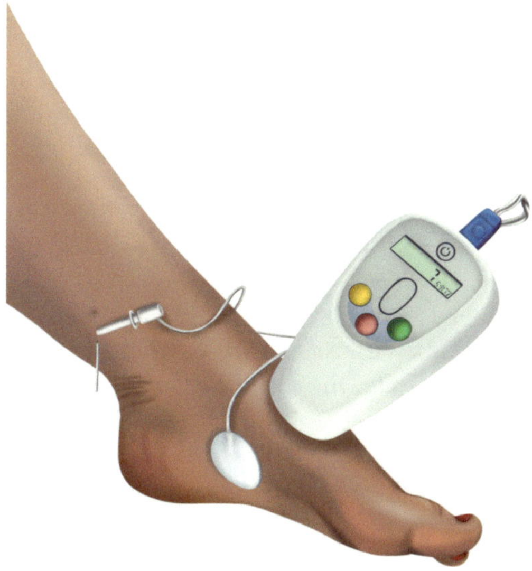

Figure 7.
Posterior tibial nerve stimulation.

home administration systems and micro implants are being developed for that sole purpose [84, 88]. PTNS, too, is less costly than SNM, on average [89, 90].

2.4.1.2 Predictors of PTNS success

In an effort to identify ideal candidates for PTNS treatment in OAB, a number of investigators identified that history of prior SNM therapy correlated negatively with PTNS outcomes. On the other hand, more severe complaints of urge urinary incontinence and urinary bladder volume at first sensation (a UDS parameter) were predictors of PTNS success [90].

2.4.1.3 Efficacy of PTNS

Efficacy of PTNS as evident from review of 4 randomized controlled trials, none of which pinned comparison against SNM, showed a majority of patients were able to achieve at least 50% improvement from baseline complaint; these studies ruled out the possibility of a hypothesized placebo effect, according to the reviewers. A substantial complaint from PTNS treatment was temporary foot pain [74].

Several trials have also compared PTNS to medical treatment of OAB, including the OrBIT trial, and reported comparable if not somewhat superior results with a lower side effect profile, particularly dry mouth and constipation among other side effects associated with anticholinergic medication [85, 91, 92].

2.4.2 Transcutaneous tibial nerve stimulation

Utilizing needles applied transcutaneously to stimulate the posterior tibial nerve, this modality of treatment has been investigated for MS and OAB patients [9]. There are limited studies that demonstrate variable improvements for OAB patients with transcutaneous tibial nerve stimulation (TTNS). Perhaps its advantages stem from its safety and fairly minimal adverse events profile, and its low costs [93].

2.4.3 Transcutaneous electrical nerve stimulation

As the name suggests, this modality is applied to areas in close proximity to target internal nerves. These include the pudendal nerve, be it through transcutaneous stimulation in the vagina in a female or in the perineal region in the male, or both the pudendal and sacral nerves when applied to the sacral skin. DGN is also a form of transcutaneous electrical nerve stimulation (TENS). It is advocated as a less invasive and low-cost neuromodulation system that can also be taught to patients for self-application [5].

Multiple small-sized trials have demonstrated improvements in symptom scores and efficacy in patients with refractory OAB or MS with bladder hyperactivity. However, although it is safe, the durability of its effect has been called into question [9, 94].

3. Neuromodulation applications for urological conditions

3.1 Overactive bladder, urgency urinary incontinence and urgency-frequency syndromes

Bladder overactivity manifests in a number of urinary conditions, depending on the pathophysiology and associated conditions and symptoms. Overactive bladder (OAB), defined by a compelling frequent urge to void, is not a precession of urgency urinary incontinence (UUI), nor is it a more defined form urgency-frequency syndromes: these are all an overlapping number of conditions where evidence of overactivity of the detrusor muscle may or may not be demonstrable, but is subjectively reported by patients and often objectively measurable.

The treatment for these conditions is mainly conservative and medical, be it targeting the bladder muscle or the other offending factors that lead to the overactivity, followed by intradetrusor botulinum injections, which has attained a more defined role in the OAB treatment scheme. SNM is an established mode of treatment for cases of OAB, UUI and urgency-frequency syndromes that are refractory to medical treatment, and despite arguments and established results and testaments, is yet to be designated a more primary or first line place in the treatment of these conditions [95].

3.1.1 Mode of effect in OAB

It has been shown that SNM has an established modulatory effect both on micturition reflexes and higher brain centers. The SNM electrical charging of sacral roots alters neural activity, stimulating somatic afferents that signal to higher brain centers and in part restore normal control over the bladder while also inhibiting certain sensory pathways to suppress reflex bladder hyperactivity. From animal models, evidence suggests this effect is achieved through SNM's inhibition of abnormal sensory input from the pudendal nerve and neuropathological C-fibers, affecting release of μ-opiods and glutamate and suppressing bladder reflexes [16].

3.1.2 SNM efficacy in OAB

Efficacy of SNM is perhaps most studied and evidently reported in refractory OAB [96]. Analysis of five trials have analytically shown significantly higher success rates for SNM in treatment of OAB compared to standard medical treatment, and equally as efficacious as intradetrusor botulinum injections with less side effects associated with the latter including risk of post-injection urinary retention and urinary tract infections [41, 74].

In one prospectively conducted multicenter trial on OAB patients, the 5-year success rate of SNM was 67%, with the most common adverse event or reason for failure demonstrated to be an undesirable change in stimulation, followed by site pain and ineffectiveness of treatment [97]. The InSite trial reported on one of the longest prospective follow-ups for SNM implants for refractory OAB. At 36-months follow-up, 83% of implants were found to have sustained efficacy [68].

3.2 Non-obstructive urinary retention and Fowler's syndrome

Non-obstructive urinary retention (NOUR) is one of the main indications for SNM therapy. It denotes an unidentifiable mechanical cause that may obstruct urinary outflow from the urinary bladder, resulting in urinary retention. It may be the result of an established neurological disease, as is the case in the acute phase of spinal shock after spinal cord trauma, or in a minority of MS patients. Neither of these conditions are indicated for SNM treatment. However, chronic or recurrent urinary retention in a "neurologically-intact" patient is.

One form of NOUR is termed Fowler's syndrome after the neurophysiologist Professor Clare J. Fowler who first described it in 1985. It is a cluster of symptoms and findings identified in a typically young woman with unexplained urinary retention, increased electromyographic activity of the external urinary sphincter and its failure to relax, and some associations to other female syndromes have been described including polycystic ovaries. Application of SNM in these patients has been shown to restore normal voiding activity [98].

3.2.1 Mode of effect

Researchers have used a number of animal models to establish the mode of effect SNM exerts in NOUR and Fowler's. Basic science evidence suggests that by blocking the inhibitory effect that abnormal afferent activity from the external urethral and anal sphincters has on micturition, restoration of the ability of the patient to void occurs. This stimulation is through blockade of the pudendal nerve's stimulatory effect of the micturition reflex [99].

3.3 Neurogenic lower urinary tract dysfunction

Lower urinary tract symptoms resulting from neurological disease are varied, and thus, determination of these symptoms and assessment is necessary before consideration for neuromodulation as not all symptoms would be ideally treated using this modality. Neurological diseases that have documented voiding dysfunction elements include SCI, MS, Parkinson's disease, cerebrovascular accidents, and diabetic neuropathy. Congenital neurologic disorders such myelomeningoceles are becoming apparent causes of voiding dysfunction in adults and SNM candidates, as management of these pediatric disorders improves, and these patients grow into the adult population [9].

Previously thought to lack efficacy in neurogenic LUTD because of lack of an intact nervous system, SNM is emerging as an efficacious therapeutic modality for this population of patients especially in reducing incontinence episodes [9, 100–104]. The concept of neural remodeling as a hypothesized effect of SNM has also been visited as a potential role in neurogenic LUTD, particularly in acute spinal shock phases [9, 104].

The ICS recommends SNM as an option for control of urinary symptoms in patients with stable neurological conditions who are at a low risk of developing upper tract deterioration from controlled voiding [4]. It is thus important to stress the need for proper assessment and continued evaluation of these patients as urinary retention, acute or chronic, could have consequences including urinary tract infection and renal failure [9].

3.3.1 Spinal cord injury

SCI, especially complete transection, has long been accepted as a contraindication for sacral neuromodulation on the basis of a disturbed neural circuit. However, numerous reports have been reviewed that show promising results for SNM in the management of neurologically-stable SCI patients, even those with complete disruption [105]. In the acute phase of spinal shock where the bladder is atonic, SNM has been found to facilitate neurogenic remodeling as researchers theorize and demonstrate sustained SNM effects and remodeling in the brain [9, 104].

In a review of eight studies where SNM was employed in the management of lower urinary tract dysfunction in SCI patients, the success rate of the test phase was a shy 45%, but that later translated into a 75% success rate once the screened patients proceeded with IPG implantation. The treatment was well-tolerated and safe without any unexpected adverse events [106].

3.3.2 Multiple sclerosis

MS is of special interest to neuro-urologists as the disease manifests with a spectrum of urinary symptoms and progresses with different patterns in this spectrum along the course of the disorder as well. Demyelination, the pathological hallmark of MS, eventually affects lower urinary tract nerves, resulting in dysfunction. Up to 80% of patients show neuro-urological symptoms within 10 years of diagnosis, most frequently bladder overactivity. As a matter of fact, voiding dysfunction is the first sign of the disease in up to 10% of patients [107].

Though not FDA approved, neuromodulation has been applied in MS patients for years, and its efficacy has been repeatedly demonstrated. SNM and PTNS have been shown in a number of series to decrease urinary symptoms and improve the quality of life of MS patients who demonstrate bladder overactivity; however, although SNM is approved for NOUR, it has not shown any benefit for MS patients demonstrating "hypoactive" urinary bladders with retention [107, 108].

What remains an important issue for MS patients being considered for SNM is appropriate patient counseling and communication with their treating physician or neurologist to assess the need for MRI examination in the future as well as stability of the disease, as disease progression and relapse would negatively affect the SNM outcomes [9, 105, 107].

3.3.3 Diabetic cystopathy

Diabetic cystopathy is a condition that describes the neuromuscular effect long-standing diabetes has on the urinary bladder. Part of the condition stems from diabetic neuropathy, while another part may stem from vasculopathy affecting the detrusor muscle itself. In the application of neuromodulation to the control of overactivity symptoms resulting from diabetic cystopathy, promising results from series were overshadowed by a substantially higher than average rate of infections (17%) compared to the accepted average, as would be expected from any foreign body implantation in diabetic patients especially those with poor glycemic control [105].

3.4 Special populations and effects

3.4.1 CPPS and IC/BPS

Chronic pelvic pain syndrome in males and its predominantly female counterpart interstitial cystitis/bladder pain syndrome are chronic conditions of pelvic pain and voiding dysfunction with a poorly understood etiology [109]. Off-label use of SNM in the treatment of these disorders is established with significant results, and similar to its unknown etiology, the way SNM provides subjective and objective improvements in bladder pain syndrome for example is yet to be clearly defined, with obvious differences in outcomes between IC/BPS and non-IC/BPS CPPS [110].

Many theories have been suggested for this mode of effect, from restoration of balance between excitatory and inhibitory signals in the pelvic plexus at different spinal levels as well as SNM's modulatory effect on bladder function and in turn pain. Another issue for consideration is the bilateral or multiple sacral root involvement in bladder and pelvic pain disorders, thus S3 stimulation may be insufficient to providing symptomatic relief, and some researchers have demonstrated efficacy of bilateral stimulation [14].

A multitude of studies and researchers are reporting on promising results for SNM in symptomatic management of CPP disorders, demonstrating improvements in pain indices and quality of life measures particularly relating to improvements in sleep, social life and sexual activity [110, 111]. With 10% of patients of IC/BPS reaching a severe stage refractory to conservative and other modes of management, SNM has found an emerging role in the therapeutic void for this condition. Success rates of SNM in IC/BPS have been reported to be high, north of 80% in some series, with apparent and significant objective improvements in pelvic pain and specific interstitial cystitis symptom scores as well as improvements in daytime frequency, nocturia, urinary urgency, and average voided volume [112].

The ICS based on grade C evidence released a level III recommendation that designates SNM as an option for patients who are deemed non-responsive to conservative treatment measures of IC/BPS and non-IC CPPS [4]. However, large randomized controlled trials are lacking, perhaps in part due to the mixed spectrum of CPP disorders, both pathologically and symptomatically, heterogenous patient population, and unclear etiologies, and poorly understood differences in outcomes between the disorders [109, 110, 113].

3.4.2 Sexual function

The effects of neuromodulation, particularly SNM, on improving sexual function among female patients, and male patients to an extent, are becoming more evident in the literature [114]. Dysfunction of the pudendal nerve, an important nerve in sexual stimulation, has been demonstrated in both refractory OAB and NOUR [115].

In a cohort of female patients who received SNM implants for OAB, urgency-frequency syndrome or NOUR, improvements in both female sexual function index and quality of life indices were reported, though they were not correlated [116]. In another study on SCI female patients who had sexual dysfunction, there was a demonstratable improvement in the female sexual distress scale after neuromodulation therapy [117].

The argument is whether the improvements SNM provides with regards to urinary symptoms allows for a better sexual experience and confidence among patients or does SNM's effect on the pelvic floor musculature rejuvenise sexual function.

This argument is important in current applications and future considerations of neuromodulation for the treatment of sexual dysfunction. This was demonstrated in reviews of studies where sacral neuromodulation was employed in the treatment of neurogenic lower urinary tract symptoms and had demonstratable and maintainable improvements in erectile function indices to almost normal levels in a majority of patients after up to 3 years of follow-up [118].

On the contrary, another study assessing for pudendal nerve dysfunction in female patients who received SNM for refractory OAB or NOUR showed nonsignificant improvement in sexual dysfunction indices, and the authors found that these improvements as well as others in quality of life measures were in part due to improvements in urinary function; this finding was supported by a recent review [115, 119].

3.4.3 Neuromodulation in children and adolescents

Scarce data, changing anatomy and somatic growth, physical activity, high reoperation rates, and neurologic instability and disease progression: all are valid arguments against application of SNM in children and adolescents. However, data is emerging on its off-label use, with modest responses. In a single center experience on eight children and adolescents with congenital lumbosacral and traumatic spinal cord defects and lower urinary tract dysfunction, the initial response rate to SNM application was 85%. This translated into a sustained efficacy in 50% of patients on 14-month follow-up, and three patients were able to abandon self-catheterization completely. These results, although on a heterogenous and small cohort of young patients, are promising and could defy the current status quo [120, 121].

Nevertheless, based on lack of evidence and limited studies, the ICS best practice statement stressed that the safety of SNM in this population cannot be established, highlighting the technical challenges associated with anatomical variations and difference in children and effects of somatic growth [4].

4. Future directions and research

4.1 Further evaluation of effects of neuromodulation in urology

Basic science research is still ongoing and perhaps still early in deciphering the exact mechanism of action of neuromodulation in restoring and normalizing bladder function. The different levels of speculated effect, in higher brain and spinal centers and in the more distal micturition pathways and reflex arcs make for a vast field of investigation, as well as the interplay of different neural and cellular messengers.

A better and clearer understanding of all factors involved would definitely allow for the optimization of patient outcomes, including most suitable candidates, duration of symptoms, and required concomitant medication, if any, that would maximize the benefit from different neuromodulation modalities. This is of particular importance when conflicting data on different effects on receptor pathways and modulated areas in the brain continue to emerge, and the definition and descriptions of the mechanisms of action are updated.

4.2 Rechargeable and MRI-compatible systems

SNM, like any battery system, faces depletion. Thus, a rechargeable system is one of special appeal. Perhaps one of the most appealing arguments for upcoming rechargeable systems is the fact it may potentially eliminate replacement surgery. The Relax-OAB study investigated the Axonics r-SNM system, a rechargeable SNM system granted post-marketing permission in Europe in 2016 and is under FDA assessment. Designed to last 15 years with charging requirements for 2 hours every 1–3 weeks, it has shown comparable objective improvements of up to 91% [83, 122, 123]. The Axonics system and the next generation InterStim Micro could revolutionize sacral neuromodulation durability.

The growing need for MR-compatible systems is not a wishful thought, but in the face of evolving biomechanical technology and a growing population that needs both SNM and regular MRI assessment, it seems sensible that the development of such devices is just a matter of time [14].

4.3 Closed-loop neuromodulation

Casually described as a system that "listens to the patient" closed-loop or functional stimulation is a mode of conditional electrical stimulation that is being investigated as a potential neuro-prosthesis that senses bladder fullness, detects bladder contractions, and eventually modulates an electrical response "blindly" without the patient having to actively control their micturition habits. To date there are a number of animal and limited human trials on a set of intelligent electrodes specifically designed to fulfill this purpose. The advantages of such a system are numerous, mainly bypassing chronic stimulation and subsequent bladder muscle fatigue through improvements in warning time for impending bladder contractions, as well as a more natural control on voiding and improved SNM battery life [83]. Many investigators have also looked into improved neurological and bladder pressure sensors as a modality for functional stimulation.

4.4 Expanding indications and revisiting limited applications

Thirty years into its first reintroduction, it is still surprising how limited the indications for SNM in particular remain in the face of accumulating evidence, albeit from small trials restricted by a small pool of patients and candidates. Off-label use of SNM in chronic pelvic pain syndromes, pregnant women, children and neurogenic bladder patients should be the priority of authoritarian bodies to promote research and insight especially when treatment of such conditions could have remarkable effects on the quality of life of those affected [124].

4.5 Dorsal genital nerve stimulation

Though an existing technology, this direct PNS variation has further potential to modulate the combined sacral nerve roots that the former effects without the need of a sacral lead. Utilizing a percutaneous prepubic electrode placed on the clitoris to temporarily deliver electric stimulation and subsequently modulate the dorsal genital nerve, the anterior terminal branch of the pudendal nerve, this technology has been tested in small scale trials with promising results.

Hypothesized to exert its effect through inhibition of bladder efferents, particularly parasympathetic pathways via vesical ganglia and detrusor smooth muscle, the dorsal genital nerve is stimulated using an external pulse generator, and has been shown to reduce urgency incontinence episodes in a number of patient cohorts. However, the device is still not appealing due to lead migration and difficult controls, improvements on which would surely stir further interest among physicians and patients alike [82].

5. Conclusion

Urological applications of neuromodulation are both established and evolving and are among the most dynamic fields for this modality of electrical stimulation. The safety and efficacy of sacral neuromodulation and posterior tibial nerve stimulation in refractory overactive bladder syndrome are high. Other indications of sacral neuromodulation include non-obstructive urinary retention including Fowler's syndrome and urgency incontinence as well as frequency-urgency syndromes. Minimally invasive and broader neuromodulation targets provide an opportunity for improving neuromodulation outcomes, as well as potential advances in the device itself.

Acknowledgements

Ms. Anna Forkavets has assisted in the creating of the illustrated figures throughout the chapter.

Conflict of interest

Dr. Al-Shaiji has received an honorarium for Medtronic sponsored lectures but no financial support for this chapter. The other authors have no conflicts of interest to declare.

Author details

Said M. Yaiesh[1]*, Abdullatif E. Al-Terki[2] and Tariq F. Al-Shaiji[2]

1 Mubarak Al-Kabeer Hospital, Kuwait City, Kuwait

2 Amiri Hospital, Kuwait City, Kuwait

*Address all correspondence to: syaiesh@hotmail.com

References

[1] Li LF, Ka-Kit Leung G, Lui WM. Sacral nerve stimulation for neurogenic bladder. World Neurosurgery. 2016;**90**: 236-243

[2] Schmidt RA. Applications of neurostimulation in urology. Neurourology and Urodynamics. 1988;7:585-592. DOI: 10.1002/nau.1930070607

[3] Tanagho EA, Schmidt RA. Electrical stimulation in the clinical management of the neurogenic bladder. The Journal of Urology. 1988;**140**(6):1331-1339

[4] Goldman HB, Lloyd JC, Noblett KL, Carey MP, Castano Botero JC, Gajewski JB, et al. International continence society best practice statement for use of sacral neuromodulation. Neurourology and Urodynamics. 2018;**37**(5):1823-1848

[5] Janssen DA, Martens FM, de Wall LL, van Breda HM, Heesakkers JP. Clinical utility of neurostimulation devices in the treatment of overactive bladder: Current perspectives. Medical Devices (Auckland, N.Z.). 2017;**10**:109-122

[6] Brindley GS. An implant to empty the bladder or close the urethra. Journal of Neurology, Neurosurgery, and Psychiatry. 1977;**40**(4):358-369

[7] Brindley GS, Polkey CE, Rushton DN, Cardozo L. Sacral anterior root stimulators for bladder control in paraplegia: The first 50 cases. Journal of Neurology, Neurosurgery, and Psychiatry. 1986;**49**(10):1104-1114

[8] Sauerwein D, Ingunza W, Fischer J, Madersbacher H, Polkey CE, Brindley GS, et al. Extradural implantation of sacral anterior root stimulators. Journal of Neurology, Neurosurgery, and Psychiatry. 1990;**53**(8):681-684

[9] Powell CR. Neuromodulation for neurogenic bladder. Current Bladder Dysfunction Reports. 2013;**8**(4):282-288

[10] Daneshgari F, Moy ML. Current indications for neuromodulation. The Urologic Clinics of North America. 2005;**32**(1):37-40, vi

[11] Al-zahrani AA, Elzayat EA, Gajewski JB. Long-term outcome and surgical interventions after sacral neuromodulation implant for lower urinary tract symptoms: 14-year experience at 1 center. The Journal of Urology. 2011;**185**(3):981-986

[12] Elterman DS, Chughtai B, Vertosick E, Thomas D, Eastham J, Sandhu J. Trends and clinical practice patterns of sacral neuromodulation for overactive bladder. Female Pelvic Medicine & Reconstructive Surgery. 2018;**24**(4):264-266

[13] Suskind AM, Dunn RL, Kaufman SR, DeLancey JO, Clemens JQ, Stoffel JT, et al. Understanding the dissemination of sacral neuromodulation. Surgical Innovation. 2013;**20**(6):625-630

[14] Laviana A, Jellison F, Kim JH. Sacral neuromodulation for refractory overactive bladder, interstitial cystitis, and painful bladder syndrome. Neurosurgery Clinics of North America. 2014;**25**(1):33-46

[15] Abello A, Das AK. Electrical neuromodulation in the management of lower urinary tract dysfunction: Evidence, experience and future prospects. Therapeutic Advances in Urology. 2018;**10**(5):165-173

[16] Malde S, Fry C, Schurch B, Marcelissen T, Averbeck M, Digesu A, et al. What is the exact working mechanism of botulinum toxin a and sacral nerve stimulation in

the treatment of overactive bladder/detrusor overactivity? ICI-RS 2017. Neurourology and Urodynamics. 2018;**37**(S4):S108-Ss16

[17] Bernstein AJ, Peters KM. Expanding indications for neuromodulation. The Urologic Clinics of North America. 2005;**32**(1):59-63

[18] Kessler TM, Wollner J, Kozomara M, Mordasini L, Mehnert U. Sacral neuromodulation for neurogenic bladder dysfunction. Urologe A. 2012;**51**(2):179-183

[19] van der Pal F, Heesakkers JP, Bemelmans BL. Current opinion on the working mechanisms of neuromodulation in the treatment of lower urinary tract dysfunction. Current Opinion in Urology. 2006;**16**(4):261-267

[20] Chancellor MB, Chartier-Kastler EJ. Principles of sacral nerve stimulation (SNS) for the treatment of bladder and urethral sphincter dysfunctions. Neuromodulation. 2000;**3**(1):16-26

[21] Ren J, Chew DJ, Thiruchelvam N. Electrical stimulation of the spinal dorsal root inhibits reflex bladder contraction and external urethra sphincter activity: Is this how sacral neuromodulation works? Urologia Internationalis. 2016;**96**(3):360-366

[22] Su X, Nickles A, Nelson DE. Optimization of neuromodulation for bladder control in a rat cystitis model. Neuromodulation. 2016;**19**(1):101-107

[23] Gill BC, Goldman HB. Sacral neuromodulation and alterations in brain activity—Discussing discrepancies. Nature Reviews. Urology. 2017;**14**(12):697-698

[24] Blok BF, Groen J, Bosch JL, Veltman DJ, Lammertsma AA. Different brain effects during chronic and acute sacral neuromodulation in urge incontinent patients with implanted neurostimulators. BJU International. 2006;**98**(6):1238-1243

[25] Weissbart SJ, Bhavsar R, Rao H, Wein AJ, Detre JA, Arya LA, et al. Specific changes in brain activity during urgency in women with overactive bladder after successful sacral neuromodulation: A functional magnetic resonance imaging study. The Journal of Urology. 2018;**200**(2):382-388

[26] Gill BC, Pizarro-Berdichevsky J, Bhattacharyya PK, Brink TS, Marks BK, Quirouet A, et al. Real-time changes in brain activity during sacral neuromodulation for overactive bladder. The Journal of Urology. 2017;**198**(6):1379-1385

[27] Zhang F, Zhao S, Shen B, Wang J, Nelson DE, Roppolo JR, et al. Neural pathways involved in sacral neuromodulation of reflex bladder activity in cats. American Journal of Physiology. Renal Physiology. 2013;**304**(6):F710-F717

[28] Li X, Liao L, Chen G, Wang Z, Deng H. Involvement of opioid receptors in inhibition of bladder overactivity induced by sacral neuromodulation in pigs: A possible action mechanism. Neurourology and Urodynamics. 2017;**36**(7):1742-1748

[29] Bandari J, Bansal U, Zhang Z, Shen B, Wang J, Lamm V, et al. Neurotransmitter mechanisms underlying sacral neuromodulation of bladder overactivity in cats. Neuromodulation. 2017;**20**(1):81-87

[30] Jiang X, Fuller TW, Bandari J, Bansal U, Zhang Z, Shen B, et al. Contribution of GABAA, glycine, and opioid receptors to sacral neuromodulation of bladder overactivity in cats. The Journal of Pharmacology and Experimental Therapeutics. 2016;**359**(3):436-441

[31] El-Azab AS, Siegel SW. Sacral neuromodulation for female pelvic floor

disorders. Arab Journal of Urology. 2019;**17**(1):14-22

[32] Thornton JS. Technical challenges and safety of magnetic resonance imaging with in situ neuromodulation from spine to brain. European Journal of Paediatric Neurology. 2017;**21**(1):232-241

[33] Lloyd JC, Gill BC, Pizarro-Berdichevsky J, Goldman HB. Removal of sacral nerve stimulation devices for magnetic resonance imaging: What happens next? Neuromodulation. 2017;**20**(8):836-840

[34] Yaiesh SM, Al-Terki AE, Al-Shaiji TF. Safety of sacral nerve stimulation in pregnancy: A literature review. Neuromodulation. 2016;**19**(7):770-779

[35] Mahran A, Soriano A, Safwat AS, Hijaz A, Mahajan ST, Trabuco EC, et al. The effect of sacral neuromodulation on pregnancy: A systematic review. International Urogynecology Journal. 2017;**28**(9):1357-1365

[36] Gahzi AA, Elterman DS, Hassouna M. Sacral neuromodulation in patients with a cardiac pacemaker. International Neurourology Journal. 2016;**20**(3):270-272

[37] Nobrega RP, Solomon E, Jenks J, Greenwell T, Ockrim J. Predicting a successful outcome in sacral neuromodulation testing: Are urodynamic parameters prognostic? Neurourology and Urodynamics. 2018;**37**(3):1007-1010

[38] Nguyen LN, Bartley J, Killinger KA, Gupta P, Lavin J, Khourdaji A, et al. Does sex matter? A matched pairs analysis of neuromodulation outcomes in women and men. International Urology and Nephrology. 2018;**50**(5):825-832

[39] Faris AER, Gill BC, Pizarro-Berdichevsky J, Dielubanza E, Clifton MM, Okafor H, et al. Impact of age and comorbidities on use of sacral neuromodulation. The Journal of Urology. 2017;**198**(1):161-166

[40] Jairam R, Drossaerts J, van Koeveringe G, van Kerrebroeck P. The impact of duration of complaints on successful outcome of sacral neuromodulation. Urologia Internationalis. 2017;**99**(1):51-55

[41] Banakhar MA, Al-Shaiji T, Hassouna M. Sacral neuromodulation and refractory overactive bladder: An emerging tool for an old problem. Therapeutic Advances in Urology. 2012;**4**(4):179-185

[42] van Kerrebroeck PE, Marcelissen TA. Sacral neuromodulation for lower urinary tract dysfunction. World Journal of Urology. 2012;**30**(4):445-450

[43] Banakhar M, Hassouna M. Patients with sacral neuromodulation: What are the factors affecting their therapy satisfaction? Urologia Internationalis. 2019;**103**(4):450-453

[44] Ammirati E, Giammo A, Manassero A, Carone R. Neuro-modulation in urology, state of the art. Urologia. 2019;**86**(4):177-182

[45] Bartley JM, Killinger KA, Boura JA, Gupta P, Gaines N, Gilleran JP, et al. The impact of prior back surgery on neuromodulation outcomes: A review of over 500 patients. Neurourology and Urodynamics. 2017;**36**(6):1535-1542

[46] Bartley JM, Ramirez V, Killinger KA, Boura JA, Gupta P, Gaines N, et al. Outcomes of sacral neuromodulation in patients with prior surgical treatment of stress urinary incontinence and pelvic organ prolapse. Female Pelvic Medicine & Reconstructive Surgery. 2017;**23**(1):8-12

[47] Hassouna MM, Sadri H. Economic evaluation of sacral neuromodulation

in overactive bladder: A Canadian perspective. Canadian Urological Association Journal. 2015;**9**(7-8):242-247

[48] Bertapelle MP, Vottero M, Popolo GD, Mencarini M, Ostardo E, Spinelli M, et al. Sacral neuromodulation and botulinum toxin a for refractory idiopathic overactive bladder: A cost-utility analysis in the perspective of Italian healthcare system. World Journal of Urology. 2015;**33**(8):1109-1117

[49] Harvie HS, Amundsen CL, Neuwahl SJ, Honeycutt AA, Lukacz ES, Sung VW, et al. Cost-effectiveness of sacral neuromodulation versus onabotulinumtoxin A for refractory urgency urinary incontinence: Results of the ROSETTA randomized trial. Journal of Urology. 2019;**203**:969-977. DOI: 101097ju0000000000000656

[50] Chughtai B, Clemens JQ, Thomas D, Sun T, Ghomrawi H, Sedrakyan A. Real world performance of sacral neuromodulation and onabotulinumtoxin A for overactive bladder: Focus on safety and cost. The Journal of Urology. 2020;**203**(1):179-184

[51] Amend B, Khalil M, Kessler TM, Sievert KD. How does sacral modulation work best? Placement and programming techniques to maximize efficacy. Current Urology Reports. 2011;**12**(5): 327-335

[52] Al-Shaiji TF, Malallah MA, Yaiesh SM, Al-Terki AE, Hassouna MM. Does psychological disturbance predict explantation in successful pelvic neuromodulation treatment for bladder dysfunction? A short series. Neuromodulation. 2018;**21**(8):805-808

[53] Marcelissen TA, Leong RK, Nieman FH, van Lankveld JJ, van Kerrebroeck PE, de Wachter SG. Psychological and psychiatric factors as predictors for success in sacral neuromodulation treatment. BJU International. 2011;**108**(11):1834-1838

[54] Alabbad A, Abdo E, Hassouna M. Is radiation exposure during sacral neuromodulation within safety limits? Canadian Urological Association Journal. 2019;**13**(3):E95-Ee6

[55] Shakuri-Rad J, Cicic A, Thompson J. Prospective randomized study evaluating ultrasound versus fluoroscopy guided sacral InterStim(R) lead placement: A pilot study. Neurourology and Urodynamics. 2018;**37**(5):1737-1743

[56] Doublet JD, Sotto A, Escaravage L, Verine JL, Conquy S, Cariou G, et al. Guidelines from the infectious disease Committee of the French Association of urology and the Neuro-urology committee of the AFU: Antibiotic prophylaxis for sacral neuromodulation. Progrès en Urologie. 2013;**23**(10):849-855

[57] El-Azab AS, Siegel SW. Specific tips for general controversies in sacral neuromodulation. Current Urology Reports. 2016;**17**(11):79

[58] Sun AJ, Harris CR, Comiter CV, Elliott CS. To stage or not to stage?—A cost minimization analysis of sacral neuromodulation placement strategies. Neurourology and Urodynamics. 2019;**38**(6):1783-1791

[59] Deveneau NE, Greenstein M, Mahalingashetty A, Herring NR, Lipetskaia L, Azadi A, et al. Surface and boney landmarks for sacral neuromodulation: A cadaveric study. International Urogynecology Journal. 2015;**26**(2):263-268

[60] Gorissen KJ, Bloemendaal AL, Prapasrivorakul S, Gosselink MP, Jones OM, Cunningham C, et al. Dynamic article: Permanent sacral nerve stimulation under local anesthesia:

Feasibility, best practice, and patient satisfaction. Diseases of the Colon and Rectum. 2015;**58**(12):1182-1185

[61] Jairam R, Drossaerts J, Marcelissen T, van Koeveringe G, van Kerrebroeck P. Onset of action of sacral neuromodulation in lower urinary tract dysfunction-what is the optimal duration of test stimulation? The Journal of Urology. 2018;**199**(6):1584-1590

[62] Lee C, Pizarro-Berdichevsky J, Clifton MM, Vasavada SP. Sacral neuromodulation implant infection: Risk factors and prevention. Current Urology Reports. 2017;**18**(2):16

[63] Hubsher CP, Jansen R, Riggs DR, Jackson BJ, Zaslau S. Sacral nerve stimulation for neuromodulation of the lower urinary tract. The Canadian Journal of Urology. 2012;**19**(5):6480-6484

[64] Thompson JH, Sutherland SE, Siegel SW. Sacral neuromodulation: Therapy evolution. Indian Journal of Urology. 2010;**26**(3):379-384

[65] Wollner J, Hampel C, Kessler TM. Surgery illustrated—Surgical atlas sacral neuromodulation. BJU International. 2012;**110**(1):146-159

[66] Matzel KE, Chartier-Kastler E, Knowles CH, Lehur PA, Munoz-Duyos A, Ratto C, et al. Sacral neuromodulation: Standardized electrode placement technique. Neuromodulation. 2017; **20**(8):816-824

[67] Jairam R, Marcelissen T, van Koeveringe G, van Kerrebroeck P. Optimal lead positioning in sacral neuromodulation: Which factors are related to treatment outcome? Neuromodulation. 2017;**20**(8):830-835

[68] Noblett K. Neuromodulation and female pelvic disorders. Current Opinion in Urology. 2016;**26**(4):321-327

[69] Banakhar M, Hassouna M. Sacral neuromodulation for genitourinary problems. Progress in Neurological Surgery. 2015;**29**:192-199

[70] Al-Shaiji TF, Banakhar M, Hassouna MM. Pelvic electrical neuromodulation for the treatment of overactive bladder symptoms. Advances in Urology. 2011;**2011**:757454

[71] Carmel ME, Vasavada SP, Goldman HB. Troubleshooting sacral neuromodulation issues. Current Urology Reports. 2012;**13**(5):363-369

[72] Powell CR. Troubleshooting Interstim sacral neuromodulation generators to recover function. Current Urology Reports. 2018;**19**(10):86

[73] Noblett K, Benson K, Kreder K. Detailed analysis of adverse events and surgical interventions in a large prospective trial of sacral neuromodulation therapy for overactive bladder patients. Neurourology and Urodynamics. 2017;**36**(4):1136-1139

[74] Tutolo M, Ammirati E, van der Aa F. What is new in neuromodulation for overactive bladder? European Urology Focus. 2018;**4**(1):49-53

[75] Peters KM, Killinger KA, Gilleran JP, Bartley J, Wolfert C, Boura JA. Predictors of reoperation after sacral neuromodulation: A single institution evaluation of over 400 patients. Neurourology and Urodynamics. 2017;**36**(2):354-359

[76] Myer ENB, Petrikovets A, Slocum PD, Lee TG, Carter-Brooks CM, Noor N, et al. Risk factors for explantation due to infection after sacral neuromodulation: A multicenter retrospective case-control study. American Journal of Obstetrics and Gynecology. 2018;**219**(1):78.e1-78.e9

[77] Marcelissen TA, Leong RK, Serroyen J, van Kerrebroeck PE,

de Wachter SG. The use of bilateral sacral nerve stimulation in patients with loss of unilateral treatment efficacy. The Journal of Urology. 2011;**185**(3):976-980

[78] Yuan AS, Almodovar JL, Erekson E. Neurologic injury after sacral neuromodulation. Female Pelvic Medicine & Reconstructive Surgery. 2019;**25**(2):e45-e46

[79] Kinman CL, Hobson DTG, Agrawal A, Vyleta MS, Francis SL. Retroperitoneal hemorrhage after sacral neurostimulator placement for urgency urinary incontinence. Female Pelvic Medicine & Reconstructive Surgery. 2017;**23**(4):e29-e31

[80] Shannon MB, Gupta N, Eberhardt J, Farooq AV. Broken sacral neuromodulation lead migration into the sigmoid colon: A case report. Female Pelvic Medicine & Reconstructive Surgery. 2018;**24**(6):e49-e50

[81] Peters KM, Feber KM, Bennett RC. Sacral versus pudendal nerve stimulation for voiding dysfunction: A prospective, single-blinded, randomized, crossover trial. Neurourology and Urodynamics. 2005;**24**(7):643-647

[82] Marinkovic SP. New technologies in the management of overactive bladder: Current research and future prospects. Therapeutic Advances in Urology. 2019;**11**:1756287219844669

[83] Jaqua K, Powell CR. Where are we headed with neuromodulation for overactive bladder? Current Urology Reports. 2017;**18**(8):59

[84] Gupta P, Ehlert MJ, Sirls LT, Peters KM. Percutaneous tibial nerve stimulation and sacral neuromodulation: An update. Current Urology Reports. 2015;**16**(2):4

[85] Sherif H, Abdelwahab O. Posterior tibial nerve stimulation as treatment for the overactive bladder. Arab Journal of Urology. 2013;**11**(2):131-135

[86] Peters KM, Carrico DJ, Wooldridge LS, Miller CJ, MacDiarmid SA. Percutaneous tibial nerve stimulation for the long-term treatment of overactive bladder: 3-year results of the STEP study. The Journal of Urology. 2013;**189**(6):2194-2201

[87] MacDiarmid SA, Peters KM, Shobeiri SA, Wooldridge LS, Rovner ES, Leong FC, et al. Long-term durability of percutaneous tibial nerve stimulation for the treatment of overactive bladder. The Journal of Urology. 2010;**183**(1):234-240

[88] Maurelli V, Petta F, Carsillo G, Miano R, Lamorte F, Perugia C, et al. What to do if percutaneous tibial nerve stimulation (PTNS) works? A pilot study on home-based transcutaneous tibial nerve stimulation. Urologia. 2012;**79**(Suppl 19):86-90

[89] Martinson M, MacDiarmid S, Black E. Cost of neuromodulation therapies for overactive bladder: Percutaneous tibial nerve stimulation versus sacral nerve stimulation. The Journal of Urology. 2013;**189**(1):210-216

[90] Rostaminia G, Chang C, Pincus JB, Sand PK, Goldberg RP. Predictors of successful percutaneous tibial nerve stimulation (PTNS) in the treatment of overactive bladder syndrome. International Urogynecology Journal. 2019;**30**(10):1735-1745

[91] Peters KM, Macdiarmid SA, Wooldridge LS, Leong FC, Shobeiri SA, Rovner ES, et al. Randomized trial of percutaneous tibial nerve stimulation versus extended-release tolterodine: Results from the overactive bladder innovative therapy trial. The Journal of Urology. 2009;**182**(3):1055-1061

[92] Vecchioli-Scaldazza C, Morosetti C, Berouz A, Giannubilo W, Ferrara V.

Solifenacin succinate versus percutaneous tibial nerve stimulation in women with overactive bladder syndrome: Results of a randomized controlled crossover study. Gynecologic and Obstetric Investigation. 2013;**75**(4):230-234

[93] Booth J, Connelly L, Dickson S, Duncan F, Lawrence M. The effectiveness of transcutaneous tibial nerve stimulation (TTNS) for adults with overactive bladder syndrome: A systematic review. Neurourology and Urodynamics. 2018;**37**(2):528-541

[94] Gross T, Schneider MP, Bachmann LM, Blok BF, Groen J, Hoen LA, et al. Transcutaneous electrical nerve stimulation for treating neurogenic lower urinary tract dysfunction: A systematic review. European Urology. 2016;**69**(6): 1102-1111

[95] Bartley J, Gilleran J, Peters K. Neuromodulation for overactive bladder. Nature Reviews. Urology. 2013;**10**(9): 513-521

[96] Sukhu T, Kennelly MJ, Kurpad R. Sacral neuromodulation in overactive bladder: A review and current perspectives. Research and Reports in Urology. 2016;**8**:193-199

[97] Siegel S, Noblett K, Mangel J, Bennett J, Griebling TL, Sutherland SE, et al. Five-year followup results of a prospective, multicenter study of patients with overactive bladder treated with sacral neuromodulation. The Journal of Urology. 2018;**199**(1):229-236

[98] Osman NI, Chapple CR. Fowler's syndrome—A cause of unexplained urinary retention in young women? Nature Reviews. Urology. 2014;**11**(2): 87-98

[99] Li X, Uy J, Yu M, Li S, Theisen K, Browning J, et al. Sacral neuromodulation blocks pudendal inhibition of reflex bladder activity in cats: Insight into the efficacy of sacral neuromodulation in Fowler's syndrome. American Journal of Physiology. Regulatory, Integrative and Comparative Physiology. 2018;**314**(1):R34-R42

[100] Roth TM. Sacral neuromodulation and lower urinary tract dysfunction in cerebral palsy. International Urogynecology Journal and Pelvic Floor Dysfunction. 2007;**18**(5):567-569

[101] Kessler TM, La Framboise D, Trelle S, Fowler CJ, Kiss G, Pannek J, et al. Sacral neuromodulation for neurogenic lower urinary tract dysfunction: Systematic review and meta-analysis. European Urology. 2010;**58**(6):865-874

[102] Spinelli M, Malaguti S, Giardiello G, Lazzeri M, Tarantola J, van den Hombergh U. A new minimally invasive procedure for pudendal nerve stimulation to treat neurogenic bladder: Description of the method and preliminary data. Neurourology and Urodynamics. 2005;**24**(4):305-309

[103] Peters KM, Kandagatla P, Killinger KA, Wolfert C, Boura JA. Clinical outcomes of sacral neuromodulation in patients with neurologic conditions. Urology. 2013;**81**(4):738-743

[104] Sievert KD, Amend B, Gakis G, Toomey P, Badke A, Kaps HP, et al. Early sacral neuromodulation prevents urinary incontinence after complete spinal cord injury. Annals of Neurology. 2010;**67**(1):74-84

[105] Barboglio Romo PG, Gupta P. Peripheral and sacral neuromodulation in the treatment of neurogenic lower urinary tract dysfunction. The Urologic Clinics of North America. 2017;**44**(3):453-461

[106] Hu M, Lai S, Zhang Y, Liu M, Wang J. Sacral neuromodulation for

lower urinary tract dysfunction in spinal cord injury: A systematic review and meta-analysis. Urologia Internationalis. 2019;**103**(3):337-343

[107] Rahnama'i MS. Neuromodulation for functional bladder disorders in patients with multiple sclerosis. Multiple Sclerosis. 2019:1-7

[108] Abboud H, Hill E, Siddiqui J, Serra A, Walter B. Neuromodulation in multiple sclerosis. Multiple Sclerosis. 2017;**23**(13):1663-1676

[109] Roy H, Offiah I, Dua A. Neuromodulation for pelvic and urogenital pain. Brain Sciences. 2018;**8**(10):180-195

[110] Mahran A, Baaklini G, Hassani D, Abolella HA, Safwat AS, Neudecker M, et al. Sacral neuromodulation treating chronic pelvic pain: A meta-analysis and systematic review of the literature. International Urogynecology Journal. 2019;**30**(7):1023-1035

[111] Polushkin AA, Isagulyan ED, Tomskiy AA, Dorokhov EV, Salyukov RV. The use of surgical neuromodulation to treat chronic pelvic pain. Zhurnal Voprosy Neĭrokhirurgii Imeni N.N. Burdenko. 2019;**83**(2):49-58

[112] Wang J, Chen Y, Chen J, Zhang G, Wu P. Sacral neuromodulation for refractory bladder pain syndrome/ interstitial cystitis: A global systematic review and meta-analysis. Scientific Reports. 2017;**7**(1):11031

[113] Tam J, Loeb C, Grajower D, Kim J, Weissbart S. Neuromodulation for chronic pelvic pain. Current Urology Reports. 2018;**19**(5):32

[114] de Oliveira PS, Reis JP, de Oliveira TR, Martinho D, e Silva RP, Marcelino J, et al. The impact of sacral neuromodulation on sexual dysfunction. Current Urology. 2019;**12**(4):188-194

[115] Parnell BA, Howard JF Jr, Geller EJ. The effect of sacral neuromodulation on pudendal nerve function and female sexual function. Neurourology and Urodynamics. 2015;**34**(5):456-460

[116] Banakhar M, Gazwani Y, Kelini ME, Al-Shaiji T, Hassouna M. Effect of sacral neuromodulation on female sexual function and quality of life: Are they correlated? Canadian Urological Association Journal. 2014;**8**(11-12):E762-E767

[117] Lombardi G, Mondaini N, Macchiarella A, Cilotti A, del Popolo G. Clinical female sexual outcome after sacral neuromodulation implant for lower urinary tract symptom (LUTS). The Journal of Sexual Medicine. 2008;**5**(6):1411-1417

[118] Lombardi G, Musco S, Kessler TM, Li Marzi V, Lanciotti M, del Popolo G. Management of sexual dysfunction due to central nervous system disorders: A systematic review. BJU International. 2015;**115**(Suppl 6): 47-56

[119] Khunda A, McCormick C, Ballard P. Sacral neuromodulation and sexual function: A systematic review and meta-analysis of the literature. International Urogynecology Journal. 2019;**30**(3):339-352

[120] Sharifiaghdas F. Sacral neuromodulation in congenital lumbo-sacral and traumatic spinal cord defects with neurogenic lower urinary tract symptoms: A single-center experience in children and adolescents. World Journal of Urology. 2019;**37**(12):2775-2783

[121] Apostolidis A. Is there enough evidence to support sacral neuromodulation as a viable treatment option in children and adolescents with neurogenic lower urinary tract dysfunction? World Journal of Urology. 2019;**37**(12):2811-2812

[122] Blok B, van Kerrebroeck P, de Wachter S, Ruffion A, van der Aa F, Jairam R, et al. Three month clinical results with a rechargeable sacral neuromodulation system for the treatment of overactive bladder. Neurourology and Urodynamics. 2018;**37**(S2):S9-S16

[123] Elterman DS. The novel Axonics(R) rechargeable sacral neuromodulation system: Procedural and technical impressions from an initial north American experience. Neurourology and Urodynamics. 2018;**37**(S2):S1-S8

[124] Moore CK, Rueb JJ, Derisavifard S. What is new in neuromodulation? Current Urology Reports. 2019;**20**(9):55

Chapter 12

Caudal Traction as a Pathogenetic Mechanism of Chiari Malformation Type I

Miguel Bautista Royo-Salvador, Marco Fiallos-Rivera and Horia Salca

Abstract

Despite the important achievements made with respect to our understanding of their clinical and image features, Chiari malformations are the result of etiopathogenetic mechanisms still sunk into mystery, while most of the efforts to dissipate it are isolated attempts that deal with rather late, secondary pathogenetic events, such as the reduction of the posterior fossa volume, the crowdedness of its contents or the disturbances of the cerebrospinal fluid flow at the level of the foramen magnum. Nevertheless, until new research will shed light onto many of these processes, the actual partial, fragmented knowledge can be structured in a much more reliable manner if one holds the theory of caudal traction as a guiding principle. We present a potential pathogenesis that could culminate into an abnormal axial tension throughout the spinal cord, as well as some image and therapeutic features found during our clinical practice, testifying in favor of this relentless caudal traction.

Keywords: Chiari malformation, tonsillar descent, hindbrain, spinal cord, caudal traction

1. Introduction

The commonest variant of Chiari malformations, the one that has been labeled "type I," including some recently derived variants (type 0, type 1.5), is unique among the central nervous system abnormalities by its capacity to elicit just as much apprehension within the community of patients, as bewilderment among the clinicians. Its ominous relationship with sudden death, as well as its resemblance with the tonsillar herniation seen in terminal stages of brain tumors, intracranial hemorrhage, and other space-occupying lesions, would very well serve to explain many of these feelings. Nevertheless, their deeper reason seems rather to be the apparent mystery that clouds its pathogenesis, hindering many attempts at agreement among the authors involved in its investigation.

Notwithstanding, an attentive eye can discover interesting pathogenetic clues issued from recent research that one only has to pin up at the right spots on an older scaffold initiated long ago by some intuitive theories that started to explore into these matters even from the discovery of the hindbrain malformation: while Hans Chiari favored hydrocephalus as the cause of tonsillar descent, Julius Arnold proposed the concept that cord tethering at the level of the associated myelomeningocele determines a caudal traction along the spinal cord that ends in the tonsillar descent of Chiari malformation type II [1].

This is why every effort to unveil the origin and the mechanisms of formation of Chiari malformation type I should be greatly welcomed. It is very likely that the same can be extrapolated to the less common Chiari malformation type II, which could be just a more severe form of the same deformity, caused by more intense but qualitatively similar pathogenetic alterations. The unifying theory that follows is merely the result of attentive, scrupulous efforts to acknowledge valuable data in the middle of puzzling research results and connect them orderly in a logical explanation of the mechanisms likely to be involved in the production of Chiari malformation type I.

The concept of caudal traction as we use it through the following lines should not be understood merely from a physical point of view, as a purely mechanical force, as it refers to a biological system with certain viscoelastic properties and an intrinsic capacity to develop a reaction to any force acting upon it. The development of the human body is a continuous interplay of genetic, molecular, biochemical, and mechanical changes that result in a more or less dynamic structure and function. Absolutely all human beings, as well as other vertebrate species, are subjected to this phenomenon of caudal traction, which is a necessary part of the development of the spinal cord and brainstem, as they grow by lengthening, distinctly from the forebrain and cerebellum, which do it by expansion. In fact, the notion of caudal traction points to a group of deformities of the nervous system and its surrounding tissues, identifiable on diagnostic images and likely to result from this longitudinal growth of its caudal segments during development; they may be discovered at various stages during this process or even later, during adulthood, which is by no means a cease of it, but merely a continuation, as an involution—apparently a reversed process, but in fact an ongoing, caudal traction at a deep structural level of the involved neural organs. After all, the definition and understanding of this dynamic concept will certainly improve in parallel with the abilities of the diagnostic tools that we shall be able to use in these patients.

After an initial presentation of this new pathogenetic theory, we will follow with a second part where we shall bring into view some conditions quite likely to be produced by means of a mechanism of caudal traction and which are frequently associated with Chiari malformation type I. The third part of this chapter will deal with the clinical arguments of our demonstration, presenting a range of suggestive, but often neglected proofs of this pathogenesis, which we meet during the diagnosis and treatment of these patients.

2. Embryology of asynchronism

It is very likely that the events that eventually lead to Chiari malformations take place at a very early stage during embryogenesis; a plausible idea if one takes as an example the defects of neural tube closure, related in some way to our problem, as we know well enough that during their evolution, some of them can cause a Chiari malformation type II—and the future will probably show that the relationship between these conditions is not limited to this (and caudal traction could be the link). If some parallel, very early, processes, related but not identical to neurulation abnormalities, would finally result in a Chiari malformation type I, it means that actually all purported etiopathogenetic mechanisms of this condition are in fact late secondary features that simply result from the abnormal development of the cranio-cervical junction. Most importantly, both the small volume of the posterior fossa and the disturbances of cerebrospinal fluid circulation across the foramen magnum would be such *effects* wrongly converted in *causes* by the most prevalent theories that try to explain at present the genesis of Chiari malformations.

This concept of very early pathogenesis of Chiari malformation type I has also another important consequence in the way we should try to understand it: most, if not all of the morphological and mechanical changes involved in its generation take place in the diminute body of a human embryo, then fetus, and then child (probably of a comparatively decreasing magnitude throughout these stages), even though the diagnosis will eventually be secured only at an adult age. This invalidates many recent research results and actual misconceptions based on mature or adult human anatomy and physiology.

Perhaps Chiari malformation type I is the best example of the meaning of Lewis Wolpert's famous phrase "It is not birth, marriage, or death, but gastrulation which is truly the most important time in your life" [2], as indeed, the events that finally lead to its development seem to originate during gastrulation (third week postfertilization), that is, at a much earlier stage of embrionary development than that stated by all theories invoked nowadays.

Thus, the primordium of the central nervous system divides along its freshly defined anterior-posterior axis into four regions, corresponding to the future forebrain, midbrain, hindbrain, and spinal cord [3], well in advance of any significant differences in shape or length among them. Interestingly, while the first two limits are represented by discrete junctional areas that function as organizing centers for nearby neural territories—the so-called anterior neural ridge between the forebrain and midbrain and the isthmic organizer between the midbrain and anterior hindbrain [4]—there is no specific anatomical hint as to the precise location of the posterior hindbrain-spinal cord transition [3]; moreover, its final position depends on quite sophisticated but also delicate mechanisms involving a negative feedback loop between retinoic acid signaling, Cdx4 transcription factor, and the Cyp26 enzyme involved in the degradation of retinoic acid [3, 5]. Despite its importance for all future development of the nervous system, this hindbrain-spinal cord transition is exposed to be moved cranially or caudally by various alterations in these complex, interconnected signaling pathways [3, 5]. For example, experimental loss of Cdx4 function in zebrafish led to caudal displacement of the transition as far as that corresponding to two somites inside the spinal cord territory. As a consequence, the hindbrain-spinal cord transition along the developing neural tube will be matched to a different mesodermal counterpart, belonging to the first pairs of somites, either occipital or cervical. In this way, it becomes easy to figure out how an alteration of the Cdx4 gene or an equivalent disturbance of retinoic acid signaling could displace the transition caudally and place the junction between the developing brainstem and the spinal cord at the level of the future atlas, while the cerebellum might be expected to expand until the same area well below the occipital foramen. In fact, maternal administration of exogenous retinoic acid has been used to produce Chiari malformations in an experimental model in hamsters [6].

By and large, the tonsillar descent seen in Chiari malformation type I would thus be the result of delicate molecular abnormalities that occur early in a critical area of the future body plan, representing the precise border separating the head, with a neural-driven expansile growth in three directions, from the spine, with a somatic-driven tensile growth in one predominant direction (**Figure 1**). This is why its developmental importance and pathological associations and consequences are so complex and puzzling in their diversity, far outweighing the apparent trivial significance that it still has in the eyes of many clinicians.

Of course, it is difficult to apply such an ultra-early pathogenesis involving molecular and genetic signaling pathways to what we actually think and know about Chiari malformation type I, but here we have again a point where an analogy with Chiari malformation type II is quite welcome. Since Julius Arnold's days, it was already supposed that a myelomeningocele would "tether" the growing child's

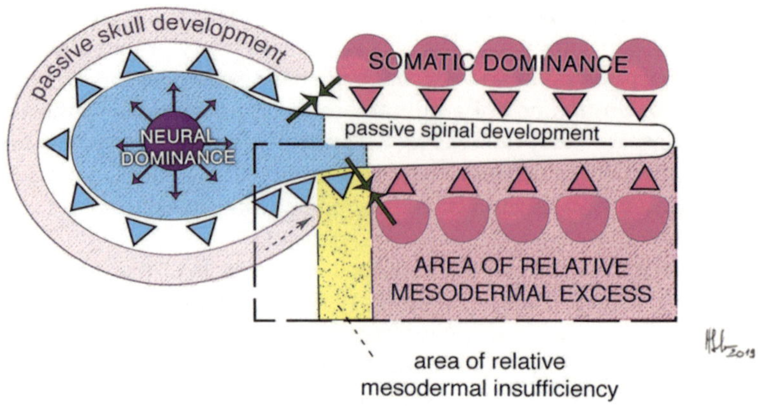

Figure 1.
The interplay of molecular and growth influences that grant a special importance to the cranio-cervical junction.

spinal cord and thus determine a progressive caudal traction on the cerebellum and the tonsillar descent through the occipital foramen. The concept of "tethering" involves both a pathological lesion that fixes the spinal cord to the vertebral column at some point and an uncompensated load, either in the form of continuous growth, repetitive forward flexion movements, or a fracture-dislocation with sudden cord traction. In fact, there is also a third, mandatory component, the lack of an adequate adaptive reaction of the body, which may be due to the overwhelming intensity, suddenness, or persistence of the pull. Now, all these features can yet be expressed in another way if we view tethering more generally, as a relative shortness of the spinal cord, underlying both Chiari malformation types I and II, with the mention that in the former, there is absolutely nothing of spinal cord tethering.

Therefore, patients with Chiari malformation type I would tend to have relatively shorter spinal cords because the neural territory assigned to the formation of the future spinal cord is reduced with respect to the nearby somitic mesoderm, a disproportion that will result in a continuous spinal cord tension during growth, as the neural tissue will always be "one step behind" its mesodermal counterpart (**Figure 1**).

Interestingly, similar arguments in favor of these pathogenetic mechanisms have come from the other side of the problem, that is, from attempts to explain a supposedly defective development of the mesodermal tissue composing the prospective vertebral column, resulting in idiopathic scoliosis: the so-called "Roth-Porter theory" invokes exactly the same "asynchronism" between the spinal cord and spine during growth [7–9], reflected in the tridimensional deformity of idiopathic scoliosis in a much more visible manner [10] than in the case of Chiari malformation type I, but we shall develop more of these aspects later.

Just as a collateral observation, here we should mention that retinoic acid was also suspected as a pathogenetic factor in adolescent idiopathic scoliosis [11].

By the way, given its role of mechanical support, the development of osseous tissue has always been regarded as being associated to the creation and maintenance of tensile or compressive forces in the neighboring tissues. Thus, the development of the cranial vault by intramembranous ossification seems to proceed by means of tensile forces created in the sutures by the growth of the underlying brain [12]. Just in the same way, it should not be surprising that the growing vertebral column could exert a barely perceptible but relentless, tensile force that by some yet unknown mechanism stimulates the growth of the contained spinal cord accordingly.

Well, this would be exactly the Achilles' heel in individuals with Chiari malformation type I, as they are exposed more than normal people to a deficiency of the homeostatic mechanisms that maintain coupled the growth of the two structures. In selected cases, this uncoupling can occur also in the absence of a tonsillar descent or with a minimal one, so that its pathological consequences do not require the 5 mm of descent that most authors use to define Chiari malformations.

3. Illustrative associations

Without pretending to be exhaustive, Chiari malformation type I is associated with a few pathological conditions that could be explained by similar mechanisms involving genetic and molecular abnormalities followed by an axial traction throughout the spinal cord and the brainstem. But before all, in order to have a crystal clear vision of these associations, we have to rule out any tonsillar descent that is obviously secondary to compressive forces from above, as in benign intracranial hypertension, hydrocephalus of any etiology, craniosynostosis, or Paget disease of the bone and other conditions with calvarial thickening, as these are not real instances of Chiari malformation [1] and only compound the problem unnecessarily: one should better consider them as merely secondary tonsillar descents in specific clinical contexts that require only the treatment of the primary pathology and nothing more, just as is always done in the posterior fossa tumors, the deadliest cause of downward displacement of the cerebellar tonsils, where nobody disputes the foremost therapeutic objective. Nevertheless, if really and honestly open-minded, one has to acknowledge that perhaps every tonsillar descent is secondary to a pathological process, even though in most cases its nature is still unknown. But in the actual state of knowledge, we should better consider as "Chiari malformation type I" only the apparently *primary* and *congenital* cases of tonsillar displacement, just keeping in mind that both features can still be open to debate in any particular case.

Malformations of the occipito-cervical junction, representing a diverse and complex group of pathological conditions and related deformities, are often multiple in the same patient and many times occur in conjunction with Chiari malformation type I—with as many as 38–40% of hindbrain herniations in cases of atlas assimilation combined with Klippel-Feil syndrome [13]. In these patients, the abnormal fusions involving the occiput, atlas, and other cervical vertebrae would most probably be generated by defects in the functions of Hox and Pax-1 genes at different levels in the occipital and cervical somites [14] at a more delayed stage than those mentioned above. A possible explanation could be that the genetic and molecular alterations are more severe and thus extend their effects over segmentation and resegmentation of the somites and specification of the sclerotomes, not only affecting the hindbrain-spinal cord boundary as we have mentioned. A second possibility might be that the anomalous establishment of this boundary creates the conditions for a defective feedback from the neural counterpart to the mesoderm, disturbing these molecular pathways and secondarily the formation of cervical vertebrae. And we could add to these qualitative alterations the obvious quantitative one: if too much mesodermal tissue has been wrongly assigned to build the prospective spine, it goes without saying that the amount of tissue left for building the skull will be insufficient (**Figure 1**). The consequences of this relative lack of occipito-cervical mesodermal tissue will be distinct from those of the lack of spinal cord progenitor tissue, as the prospective growth of this segment of somitic mesoderm will be governed by the underlying hindbrain which, as far as we know, is very strictly divided in rhombomeres with distinct features, as opposed to the monotony of the spinal cord organization in these early stages. Their feedback over their corresponding (and quantitatively defective) mesodermal counterpart will put quite stressful limits on the availability of compensatory mechanisms and thus determine an abnormal formation of the osseous and ligamentous elements of the occipito-cervical junction.

The same could happen also at more cranial levels, corresponding to the first occipital rhombomeres, where the same disproportion between the neural tissue contained within and the nearby mesoderm that receives its developmental induction would produce the deformities of basilar impression, platybasia, brainstem kinking, and retroflexed odontoid, found in 7.7% of our patients with Chiari malformation type I (Royo-Salvador et al., unpublished data). All these osseous anomalies could probably be explained by the interplay of discrete but persistent compressive and tensile forces developed among occipito-vertebral mesodermal segments during their development, secondarily to the mentioned genetic and molecular defects, recording somehow to the tenets of the Hueter-Volkmann law as applied to the spine [15].

At the same time, the disproportion between the contained, apparently hypertrophic hindbrain and the corresponding scarcely available mesodermal tissue will create the conditions for what Roth described in 1986 with such a brilliant intuition as "cranio-cervical growth collision" [16]: the impaction of the developing hindbrain against the growing vertebral column, which surpasses and deforms the insufficient occipito-cervical junction mesodermal primordium (the former from the inside, the latter from below (**Figure 1**)), accentuating the tonsillar descent, enlarging the occipital foramen, and leaving too little room for the formation of the occipital bone. It is amazing how the actual general opinion is able to conceive only this last developmental step [1, 17], but yes, finally, there is a para-axial mesodermal insufficiency associated with the Chiari malformations, but it is an associated phenomenon, somehow delayed and of secondary importance.

Among cranio-cervical junction malformations, a special mention deserves odontoid retroflexion, as it is a bony deformity that although it is less known and more imprecisely defined, it was found to be more marked and more common in children and adults with Chiari malformation type I than in normal controls [18, 19]. Moreover, in children with Chiari malformation type I, a study found it was correlated with the presence of syringomyelia and with a lower position of the *obex* [18]—that is, with a more intense cranio-caudal distortion of the brainstem. The pathogenesis of odontoid retroflexion seems more clearly related to an abnormal caudal traction exerted by the growing cervical spine than that of other occipito-cervical junction malformations, its mechanism of action being also more prolonged, as the dental central synchondrosis that connects the odontoid to the body of the axis can persist until the age of 8 years [13], being thus exposed to this axial strain, transmitted through the occipito-cervical dura mater and neighboring ligaments and membranes. But the most important detail that these studies on odontoid retroflexion provide is that they prove indirectly that the cerebellar tonsils were *pulled* and not *pushed* into the cervical funnel—in other words, that traction overrides compression at least in these cases—because if the opposite were true, the odontoid had been displaced anteriorly in patients with Chiari malformation type I, as a result of the "overcrowding" of the posterior fossa [18].

Since long ago, observations were published on the frequent association between Chiari malformation type I and idiopathic scoliosis [20], even though no coherent explanation of this fact has ever been provided. As a specific point, we have to insist that the presence of syringomyelia is not really necessary, as many have thought so far. Among our patients, Chiari malformation type I was associated with idiopathic scoliosis in 78.8% of cases, out of which only 52.1% also had idiopathic syringomyelia (Royo-Salvador et al., unpublished data). Instead, a common pathogenesis, based on an abnormal caudal traction, seems more likely to be involved: in fact, as we mentioned before, the concept of "neuro-vertebral growth asynchrony" was coined in the realm of idiopathic scoliosis and constitutes the mainstay of the Roth-Porter pathogenetic theory [7–9], which uses various mechanical experimental models to demonstrate that an uncoupling of the growth velocity between the spine and spinal cord makes the latter to lag behind, putting tension on the posterior elements which will grow at a slower pace (here we come once again in close contact to the Hueter-Volkmann law), so that the anterior elements will grow too much and the vertebral bodies, "tethered" posteriorly, will start to rotate around an axis represented by the spinal cord itself and will deviate to one side as they grow restrained in this way, thus creating the scoliotic curve [21]. It is not difficult to imagine how a similar mechanism of caudal traction would produce both a Chiari malformation type I and an idiopathic scoliosis if this intrinsic "tether" acted continuously over the vertebral column and spinal cord throughout their development and associated longitudinal growth, a fact especially conceivable if, following the mentioned alterations in the definition of the hindbrain-spinal cord boundary, there is a relative excess of mesenchymal tissue composing the sclerotomes of the future thoracic spine, even though it would be much later that this unbalanced tissue distribution would become manifested, during the growth spurt of the adolescence.

Last but not the least, among enlightening pathological associations of Chiari malformation type I is the tethered cord syndrome, maybe the most interesting of all, the most difficult to explain, and nevertheless, the most important, as it forms a bridge between Chiari malformation types I and II. In fact, this association should be better regarded as a separate third category of Chiari malformations, taking into account the different mechanism of relative spinal cord "shortening": if in Chiari malformation type I this originated in a caudal displacement of the hindbrain-spinal cord boundary and in Chiari malformation type II, in the traction exerted by a caudal myelomeningocele on the growing spinal cord, here there is an abnormal *filum terminale*, short, thickened, and/or lipomatous that hampers the spinal cord longitudinal growth and that alters the coupling between vertebral and neural growth. Among our patients, the level of the *conus medullaris* was below the L1 L2 disk in as many as 20.9%, and most interestingly, it was statistically correlated with the degree of tonsillar descent (Royo-Salvador et al., unpublished data).

Now of course, if one accepts that the pathogenesis of Chiari malformations includes a common pathway of relative shortening of the spinal cord with respect to the vertebral column, of various etiologies that can be grouped into these three large groups, an important question comes about: why not any patient with this relative spinal cord shortening has a tonsillar descent? Well, the answer is quite simple, because, as we have already pointed out, there is another decisive factor that will eventually determine the occurrence or not of a Chiari malformation: the adequacy of the neural tissue reaction to the tensile forces developed as a consequence of the growth asynchrony. In other words, the tonsils will descend only if this homeostatic mechanism doesn't function properly for one reason or another; moreover, any degree of tonsillar descent and of brainstem and fourth ventricle distortion should be possible in every one of the three main etiopathogenetic groups mentioned, so it should be time that we stop associating Chiari malformation type II only to myelomeningocele and instead, consider, for example, three degrees of tonsillar descent, perhaps labeled as Chiari malformation types 1, 1.5, and 2 (even four if a Chiari malformation type 0 were added) and defined with clear-cut morphological criteria, including measures of brainstem elongation and fourth ventricle distortion [22].

4. Clinical arguments

Magnetic resonance imaging, if scrutinized really carefully, can provide much more information than just detect Chiari malformation type I. Early on, we mentioned the special meaning that a retroflexed odontoid can get as a proof of caudal traction applied on the occipito-cervical junction (**Figure 2**).

In many Chiari malformation type I patients, we can ascertain a descent not only of the cerebellar tonsils but seemingly of the whole cerebellum, as there is a readily identifiable difference of width of subarachnoid spaces above and behind the cerebellum, a feature that others have labeled "obliteration of retrocerebellar cerebrospinal fluid spaces" [17] following a different interpretation; of course, if a diminished posterior fossa volume were the cause of the tonsillar descent, there would be no free subarachnoid space visible underneath the tentorium as we see in many patients (**Figure 3**).

But maybe the most spectacular image testimony of the mechanisms mentioned above is the feature that we called "tense spinal cord," which has also been described in relation to idiopathic scoliosis [9] but that we could identify in many patients with Chiari malformation type I with or without scoliosis: in sagittal cuts, the spinal cord does not follow closely to the curves of the spinal canal, but instead, it takes the shortest route within the canal and is thus more or less straightened, in some cases even stuck on the concave side of the lordotic or kyphotic curve of the spinal canal (**Figure 4a**), corresponding in axial cuts to an eccentric position of the spinal cord in the canal, closer to the concave side (**Figure 4b**).

We interpret in a similar way another associated image feature, denominated "lateralized spinal cord," visible in coronal or axial cuts (**Figure 5**) and that can be understood as a marker of tension through the spinal cord if one keeps in mind Porter's experimental model [9], this time conditioned by the presence of at least a minimal degree of scoliosis. All this is even easier to figure out by neurosurgeons, because here the spine recalls the principle of functioning of the Leyla retractor system introduced by Gazi Yasargil and so often used to hold brain spatulas. In other words, a central cable in a hollow curved construct will deviate towards the concavity if subjected to axial tension, and in the vertebral column, this can happen either in the sagittal plane, in the coronal plane, or in both.

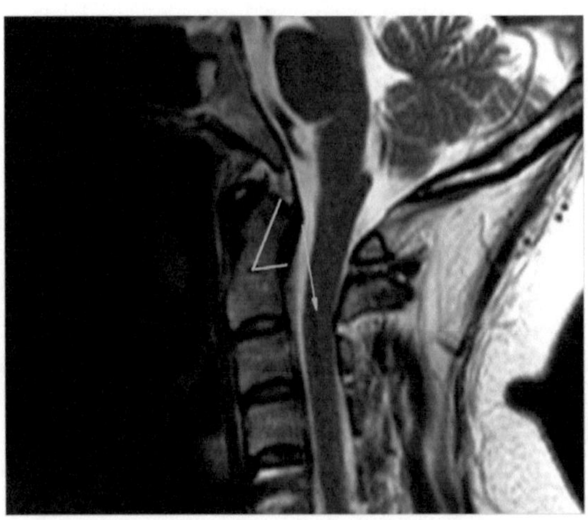

Figure 2.
The causative vector of a retroflexed odontoid is likely parallel to the caudal traction (arrow).

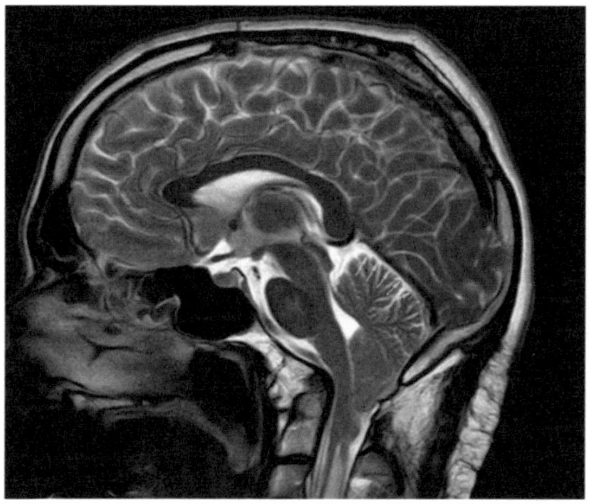

Figure 3.
Increased subarachnoid spaces between the tentorium and the cerebellum reflect the global displacement of the latter towards the foramen magnum.

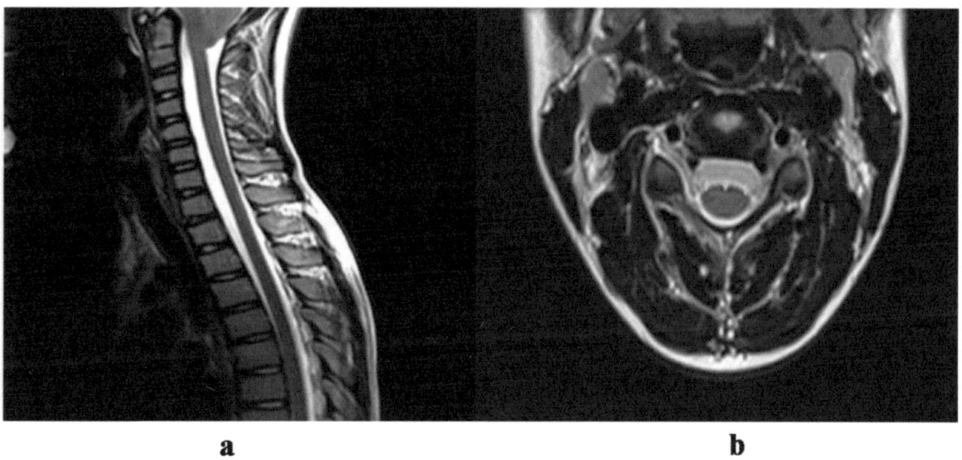

Figure 4.
Tense spinal cord in a sagittal cut (a) and an axial one (b). The spinal cord travels closer to the concavity of the curves and occupies an eccentric downward position in axial images (arrows).

As an expected consequence of an incomplete understanding of the etiopathogenesis of Chiari malformation type I, its surgical treatment seems the unhappy heir of a mysterious real estate, haunted by dreadful ghosts such as sleep apnea and sudden death. If in some cases it is indeed elementary caution and justified to do no treatment at all, as the tonsillar descent is merely an asymptomatic deformity discovered incidentally, in many other instances, the patients are left to struggle with their own despair as the obvious symptoms and signs they present are not recognized as such by the neurosurgeons in charge. And the reverse is also true: when an active treatment is chosen, it consists usually of suboccipital craniectomy, C1 laminectomy, and duraplasty, which is equivalent to performing an en bloc resection with healthy borders followed by radiotherapy and chemotherapy for a tumor of unknown behavior (not to mention the tonsillar resection added at times). Well, some minimalizing technical advances have been proposed, like leaving the dura mater or the atlas intact, but their problem rests in not getting to the heart of the matter—so, they might lack the desired efficacy. Recent efforts

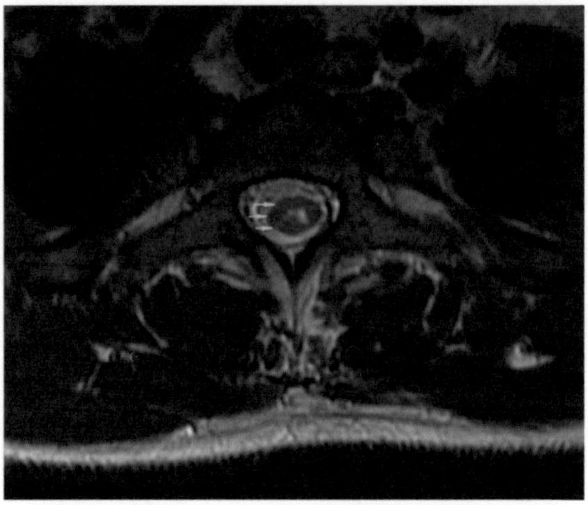

Figure 5.
Lateralized spinal cord deviated towards the left inside the spinal canal.

complicating more this subject have tried to define instances of cranio-cervical or atlantoaxial instability that supposedly would require complicated and risky procedures applied without firstly securing more confidently a diagnosis of genuine instability—one that is perfectly plausible in selected cases of traumatic spine injury.

Many of the delusions and mishaps issued from the actual therapeutic strategy applied to Chiari malformation type I could be avoided if, taking into account patiently all the facts presented above, one should switch his or her vision from the actual obsession to perform a *circumferential* decompression of the tonsils squeezed against the elongated brainstem to an objective of a rather *longitudinal* or *axial* release of the deformity that affects not only the brainstem-spinal cord junction but the whole of the brainstem *and* the spinal cord starting at the level of the *dorsum sellae*—upper end of the notochordal-influenced growth and somitic division of the mesoderm—until the very tailbone that at earlier stages was the advancing front of axial somatic growth and a possible regulator and intermediate of the coupling between the vertebral and spinal cord growth.

The most logical initial step for interfering with this pathogenesis, considering caudal traction as a final common pathway of multiple etiologies, would be to interrupt this unique route of producing damage to the brain, spinal cord, and spine itself. Technically, this is straightforward if done at the caudal end of the tense spinal cord instead of a frontal attack upon the delicate, impacted cranio-cervical junction. This should consist of a *filum terminale* release by means of the best available technique. A bonus of this approach is that it eliminates the concerns of a possible worsening of a hidden cranio-cervical instability. Its guarantee of success in releasing the conflict between the tonsils, brainstem-spinal cord junction, and occipital foramen stands in the continuous process of spinal growth which produced the progressive lengthening of the cord throughout the intrauterine life and childhood, by adding up collagen and elastin fibers to the complex tridimensional network that conforms the *pia mater* and holds the spinal cord connected mechanically with the vertebral column during its growth and movements. During adulthood, as we have already mentioned, although growth eventually stops, the axial tension is maintained by ongoing processes of degeneration and atrophy which paradoxically, instead of reverting it, will convert the mentioned *neuro-vertebral asynchrony* into a lifelong feature of the human body.

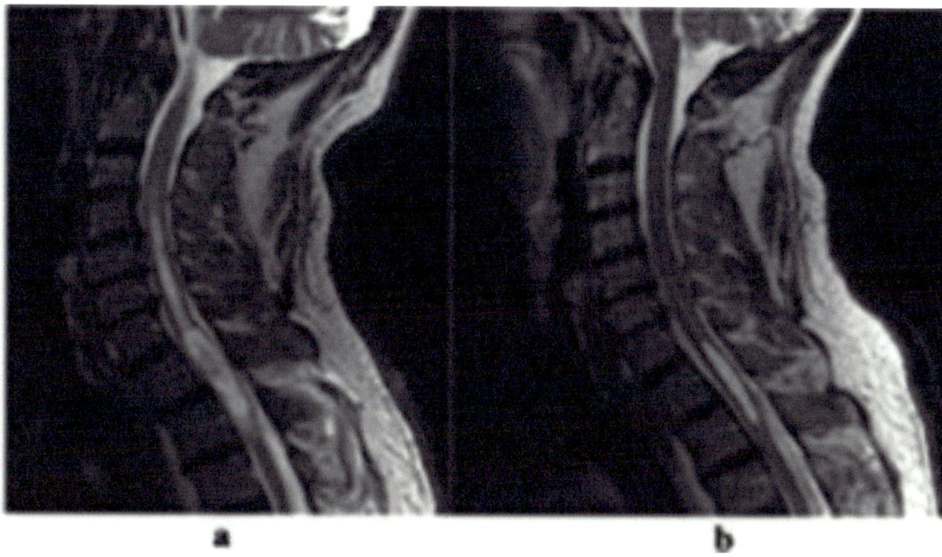

Figure 6.
Preoperative (a) and postoperative (b, at 30 months) magnetic resonance images of a 56-year-old male patient with Chiari malformation type 0, operated of filum terminale sectioning; the improvement of his idiopathic syringomyelia, visible also in a previous control (not shown), is now quite obvious, pointing to caudal traction as a possible mechanism.

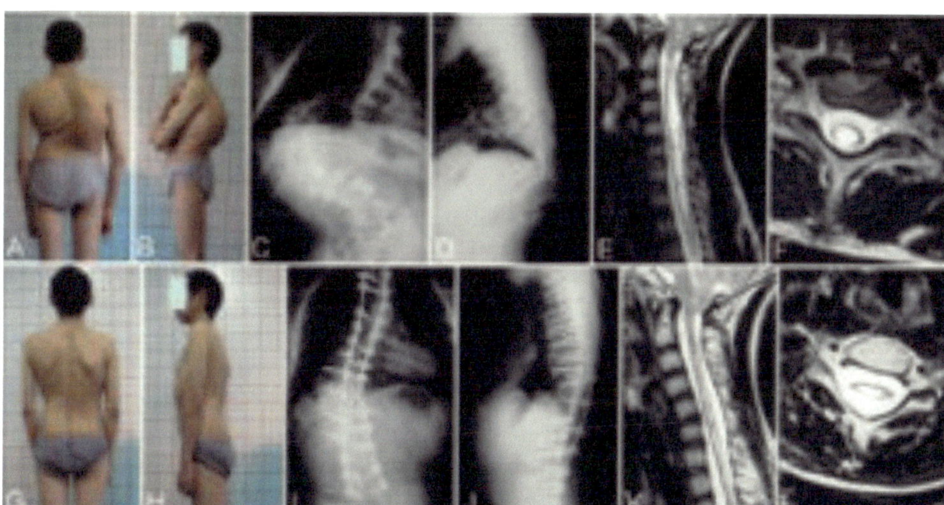

Figure 7.
Preoperative (A–F) and postoperative (G–L, at 3 months) photographs, radiographs, and magnetic resonance images of a 17-year-old male patient with Chiari malformation type I, idiopathic syringomyelia, and severe scoliosis, operated of spinal resection and instrumentation, with marked improvement of his syringomyelia (with permission from Wang et al. [25]).

Of course, the actual surgical approach of suboccipital craniectomy *does* lead to the completion of a similar release of longitudinal spinal tension but at a much higher cost and with much more risk of potential complications; moreover, it might be less efficient, because in the cervical spine, the stronger and more numerous dentate ligaments limit more the stress release than in the lumbar region.

Interestingly, against all odds, some subtle developments occurred in recent years in the surgical treatment of Chiari malformation type I, proving that more

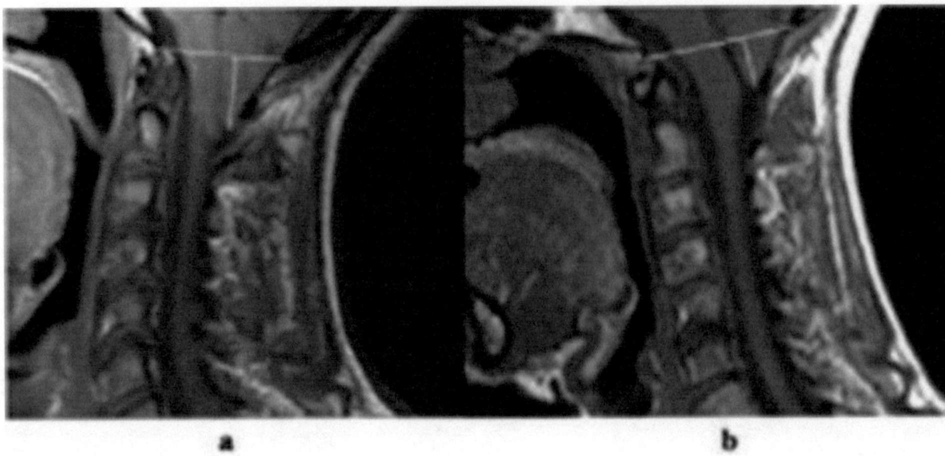

Figure 8.
Preoperative (a) and postoperative (b, at 7 years) magnetic resonance images of a 49-year-old female patient with Chiari malformation type I, operated of filum terminale *sectioning, with impressive improvement of the tonsillar descent from 17 to 13 mm with respect to McRae's line (measured in the cuts with maximal descent).*

and more clinicians are starting to accept that maybe suboccipital craniectomy is not the only surgical solution to this condition. For this reason, we can present here three "surgical" testimonies in favor of the theory of caudal traction, as follows:

1. In fact, it is suboccipital craniectomy itself that opened these new perspectives when in the hands of some fearless teams [23, 24]; it started to be used for treating patients with syringomyelia without tonsillar descent, with encouraging results, but they did not realize their meaning not even when they discovered that in these children, there were image features suggesting a caudal elongation of the brainstem with displacement of the obex and increased diameter of the *foramen magnum*, as occurs also in Chiari malformation type II [24]. In **Figure 6** we show a similar example from our series of patients, where sectioning the *filum terminale* determined a marked improvement of a cervicothoracic syringomyelia in a case of Chiari malformation type 0.

2. Another ingenious team discovered that if they performed idiopathic scoliosis correction by a technique of posterior vertebral column resection with spine shortening and instrumentation after applying compressive forces, the cerebrospinal fluid flow at the level of the *foramen magnum* improved in patients with Chiari malformation type I and syringomyelia, and in many of them, even the latter diminished in size [25]. Obviously, scoliosis surgery by no means could have accomplished any *circumferential decompression* of the occipital foramen but a release of the tension in the brainstem and tonsils (or, as we stated above, a welcome *longitudinal decompression*) (**Figure** 7).

3. Yet the most important testimony came from the hands of a group which operated 318 patients presenting both tethered cord syndromes defined according to very exigent criteria and Chiari malformation type I or low-lying cerebellar tonsils of 0–4 mm descent (that we consider as being also Chiari malformation type I, together with more and more authors [1]), but the technique used was not suboccipital craniectomy, but sectioning of the *filum terminale* by means of an L4 laminectomy. Their results were excellent, both concerning the clinical picture and various morphometric criteria of the posterior fossa contents,

demonstrating that the hindbrains of these patients were abnormally descended preoperatively and improved their position after the indirect surgery and applied to the other end of the spinal cord [22]. In **Figure 8** we present pre- and postoperative images of one of our cases, with a significant ascent of the tonsils after the filum terminale release.

5. Final remarks and future directions

In the actual state of knowledge, it is imperative to recognize that the development of the hindbrain and the spinal cord is a complex process regulated by genetic, molecular, mechanical, endocrine, and nervous homeostatic mechanisms that compensate one for another—within certain limits—in case of imbalances and disturbances. Nevertheless, it is exactly this complexity, coupled with the elevated functional requirements that the cranio-cervical junction has to meet, that makes their union so sensitive to various pathogenetic factors and determines malformations among which the one known as Chiari malformation type I is the most common. According to all the arguments presented in this chapter, the final common pathway of these etiopathogenetic aggressions seems to be caudal traction, a complex biological phenomenon that by no means should be reduced to a simple mechanical force of axial pull. There is still much left to discover about the physiologic mechanisms that govern the coupling between the growth of the vertebral column and that of the spinal cord during somatic development, where maybe future research will define the roles played by the pineal gland, the subcommissural organ, and the *filum terminale*, just to cite a few of the possible actors eligible for this casting.

Author details

Miguel Bautista Royo-Salvador, Marco Fiallos-Rivera and Horia Salca*
Institute Chiari and Syringomyelia and Scoliosis of Barcelona, Spain

*Address all correspondence to: hsalca@institutchiaribcn.com

References

[1] Raybaud C, Jallo GI. Chiari I deformity in children: Etiopathogenesis and radiologic diagnosis. In: Manto M, Huisman TAGM, editors. Handbook of Clinical Neurology, (3rd series) The Cerebellum: Disorders and Treatment. Vol. 155. Amsterdam: Elsevier BV; 2018. pp. 25-48

[2] Wolpert L. The triumph of the embryo. Courier Corporation. 2008. p. 12

[3] Chang J, Skromne I, Ho RK. CDX4 and retinoic acid interact to position the hindbrain-spinal cord transition. Developmental Biology. 2016;**410**:178-189

[4] Martinez-Barbera JP, Signore M, Boyl PP, Puelles E, Acampora D, Gogoi R, et al. Regionalisation of anterior neuroectoderm and its competence in responding to forebrain and midbrain inducing activities depend on mutual antagonism between OTX2 and GBX2. Development. 2001;**128**:4789-4800

[5] Lee K, Skromne I. Retinoic acid regulates size, pattern and alignment of tissues at the head-trunk transition. Development. 2014;**141**:4375-4384

[6] Marin-Padilla M, Marin-Padilla TM. Morphogenesis of experimentally induced Arnold-Chiari malformation. Journal of the Neurological Sciences. 1981;**50**:29-55

[7] Roth M. Idiopathic scoliosis from the point of view of the neuroradiologist. Neuroradiology. 1981;**21**(3):133-138

[8] Porter RW. The pathogenesis of idiopathic scoliosis: Uncoupled neuro-osseous growth? European Spine Journal. 2001;**10**:473-481

[9] Porter RW. Can a short spinal cord produce scoliosis? European Spine Journal. 2001;**10**(1):2-9

[10] Chu WC, Lam WM, Ng BK, et al. Relative shortening and functional tethering of spinal cord in adolescent scoliosis—Result of asynchronous neuro-osseous growth, summary of an electronic focus group debate of the IBSE. Scoliosis. 2008;**3**:8. Published 2008 Jun 27. DOI: 10.1186/1748-7161-3-8

[11] Dayer R, Haumont T, Belaieff W, Lascombes P. Idiopathic scoliosis: Etiological concepts and hypotheses. Journal of Children's Orthopaedics. 2013;**7**(1):11-16

[12] Opperman LA. Cranial sutures as intramembranous bone growth sites. Developmental Dynamics. 2000;**219**(4):472-485

[13] Menezes AH. Craniocervical developmental anatomy and its implications. Child's Nervous System. 2008;**24**(10):1109-1122

[14] Pang D, Thompson DNP. Embryology and bony malformations of the craniovertebral junction. Child's Nervous System. 2011;**27**:523-564

[15] Stokes IAF. Mechanical effects on skeletal growth. Journal of Musculoskeletal & Neuronal Interactions. 2002;**2**(3):277-280

[16] Roth M. Cranio-cervical growth collision: Another explanation of the Arnold-Chiari malformation and of basilar impression. Neuroradiology. 1986;**28**:187-194

[17] Milhorat TH, Chou MW, Trinidad EM, Kula RW, Mandell M, Wolpert C, et al. Chiari I malformation redefined: Clinical and radiographic findings for 364 symptomatic patients. Neurosurgery. 1999;**44**(5):1005-1017

[18] Tubbs RS, Wellons JCIII, Blount JP, Grabb PA, Oakes WJ. Inclination of

the odontoid process in the pediatric Chiari I malformation. Journal of Neurosurgery. 2003;**98**(1 Suppl):43-49

[19] Besachio DO, Khaleel Z, Shah LM. Odontoid process inclination in normal adults and in an adult population with Chiari malformation Type I. Journal of Neurosurgery. Spine. 2015;**23**:701-706

[20] Muhonen MG, Menezes AH, Sawin PD, Weinstein SL. Scoliosis in pediatric Chiari malformations without myelodysplasia. Journal of Neurosurgery. 1992;**77**:69-77

[21] Dickson RA, Lawton JO, Archer IA, Butt WP. The pathogenesis of idiopathic scoliosis: Biplanar spinal asymmetry. Journal of Bone and Joint Surgery. British Volume (London). 1984;**66**:8-15

[22] Milhorat TH, Bolognese PA, Nishikawa M, et al. Association of Chiari malformation type I and tethered cord syndrome: Preliminary results of sectioning filum terminale. Surgical Neurology. 2009;**72**:20-35

[23] Newton EJ. Syringomyelia as a manifestation of defective fourth ventricular drainage. Annals of the Royal College of Surgeons of England. 1969;**44**:194-213

[24] Tubbs RS, Elton S, Grabb P, et al. Analysis of the posterior fossa in children with the Chiari 0 malformation. Neurosurgery. 2001;**48**:1050-1055

[25] Wang Y, Xie J, Zhao Z, Zhang Y, Li T, Si Y. Changes in CSF flow after one-stage posterior vertebral column resection in scoliosis patients with syringomyelia and Chiari malformation Type I. Journal of Neurosurgery. Spine. 2013;**18**:456-464